Design and implementation of health information systems

Design and implementation of health information systems

Edited by

Theo Lippeveld
Director of Health Information Systems, John Snow Inc.,
Boston, MA, USA

Rainer Sauerborn
Director of the Department of Tropical Hygiene and Public Health,
University of Heidelberg, Germany

Claude Bodart
Project Director, German Development Cooperation, Manila, Philippines

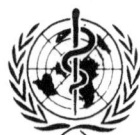

World Health Organization
Geneva
2000

WHO Library Cataloguing in Publication Data

Design and implementation of health information systems / edited by Theo Lippeveld,
Rainer Sauerborn, Claude Bodart.

    1.Information systems—organization and administration   2.Data collection—methods
    I.Lippeveld, Theo   II.Sauerborn, Rainer   III.Bodart, Claude

    ISBN 92 4 1561998   (NLM classification: WA 62.5)

Typeset in Hong Kong
Printed in France
99/12 706—Best-set/CD-COM/Granchamp-7000

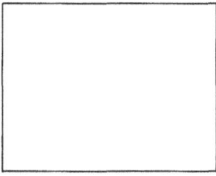

Contents

Foreword   ix

Acknowledgements   x

Chapter 1   Introduction   1
            by Rainer Sauerborn and Theo Lippeveld
            Why health information systems?   1
            Definitions   2
            What is wrong with current health information systems?   3
            Efforts to reform health information systems   5
            Review of the literature on health information systems reform   7
            Scope of the book   8
            Organization of the book   10
            References   10

Chapter 2   A framework for designing health information systems   15
            by Theo Lippeveld and Rainer Sauerborn
            Developing a "systems approach" for health information systems   15
            The health information system structure   16
            The relationship between the health information system and the
                health system at large   17
            Matching the health information system restructuring process
                with the health services system   24
            Conclusion   30
            References   31

Chapter 3   Using information to make decisions   33
            by Rainer Sauerborn
            The problem   33
            Defining information use   33
            How are decisions made?   34
            Ways to enhance the use of information in decision-making   38
            Outlook and sketch of a research agenda   46
            Conclusion   47
            References   47

Chapter 4   Identifying information needs and indicators   49
            by Claude Bodart and Laura B. Shrestha
            Introduction   49
            A general framework for defining information needs and indicators 50
            Performing a functional analysis at each management level
                of the health services system   51
            Identifying information needs   51
            Defining and classifying essential indicators   56
            Selecting essential indicators   60
            Summary   70
            References   71

Chapter 5	Assessing health information systems	73
	by Steve Sapirie	
	Introduction	73
	Assessment as a step in the development and implementation of the health information system	73
	A framework for assessing the health information system	74
	Reasons for health information system assessment	76
	Basic steps of health information system assessment	77
	Conclusion	85
	References	87
Chapter 6	Routine data collection methods	88
	by Theo Lippeveld	
	Use of routine versus nonroutine data collection methods	88
	Types of routine data collection methods	90
	Data collection instruments	95
	Data collection instruments for system management	103
	Design and implementation of routine data collection systems	105
	Conclusion	110
	References	111
Chapter 7	Nonroutine data collection methods: an overview	114
	by Rainer Sauerborn	
	Definition and classification	114
	Rapid assessment procedures	115
	Participant observation	117
	Individual interviews	117
	Focus groups	118
	WHO's rapid evaluation method	119
	Surveys	119
	Demographic surveillance systems	121
	Link between nonroutine and routine methods: triangulation	126
	References	127
Chapter 8	Data transmission, data processing, and data quality	128
	by Laura B. Shrestha and Claude Bodart	
	Introduction	128
	Data transmission	128
	Data processing	133
	Data quality	137
	Threats to data quality from poor recording and reporting	138
	Conclusion	144
	References	145
Chapter 9	Population-based community health information systems	146
	by David Marsh	
	Introduction	146
	History: population-based community approaches	150
	Rationale	154
	Development of population-based community health information systems	159
	Conclusion	170
	References	173
Chapter 10	Management of health information systems	176
	by Eckhard Kleinau	

Introduction 176
Resource requirements 176
Resource requirements for a hospital health information
system 187
Organizational rules 190
Conclusion 197
References 197

Chapter 11 Using computers in health information systems 198
by Randy Wilson
Historical overview 198
Rationale for using computers in health information
systems 199
Key issues to resolve with respect to computerization 200
Software and hardware options 205
References 211

Chapter 12 Geographic information systems 213
by Rainer Sauerborn and Marc Karam
Why are geographic information systems a useful supplement
to health information systems? 213
What are geographic information systems and how can we
use them in the context of health information systems? 214
How much do geographic information systems cost? 218
Applications of geographic information systems within health
information systems 219
Who uses maps? 221
Research agenda 222
Summary 223
References 223

Chapter 13 The context of health information system reform 225
by Theo Lippeveld
Introduction 225
Health information system reform: a policy analysis 226
Strategies for health information system reform 236
References 241

Chapter 14 Approaches to strengthening health information systems 243
by Theo Lippeveld and Steve Sapirie
Introduction 243
Restructuring routine health information systems: what
works and what does not work? 244
An agenda for further health information system development
experiences and research 250
References 252

Annexes

Annex 1 Classes of indicators and their major attributes 253
Annex 2 National lists of indicators: the trade-off between conciseness
and completeness 256
Annex 3 Health information subsystem: issue framework 258
Annex 4 Examples of assessment questions and recording formats 259
Annex 5 Examples of assessment data tables 261
Annex 6 Mother health card, Chandigarh, India 263
Annex 7 Child health register 264

Annex 8   Example of tally sheet   265
Annex 9   Hospital daily attendance sheet   266
Annex 10   Population chart of catchment area   267
Annex 11   Example of supervisory checklist   268
Annex 12   HMIS/FLCF monthly report: section on mother care activities   269
Annex 13   Data collection instrument pre-test review form   270

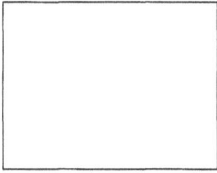

Foreword

This project was proposed by Theo Lippeveld and Rainer Sauerborn to address what was a huge gap in the health development literature: concepts and experiences in developing national health information systems.

The editors were able quickly to agree on the basic orientation and content of the book—to address the information needs of routine services management. The health professionals who were called upon to contribute chapters have extensive experience in health information systems development and use in many different situations.

Yet the task proved to be more daunting than we anticipated. There was, for instance, a need for a common conceptual framework. WHO has placed emphasis on addressing priority health and service problems, but emphasis on strengthening service performance—particularly at the peripheral level—proved to be a common principle among the contributors to this book. Only a few conceptual nuances, terms and styles of presentation required negotiation.

The development of health information systems is a fast-moving field. Not only is information technology changing rapidly, but concepts and methods for making the best use of existing data for managing health services and resources are quickly evolving. Efficiency in information management is becoming increasingly essential because of the concern for cost control in services and the way service staff spend their time. Approaches such as the use of health indicators are rapidly becoming the norm rather than the exception in order to reduce data handling, while increasing validity and timeliness. Efficient use of minimum data for managing cases, clinics and community health is essential, and it is toward this end that this book has been designed.

WHO is pleased to present this collection of health information system concepts, experiences and examples. We encourage public health administrators to react to these chapters and share with us, and with each other, new methods and techniques for health information system development and use that have proved effective in their countries.

Dr Stephen Sapirie
Director, Information for Management Program, Management Sciences for Health, Boston, USA

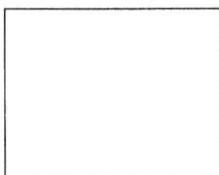

Acknowledgements

The editors wish to acknowledge the contributions of the co-authors, without whose efforts this unique volume would not have been possible. Particular thanks go to Ronald Wilson, Steve Sapirie and the Strengthening of Country Health Information team of WHO. Their careful review of the manuscripts was extremely helpful.

The Harvard Institute for International Development in Cambridge (USA) generously provided a grant to fund some of the time of the editors and other administrative costs.

The editors also wish to thank Laraine and Don Lippincott for their editorial work. Nawal Birdaha in Morocco and Sarah Newberry and Deirdre Pierotti in the USA provided copy-editing assistance.

About the editors

Theo Lippeveld, MD, MPH is currently Director of Health Information Systems at John Snow Inc., Boston, USA. Between 1985 and 1997 he was Research Associate and later on Development Advisor at the Harvard Institute for International Development. He lectured at the Harvard School of Public Health, USA, in courses on "Health Information Systems". In the last 20 years, he assisted ministries of health in health information system restructuring in Cameroon, Chad, Pakistan, Eritrea, Niger, Palestine, and recently also in Morocco.

Rainer Sauerborn, MD, MSc(MCH), MPH, DrPH is Director of the Department of Tropical Hygiene and Public Health at Heidelberg University, Germany. Until 1996, he was an Institute Associate at the Harvard Institute for International Development, USA. He lectured at the Harvard School of Public Health in courses on "Health Information Systems", "Community Epidemiology" and "Health Care Financing". In addition, he taught a course on "International Health" at Tufts University, Boston, USA, where he was an Associate Clinical Professor. His experience as a health practitioner at the district level dates back to the years 1979-1983, when he worked as a district health physician in Burkina Faso.

Claude Bodart, MD, MPH, is currently working for the German Development Cooperation in the Philippines. He has been involved in health sector reform in several Central and West African countries since 1983. Between 1994 and 1996 he served as a public health specialist in the Africa Technical Department of the World Bank in Washington, DC, USA. From 1989 to 1994, as Project Associate for the Harvard Institute for International Development, USA, he assisted the Ministry of Health of Cameroon in reorganizing the country's national health care system.

Co-authors

Steve Sapirie, DrPH, MBA, is Director of the Information for Management Program of Management Sciences for Health, Boston, MA, USA. He was formerly Chief of the Unit for Strengthening Country Health Information in the Health Situation and Trend Assessment Programme of the World Health Organization, Geneva, Switzerland. Dr. Sapirie has 30 years of experience in developing, applying and transferring methods in health planning, health programme evaluation and enhancing health information systems at global, regional and country levels.

Laura B. Shrestha, PhD, is employed by the World Bank, Human Development Department, based in Washington, DC, USA, as Operations Officer for Health, Nutrition, and Population. Ms Shrestha holds a PhD in demography from the University of Pennsylvania's Population Studies Center and a degree in economics from the University of Hawaii/East West Center. Her research interests are in the areas of monitoring and evaluation, health and mortality, and ageing.

David R. Marsh, MD, MPH is currently the Epidemiologist at the Health, Population and Nutrition Office for International Programs of Save the Children/USA. As a pediatrician and public health physician, he taught epidemiology and health systems development at the Aga Khan University, Karachi, Pakistan, and presently develops, monitors, evaluates, and documents primary health care programs in Africa, Asia, and Latin America.

Eckhard Kleinau, DrPH, MD, MS is Deputy Director for Evaluation and Management Information Systems at the BASICS Project in Arlington, VA, USA. Dr. Kleinau has more than 15 years of experience as a manager and consultant in public health and primary health care in Africa, Asia, Central America and the USA. His work includes the analysis and development of Health Management Information Systems for the World Bank and United States Agency for International Development (USAID).

Randy Wilson, MPH, is a Systems Analyst who is currently serving as the Logistics/MIS Specialist in Madagascar with the USAID-funded APPROPOP family planning support project. Over the past 20 years, his career has combined public health work and information system development in a variety of developing countries. He is one of the principal instructors in the MIS training courses organized by MSH, Boston, MA, USA.

Marc Karam, MD, was involved in tropical diseases projects in West Africa in the 1970s, in association with the University of Paris VI, France. He joined the epidemiological evaluation unit of the Onchocerciasis Control Programme in West Africa in 1980 and carried out field epidemiological studies as well as biomedical research. He subsequently joined the WHO Global Programme on AIDS in Geneva, first in the epidemiological research unit and then in the clinical research and drug development unit. He is currently in charge of certification of elimination and eradication of diseases in the Communicable Diseases cluster at WHO.

1 Introduction

Rainer Sauerborn and Theo Lippeveld

Why health information systems?

Good management is a prerequisite for increasing the efficiency of health services. The need to do more with less is especially important because the health sector faces ever increasing demands while receiving stagnant or decreasing resources.

Good management is also a prerequisite for increasing the effectiveness of health services. There is ample evidence that interventions lose a great deal of their theoretical effectiveness, also called efficacy, if they are delivered by poorly run health services (Tanner & Lemgeler, 1993; Tugwell et al., 1985). As an example, the effectiveness of polio vaccines may be diminished by breakdowns of the cold chain, incorrect assessment of the age of the child, failure to follow up on children who do not come for booster shots, and other such flaws. The challenge for health systems is to optimize the management of service delivery in a way that minimizes losses in effectiveness.

The World Health Organization (WHO) has long identified health information systems as critical for achieving health for all by the year 2000 (Mahler, 1986). A report of a WHO meeting (1987) clearly links improved management to improved health information systems: "Of the major obstacles to effective management, information support is the one most frequently cited." Unger and Dujardin (1992) and Lippeveld et al. (1992), recently stressed the need for well-designed routine information systems for ensuring that services are delivered according to standards.

For information to influence management in an optimal way, it has to be used by decision-makers at each point of the management spiral. Examples of these decision points include undertaking situational analysis, setting priorities, or implementing a programmed activity (see Fig. 1). Information is crucial at all management levels of the health services, from the periphery to the centre. It is crucial for patient/client management, for health unit management, as well as for health system planning and management. This means that not only policymakers and managers need to make use of information in decision making but also care providers, including doctors, health technicians, and community health workers. Unless this occurs, the considerable opportunity costs involved in set-up and maintenance of health information systems can be difficult to justify.

Helfenbein et al. (1987) rightly stated that "changing the way information is gathered, processed, and used for decision-making implies changing the way an organization operates". Or as Newbrander and Thomason

Fig. 1   *Information support to each step in the management cycle*

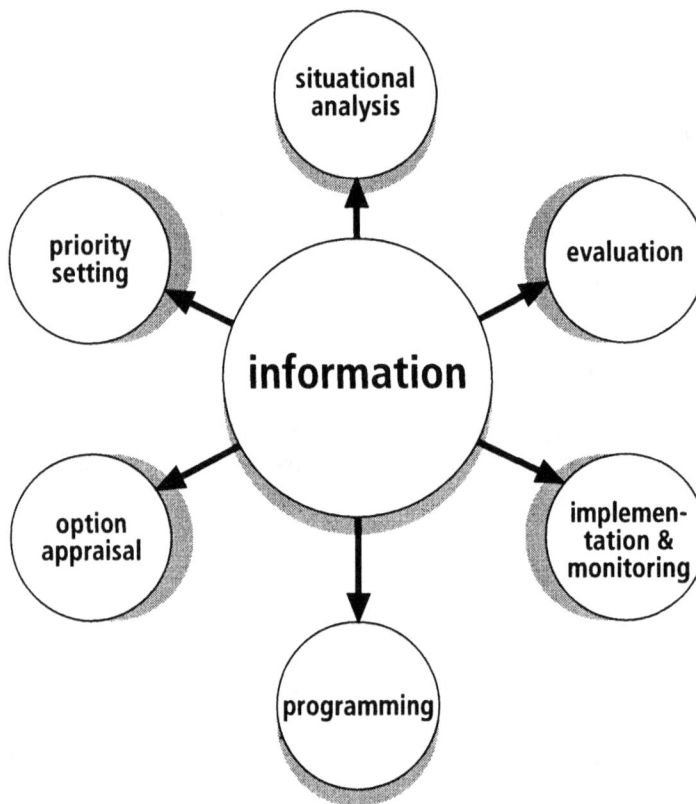

Source: modified from Green (1992)

(1988) pointed out in their article on health information systems in Papua New Guinea: "The enhanced development of the health information system has been used as the entry point for the improvement of managerial capabilities in the health system". Similarly, our hypothesis is that the development of rationally structured routine information systems, closely adapted to the information needs of health services at the district, health centre, and community levels, can potentially contribute to the overall improvement of health service management.

Definitions

A "system" is conveniently defined as any collection of components that work together to achieve a common objective. The objective in the case of a health information system then is to improve health services management through optimal information support. We define "information" as a meaningful collection of facts or data.

While consensus on the definition of "system" and "information" is quickly established, defining the term "health information system" is less obvious. At the outset, health information systems were oriented to collect information on diseases ("surveillance") and on health service output. While these functions are certainly important, we prefer to start from the definition of information systems as commonly used in industry. Hurtubise (1984) describes them as systems that provide specific information support to the decision-making process at each level of an organization. The ultimate objective of health information systems is therefore not "to gain information" but "to improve action". Applied to the health sector, we can now define health information systems as a set of components and procedures organized with the objective of generating information which will improve health care management decisions at all levels of the health system.

The widely used term "health management information system" could be misleading, since it may suggest that there are different information systems for different functions, for example management information systems, epidemiological surveillance systems, and administrative information systems. We consider all these as "subsystems" (see also Chapter 2) of a unified health information system and therefore prefer the latter term.

In summary, health information systems integrate data collection, processing, reporting, and use of the information necessary for improving health service effectiveness and efficiency through better management at all levels of health services.

What is wrong with current health information systems?

Unfortunately, health information systems in most countries are inadequate in providing the needed management support (WHO, 1987; Lippeveld, Foltz & Mahouri, 1992). Most health care providers in developing countries equate information systems with filling endless registers with names and addresses of patients, compiling information on diseases (e.g. sex and age of patients) every week or every month, and sending out reports without adequate feedback. Furthermore, the data received are often not helpful for management decision making because they are incomplete, inaccurate, untimely, obsolete, and unrelated to priority tasks and functions of local health personnel. In other words, information systems tend to be "data-driven" instead of "action-driven" (Sandiford, Annett & Cibulskis, 1992). A large part of the data collected passes to the national level without being analysed and used, and frequently ends up on the dusty shelves of an office in the Ministry of Health (Smith, Hansen & Karim, 1988; Becht, 1986; Frere, 1987; Ho, 1985; Kiaffi, 1988; WHO, 1988a; de Kadt, 1989). Current health information systems are therefore widely seen as management obstacles rather than as tools. The reasons can be summarized in five points:

Irrelevance of the information gathered

According to a WHO Expert Committee (1994), "Many of the data recorded and reported by the health service staff are not needed for the tasks the staff perform". Data collection tends to focus on disease reporting and only partially addresses management objectives at the health unit level or at the patient/client level. Yet data that are needed are frequently not collected. For example, appropriate indicators to monitor continuity of care of individual patients or clients are rarely included in health information systems.

The common denominator of these two observations is a lack of a consensus between producers and users of data at each level of the health care system regarding the information needed.

Poor quality of data

Data requirements are frequently chosen without taking into account the technical skills of the health workers collecting the data, or the available diagnostic equipment in peripheral health facilities (Nordberg, 1988; Lippeveld, Foltz & Mahouri, 1992; Frere, 1987). For example, at the first level of care, auxiliary health staff without laboratory or X-ray facilities are required to report on diseases such as leishmaniasis, diphtheria, and peptic ulcer. Furthermore, health workers receive little if any training in data collection methods (Murthy & Patel, 1988; Kiaffi, 1988; Nordberg, 1988), and rarely have standardized instructions on how to collect the data (Frere, 1987; Foreit et al., 1988; Jaravaza et al., 1982; WHO, 1994).

Another reason data quality is low is lack of motivation among health services personnel. Since health services supervisors and peripheral health workers rarely receive feedback on the data reported to higher levels (Smith, Hansen & Karim, 1988; de Kadt, 1989; Frere, 1987; Ho, 1985; Mitchell & Cromwell, 1982), they have little incentive to ensure the quality of the collected data and to comply with reporting requirements (Smith, Hansen & Karim, 1988; Frere, 1987; Ho, 1985; Mitchell, 1983; Helfenbein et al., 1987; Stinson, 1983; Murthy & Patel, 1988).

Duplication and waste among parallel health information systems

Historically, national reporting systems, even in developed countries, are rarely the result of a coordinated effort to address information needs of health planners and managers. Often, donor agencies or national programmes within the Ministry of Health developed their own specialized information system (Mitchell & Cromwell, 1982; Lippeveld, Foltz & Mahouri, 1992; Foreit et al., 1988; WHO, 1994), mostly under pressure and with financial assistance from external donor agencies.

Designed as vertically structured "empires", these programmes replaced line managers with programme directors who managed separate categories of personnel, facilitated separate training programmes, and created separate "programme information systems" which tended to focus on one specific disease (e.g. diarrhoea), a specialized service (e.g. "family planning information systems"), or a management subsystem (e.g. "drug management information system") instead of addressing management functions in a comprehensive way. These programme information systems existed side by side and in addition to the general routine health information system, which was considered insufficient and incapable of delivering the data needed for programme management. While these separate systems could indeed provide real information support for programmatic decisions, and the quality of information generated tended to be better than that of the general information system (WHO, 1994), the net result was that routine health information systems became chaotic and bothersome (Ho, 1985; Foreit et al., 1988; Kiaffi, 1988; Murthy & Patel, 1988).

The literature reveals several design and implementation problems. Reporting and transmission within each system is usually designed with minimal involvement of the line managers and providers of the health services (Frere, 1987; Mitchell & Cromwell, 1982; Stinson, 1983). The result is that health workers are drowned in a multitude of reports to be completed every month (Ho, 1985; Murthy & Patel, 1988; Kiaffi, 1988; Stinson, 1983). Since the data are not cross-referenced among the different systems, health care providers and systems managers spend a considerable amount of time collecting redundant and overlapping information (Smith, Hansen & Karim, 1988; Ho, 1985; Foreit et al., 1988; Rodrigues and Israel, 1995). Furthermore, data transmission does not follow the hierarchical lines of communication, so that reports often do not reach their destination (Frere, 1987; Ho, 1985; Lippeveld, Foltz & Mahouri, 1992). Elimination of duplication and waste requires a unified system rather than better coordination among the existing parallel structures.

Lack of timely reporting and feedback

The process of transmitting, compiling, analysing, and presenting the data is usually so tedious that by the time a report is prepared, the data are frequently obsolete and decisions are often made without any information input. Planners and managers face deadlines and time constraints in their daily decision making. Outdated information, even if of high quality, is of low value to them. Delays in data transmission and lack of feedback at the district level are often caused by the presence of strong vertical programmes. Health facilities report data directly to national programme managers, and line managers at the district level receive outdated feedback reports, if any.

Poor use of information

Despite the evidence that much of the generated data is irrelevant, of poor quality, redundant, or obsolete, there are nonetheless some useful data sets available. Unfortunately, researchers have not adequately evaluated or documented information use, and the prevailing sentiment that information is poorly used is based mainly on anecdotal evidence.

However, a few existing studies do point to some of the culprits. For example, information use was found to be especially weak at the district, health centre, and community levels (Smith, Hansen & Karim, 1988; WHO, 1988b; de Kadt, 1989), given the centralization of many health systems and, hence, health information systems. This raises serious concerns, given the current effort to decentralize decision making and build capacity at the district level.

Dunn (1980) revealed another impediment to ensuring use of information: the difference in "culture" between data people and decision-makers, which is difficult to bridge. Consequently, planning and management staff rely primarily on "gut feelings" to formulate ad hoc decisions rather than seek pertinent data. We will explore the factors that lead to the failure to use information and provide suggestions for solving this problem in Chapter 3.

Efforts to reform health information systems

The chaotic status and inefficiency of most existing information systems in developing countries are linked to the structural weakness of the system and lack of integration in the overall health system. This can be explained by the fact that historically, as in most developed countries, information systems were not intentionally planned to provide management support to the health services in an integrated way. Foltz (1993)

5

explains: "They differ from country to country depending upon historical accident and the interests of policy makers, administrators and researchers".

The first efforts to systematically collect, analyse, and report data for improved management in developing countries were undertaken by national programme managers of vertically structured "empires", as discussed above. This was due to the fact that foreign assistance to the health sector was typically focused on programmes rather than the entire health system. Since such projects were accountable to their respective donors, information on performance had to be collected. Targeting financial resources on disease control programmes or programmes addressing a group of specific "health problems" was indeed attractive to the donors because the quantifiable success of these programmes justified the use of their funds. This vertical approach to health care delivery, and thus to health information systems, was considered even more justified in the early eighties because of the prevailing "ideology" of selective primary health care (Walsh & Warren, 1979). However, apart from their effect on health information systems, these vertical programmes were undermining the development of a sustainable primary health care-based health infrastructure. In recent years great efforts were made in many countries to integrate the Expanded Programme for Immunization, the Control of Diarrhoeal Disease Programme, onchocerciasis control, and other vertical programmes into existing health structures, thus strengthening them.

The problems with health information systems were not lost on national policymakers and donors. Many countries decided to attack the information problem at its roots and planned for a more integrated approach to improving health information systems. Comprehensive restructuring efforts in countries such as Cameroon (see Sauerborn, 1991; Berg, 1988; Weber, 1989), Chad (see Lippeveld, Foltz & Mahouri, 1992; Unger, 1989), and Pakistan (see Ministry of Health, 1994) concentrated on the routine health information system for first-level care facilities. In Cameroon, health information system restructuring was complementary to an overall reform of the health services, building on a decentralized district health system based on primary health care. In Chad and Pakistan, restructuring of the health information system was done as a separate project.

In other countries, health information systems reform was done using a more gradual approach which consisted of either the reform of subsystems, such as epidemic disease surveillance (e.g. Burkina Faso) or routine services reporting (e.g. Niger). Table 1 gives an illustrative list of countries where national health information systems reform efforts took place recently or are still underway.

The drive for the reform of health information systems coincided with a revolution in information and communications technology. The computer has made its entry even in the most reluctant ministry of health. Doctors and nurses discuss hardware, databases, and spreadsheets. Low-cost powerful microcomputers and modems can efficiently store, process, and transmit enormous amounts of data. "User-friendly" desktop publishing and graphics software permit timely, specific, and action-oriented feedback to managers at different levels of the health services. With this state-of-the-art technology combined with pressure from the computer industry, most recently created or restructured health information

Table 1 *Illustrative list of published reports on national health information systems reform projects*

Country	Reference
Bangladesh	Reynolds, 1988
Burma	Reynolds, 1988
Bolivia	Cardenas, 1992
Cameroon	Sauerborn, 1991; Berg, 1988; Weber, 1989
Chad	Lippeveld, Foltz & Mahouri, 1992; Unger, 1989; Foltz, 1993
Eritrea	Tekle et al., 1995
Ghana	Campbell, Adjei & Heywood, 1996
Nigeria	Lecky, 1991
Niger	Kiaffi, 1988
Pakistan	Ministry of Health, 1994
Papua New Guinea	Campos-Outcalt, 1991
Philippines	Magnani, 1990
Swaziland	Ministry of Health, 1990
Thailand	Reynolds, 1988

systems are computerized to various degrees. But introducing computer technology in the development of improved health information systems is not necessarily the "silver bullet" that solves the efficiency problem of the health services (Sandiford, Annett & Cibulskis, 1992). On the contrary, lack of appropriately trained staff, a hostile climate, and hardware and software maintenance problems sometimes result in the decay and obsolescence of expensive computer equipment.

Review of the literature on health information systems reform

The scientific literature on how to develop appropriate health information systems in support of basic health services is relatively scanty, despite the general consensus that these systems should be restructured. Before 1985, most of the literature on management information systems focused on the use of computer technology rather than organizational aspects of information handling, information systems for large tertiary hospitals rather than basic health services, and survey methodology rather than routine health unit-based information systems. Other publications have underlined the importance of the development of such information systems, but without detailing how they could be developed. One of these publications is the report on an international workshop on management information systems and primary heath care organized by the Aga Khan Foundation in Lisbon (Portugal) in 1987 (Wilson et al., 1988), which covers most of the issues cited. Most publications have focused on a single aspect of the development of health management information systems (see Table 2).

Somewhat more comprehensive, the publications of Stinson (1983) and Helfenbein et al. (1987) provide a fair amount of detail on available methodologies and technologies for the development of routine health unit-based information systems in developing countries, but they reached a limited target audience and date from 1983 and 1987, respectively. The Aga Khan Foundation published the Primary Health Care Management Advancement Program series (Wilson & Sapanuchart,

Table 2 *Specific aspects of health information systems development in the literature*

Aspect of health information systems	Reference
Information needs for national health planning	White, 1977; WHO, 1981; WHO, 1994
Disease surveillance systems	Klaucke et al., 1988; Thacker, Parrish & Trowbridge, 1988
Development of computerized data processing systems	Brodman, 1986; Bussell, 1993; Rodrigues & Israel, 1995
Programmatic information systems	Ho, 1985; Newbrander, Carrin & Le Touze, 1994; Pelletier, 1994
Data collection methods	Anker, 1991; Frerichs, 1988; Guhasapir, 1991; Hill, Zlotnik & Trussell 1981; Kielmann, Janovsky & Annett, 1995; Kroeger, 1983; Lanata & Black, 1991; Oranga & Nordberg, 1993; Scrimshaw et al., 1992; Seltzer, 1990; Valadez, 1991
Epidemiological techniques	Vaughan & Morrow, 1995
Community involvement	Husein et al., 1993; O'Neill, 1993; Scott, 1988
Measurement of quality of care and health information systems	Garnick et al., 1994; Roemer & Montoya-Aguilar, 1988
Politics of health information systems reform	Foltz & Foltz, 1991

1993). Conceived as a set of field guides to strengthen the quality and utility of health data organized around nine thematic modules, the Management Advancement Program series helps primary health care managers at the local level to collect and use information for managing the health services under their supervision. Also, more recently, two WHO documents on the development of district-based routine health information systems were published, the first titled *Information support for new public health action at district level* (1994), and the second, by the Pan American Health Organization titled *Conceptual framework and guidelines for the establishment of district-based information systems* (Rodrigues & Israel, 1995). The first document is a report of a WHO Expert Committee, summarizing problems and strategies related to the development of district routine health information systems. The second publication, by Rodrigues and Israel, gives an excellent treatment of the design of district-based health information systems, with a strong emphasis on computer software and hardware.

Scope of the book

This book responds to an urgent need in the public health community to gather in one publication the state of the art of designing and implementing health information systems, particularly in developing countries. It especially addresses the question of how to transform existing information systems into management support systems.

The focus is on routine health unit-based information systems. The rationale behind this approach is based on several conditions which exist in the basic health services in most developing countries. First, the problems of inefficient and chaotic data collection and use of information in peripheral health units as previously described typically apply to routine health unit-based information systems. Many government agencies and donors tend to "use . . . general and special-purpose surveys to capture data that should be part of routine reporting" (WHO, 1994). But these problems do not solely originate from the methodological attributes of routine information systems. They also reflect poor general management capability of the basic health services. Our hypothesis is that the development of rationally structured routine information systems will also contribute to the overall improvement of the management capability of the basic health services, particularly if a consensus-building design process is used. Second, routine health unit-managed information systems are the only way to generate data for patient and client management decisions. They are especially suited for routine managerial decisions, such as those related to ordering supplies, or supervision of health personnel. Considering the fact that data collection is performed mainly by health care providers as part of their health care tasks, marginal cost is low. Finally, the development of routine health information systems, compared with surveys and other nonroutine methods, has been less well described in the scientific literature.

Most of the analysis and strategies on health information systems development discussed in this book will pertain to government-managed health services because this is the most common health services system in developing countries. Yet one of the roles of the district management team is to coordinate and supervise nongovernment and private health services within the district (WHO, 1988b). We will therefore also discuss in the following chapters means and strategies to involve private sector health care services in health information systems development.

The strength of the book lies in the case material distilled from information systems which the authors have helped to design and maintain. In the last 10 years, the authors have gathered broad and varied experience in the development of health information systems through projects and advisory services in developing countries throughout the world: Bolivia, Burkina Faso, Cameroon, Chad, Costa Rica, the Democratic Republic of the Congo, Eritrea, Malawi, Niger, and Pakistan. Some of these efforts involved overall restructuring of health information systems, such as in Cameroon, Chad, Eritrea, and Pakistan. Other efforts were limited to more specific aspects of health information systems development, such as the introduction of lot quality assurance sampling as a tool to improve quality of care in Costa Rica, the use of geographic information systems in Bolivia, and production of annual feedback reports for district managers in Niger. These experiences, combined with those of the guest authors and the team of the Strengthening Country Information System unit of WHO/Geneva, provide a unique opportunity to bring together in book form lessons learned about the development of health information systems.

The book targets professionals not only in the health sector but also in related sectors involved in planning and managing health services at national and intermediate levels, particularly government health services and of nongovernmental organizations. Our focus on decentralized, district level-operated health services makes it a valuable guidebook for district health managers. The presentation of case studies and the continuous link in the text between concepts presented and actual implementation in the field are intended as a resource for teachers and students in programmes related to planning and managing health services in developing countries, and more specifically to developing health information systems.

Organization of the book

The chapters of the book have been grouped under four parts. The theme of the first part with two chapters is information for decision making. In Chapter 2, we lay the groundwork for health information systems design by providing a health services system framework closely linked to the health information systems restructuring process. Chapter 3 deals with use of information, analysing the reasons information is rarely used by decision-makers and suggesting ways and means to improve its use.

The second part of the book has six chapters examining step by step how health information systems should be structured so that they can provide information useful to decision making at all levels of the health services. Chapter 4 deals with the first step, information needs and indicators and how to define them through consensus building. In Chapter 5, the author proposes a health information system assessment methodology to identify weak elements in the existing health information system and set the agenda for the restructuring process. Chapter 6 contrasts the different routine data collection methods, while Chapter 7 gives an overview of nonroutine data collection tools. Data transmission and processing are the focus of Chapter 8, with particular emphasis on assessing and assuring data quality. Chapter 9 applies these health information systems restructuring principles to population-based community health information systems.

The three chapters of the third part of the book deal with resources and tools required for a well-functioning health information system. Chapter 10 provides a comprehensive view of the health information system resource base: staffing, training, and supervision; procurement and distribution systems of printed supplies; purchase and maintenance of hardware and software; and budgeting for recurrent health information system costs. Chapter 11 analyses the strengths and weaknesses of computer use in health information systems. Chapter 12 highlights one particular computer application: geographic information systems and their potential usefulness in health services planning and management.

Whereas the first three parts of the book provide the principles and technical content of health information systems for decision making, the two chapters of the last part are about the process of health information systems restructuring. Chapter 13 focuses on the politics of change, analysing how different interest groups and contextual factors can influence the design and implementation of new health information systems in a positive or negative way, and proposing health information systems design strategies to deal with these factors. Finally, in Chapter 14, the authors, based on their experience, summarize health information systems development approaches which almost certainly will fail, and those, on the contrary, which will lead most likely to successful health information systems restructuring. The chapter also identifies areas for future research and development experience.

References

Anker M (1991). Epidemiological and statistical methods for rapid health assessment: introduction. *World health statistics quarterly*, 44(3):94–98.

Becht JN (1986). Management information systems: lessons from evaluations of ten private voluntary organization (PVO) health programs. In *Management issues in health in the developing world*. Washington, DC, National Council for International Health: 105–112.

Berg H (1988). *Surveys and health management information systems* (prepared for the GTZ primary health care project in the North-West Province of Cameroon). Heidelberg, Heidelberg University School of Public Health.

Brodman JZ (1986). *Using microcomputers to improve decision-making in Third World governments*. Development Discussion Papers. Cambridge, MA, Harvard Institute of International Development: 1–46 (Development Discussion Papers, No. 231).

Bussell KE (1993). *Computer applications for health information systems*. Atlanta, GA, Centers for Disease Control and Prevention: 1–120.

Campos-Outcalt D (1991). Microcomputers and health information in Papua New Guinea: a two year follow-up evaluation. *Health policy and planning*, 6:348–353.

Campbell B, Adjei S, Heywood A (1996). *From data to decision making in health: the evolution of a health management information system*. Amsterdam, Royal Tropical Institute.

Cardenas CO et al. (1992). *Bolivia information system* (training manual for management of the national health information subsystem). La Paz, Ministry of Social Welfare and Public Health.

de Kadt E (1989). Making health policy management intersectoral: issues of information analysis and use in less developed countries. *Social science and medicine*, 29:503–514.

Dunn WN (1980). The two-communities metaphor and models of knowledge use: an exploratory case survey. *Knowledge*, 1:515–536.

Foltz A, Foltz W (1991). The politics of health reform in Chad. In: Perkins D, Roemer M, eds. *Reforming economic systems in developing countries*. Cambridge, MA, Harvard Institute for International Development.

Foltz AM (1993). Modeling technology transfer in health information systems—learning from the experience of Chad. *International journal of technology assessment in health care*, 1993, 9:345–361.

Foreit K et al. (1988). *Automating Ecuador's health information system*. Paper presented at the 116th Annual Meeting of the American Public Health Association, Boston: 1–7.

Frere JJ (1987). *Health and management information system for child survival project in Pakistan*. Washington, DC, Technologies for Primary Health Care Project, United States Agency for International Development: 1–23.

Frerichs RR (1988). Rapid microcomputer surveys. *Journal of tropical pediatrics*, 34:147–149.

Garnick DW, Hendricks AM, Comstock CB (1994). Measuring quality of care: fundamental information from administrative datasets. *International journal for quality in health care*, 6:163–177.

Green A (1992). *An introduction to health planning in developing countries*. Oxford, Oxford University Press.

Guhasapir D (1991). Rapid assessment of health needs in mass emergencies: review of current concepts and methods. *World health statistics quarterly*, 44:171–181.

Helfenbein S et al. (1987). *Technologies for management information systems in primary health care*. Geneva, World Federation of Public Health Associations (Issue Paper, Information for Action Series).

Hill K, Zlotnik H, Trussell J (1981). *Demographic estimation: a manual on indirect techniques*. Washington, DC, National Academy of Sciences: 1–52.

Ho TJ (1985). *Managing health and family planning delivery through a management information system*. Washington, DC, World Bank.

Hurtubise R (1984). *Managing information systems: concepts and tools*. West Hartford, CT, Kumarian Press: 1–168.

Husein K et al. (1993). Developing a primary health care management information system that supports the pursuit of equity, effectiveness, and affordability. *Social science and medicine*, 36:585–596.

Jaravaza VS et al. (1982). Unified national health information system. *Central African journal of medicine*, 28:25–170.

Kiaffi A (1988). *Rapport d'évaluation du nouveau système de collecte de données. [Report of the evaluation of a new data collection system.]* Niamey, Ministry of Public Health: 1–26.

Kielmann AA, Janovsky K, Annett H (1995). *Assessing district health needs, services, and systems: protocols for rapid data collection and analysis*. London, Macmillan Education.

Klaucke DN et al. (1988). Guidelines for evaluating surveillance systems. *Morbidity and mortality weekly report*, 37:1–18.

Kroeger A (1983). Anthropological and socio-medical health care research in developing countries. *Social science and medicine*, 17:147–161.

Lanata CF, Black RE (1991). Lot quality assurance sampling techniques in health surveys in developing countries: advantages and current constraints. *World health statistics quarterly*, 44:133–139.

Lecky MY (1991). *Strengthening and integrating the health information system for decision making in Nigeria*. Cambridge, MA, Harvard School of Public Health (Working Paper No. 2).

Lippeveld TJ, Foltz A, Mahouri YM (1992). *Transforming health facility-based reporting systems into management information systems: lessons from the Chad experience*. Cambridge, MA, Harvard Institute of International Development: 1–27 (Development Discussion Papers, No. 430).

Magnani RJ (1990). *Information systems development at the Republic of the Philippines Department of Health*. Manila, Department of Health: 1–20.

Ministry of Health of Swaziland (1990). *Swaziland outpatient health information system*. Mbabane, Ministry of Health: 1–110.

Ministry of Health of Pakistan (1994). *Health management information system for first level care facilities: instruction manual*. Islamabad, Ministry of Health.

Mitchell JB, Cromwell J (1982). Physician behavior under the Medicare assignment option. *Journal of health economics*, 1:245–264.

Mitchell M (1983). *Provincial health plan, 1983–1987*. Port Moresby, Papua New Guinea Division of Health.

Murthy N, Patel KG (1988). *A computer based information system for health and family welfare: the Bavala experiment*. Ahmedabad, Indian Institute of Management.

Newbrander W, Thomason JA (1988). Computerizing a national health system in Papua New Guinea. *Health policy and planning*, 3:255–259.

Newbrander W, Carrin G, Le Touze D (1994). Health expenditure information: what exists and what is needed? *Health policy and planning*, 9(4):396–408.

Nordberg E (1988). Household health surveys in developing countries: could more use be made of them in planning? *Health policy and planning*, 3:32–39.

O'Neill K (1993). *Community based surveillance: a critical examination of nine case studies*. London, London School of Hygiene and Tropical Medicine: 1–84.

Oranga HM, Nordberg E (1993). The Delphi panel method for generating health information. *Health policy and planning*, 8(4):405–412.

Pelletier DL, Shrimpton R (1994). The role of information in the planning, management and evaluation of community nutrition programmes. *Health policy and planning*, 9:171–184.

Reynolds J (1988). Overview: current perspectives on management information systems in primary health care. In: Wilson RG et al., eds. *Management information systems and microcomputers in primary health care*. Geneva, Aga Khan Foundation: 67–70.

Rodrigues RJ, Israel K (1995). *Conceptual framework and guidelines for the establishment of district-based information systems*. Barbados, Pan American Health Organization, Office of the Caribbean Program Coordination (document PAHO/CPC/3.1/95.1).

Roemer MI, Montoya-Aguilar C (1988). Quality assessment and assurance in primary health care. Geneva, World Health Organization: 1–78 (WHO offset publication, No. 105).

Sandiford P, Annett H, Cibulskis R (1992). What can information systems do for primary health care? An International Perspective. *Social science and medicine*, 34:1077–1087.

Sauerborn R (1991). *Propositions pour un système d'information pour le projet SESA. [Proposals for an information system for the SESA project.]* Cambridge, MA, Harvard Institute of International Development: 1–117.

Scott W (1988). Community-based health reporting. *World health statistics quarterly*, 41:26–32.

Scrimshaw NS, Gleason GR, eds. (1992). *Rapid assessment procedures— qualitative methodologies for planning and evaluation of health related programmes*. Boston, MA, International Nutrition Foundation for Developing Countries.

Seltzer JB (1990). *Handbook for conducting local rapid assessments*. Boston, Management Sciences for Health: 1–25.

Smith DL, Hansen H, and Karim MS (1988). Management information support for district health systems based on primary health care. In: Wilson RG et al., eds. *Management information systems and microcomputers in primary health care*. Geneva, Aga Khan Foundation: 89–110.

Stinson W (1983). *Information systems in primary health care*. Washington, DC, American Public Health Association, 1:1–76.

Tanner M, Lengeler C (1993). From the efficacy of disease control tools to community effectiveness. *Transactions of the Royal Society of Tropical Medicine and Hygiene*, 87:518–523.

Tekle DI et al. (1995). *Health information system assessment study: findings and recommendations*. Asmara, Ministry of Health.

Thacker BS, Parrish RG, Trowbridge FL (1988). A method for evaluating systems of epidemiological surveillance. *World health statistics quarterly*, 41:11–19.

Tugwell P et al. (1985). The measurement iterative loop: a framework for the critical appraisal of need, benefits, and costs of health interventions. *Journal of chronic diseases*, 38:339–351.

Unger JP (1989). *Evaluation du système national d'information du secteur santé. [Evaluating a national information system for the health sector.]* N'Djamena, Ministry of Public Health: 1–25.

Unger JP, Dujardin B (1992). Epidemiology's contribution to health service management and planning in developing countries: a missing link. *Bulletin of the World Health Organization*, 70:487–497.

Valadez JJ (1991). *Assessing child survival programs in developing countries: testing lot quality assurance sampling*. Cambridge, MA, Harvard University Press (Harvard Series on Population and International Health).

Vaughan JP, Morrow RH (1995). *Manual of epidemiology for district health management*. Geneva, World Health Organization.

Walsh JA, Warren KS (1979). Selective primary health care. *Social science and medicine*, 1979, 301:967–974.

Weber W (1989). *Health management information system: Bamenda, Cameroon*. Yaounde, GTZ: 1–60.

White KL et al. (1977). *Health services concepts and information for national planning and management*. Geneva, World Health Organization: 103–106 (Public Health Papers, No. 67).

Wilson R, Sapanuchart T (1993). *Primary health care management advancement programme*. Washington, DC, Aga Khan Foundation.

Wilson RG et al. (1988). *Management information systems and microcomputers in primary health care*. Geneva, Aga Khan Foundation.

World Health Organization (1981). Information support. In: *Managerial process for national health development*. Geneva, World Health Organization: 57–60 (*Health for all* series, No. 5).

World Health Organization (1987). *Report of the Interregional Meeting on Strengthening District Health Systems, Based on Primary Health Care, Harare, Zimbabwe 3–7 August 1987*. Geneva, World Health Organization: 1–42 (unpublished document WHO/SHS/DHS/87.13; available on request from Evidence and Information for Policy, World Health Organization, 1211 Geneva 27, Switzerland).

World Health Organization (1988a). *The challenge of implementation: district health systems for primary care.* Geneva, World Health Organization (unpublished document WHO/SHS/DHS/88.1; available on request from Evidence and Information for Policy, World Health Organization, 1211 Geneva 27, Switzerland).

World Health Organization (1988b). Household surveys on health and nutrition. In: Anderson JG, Aydin CE, Jay SJ, eds. *Evaluation health care information systems: methods and applications.* Thousand Oaks, CA, Sage.

World Health Organization (1994). *Information support for new public health action at the district level. Report of a WHO Expert Committee.* Geneva, World Health Organization: 1–31 (WHO Technical Report Series, No. 845).

2 A framework for designing health information systems

Theo Lippeveld and Rainer Sauerborn

Developing a "systems approach" for health information systems

The need for improved routine health information systems is unequivocal and well documented (WHO, 1986; de Kadt, 1989; Sandiford, Annett & Cibulskis 1992; Lippeveld, Foltz & Mahouri, 1992). While there is a general consensus that health information systems should be restructured, very few publications have focused on how to develop such systems.

It has even been argued that health information systems are idiosyncratic to the countries that develop them, and that no appropriate models exist that can be applied to all countries (Foltz, 1993). A health information system in a largely urban country with a literacy rate of more than 80%, a GNP per capita of more than US$1000, and mostly privately operated health services will certainly be different from one in an extremely poor country where the majority of the rural population is illiterate, and with predominantly government-managed health services. It is obvious that each country has to develop or restructure its own specific system, tailored to the prevailing socioeconomic, political, and administrative context. There are some common elements, however, which can be adapted to create more effective and efficient systems. Each health information system has, at the minimum, some sort of information-generating process whereby data are transformed into information; and to run this process, a more or less organized structure is present where persons interact with resources, such as data collection instruments, or with machines, such as computers.

This chapter intends to provide public health professionals with a "systems approach" towards the development of health information systems. How can the common elements be combined in such a way that information is or becomes a real "resource" to solve health problems at all levels of the health services system? What kind of system will generate and disseminate information to support management rather than to block it? In order to answer these questions, this chapter first examines the health information system structure and its breakdown into components. We then describe an organizational model of the health services with concentration levels from the periphery to the centre. Management functions at each level are discussed. Finally, we propose a health information systems restructuring process in six steps, carefully matching each step with the proposed health services model.

The health information system structure

In order to explain the conceptual link between health information systems and the health services system at large, we start from the generic definition of a management information system, as we previously indicated in Chapter 1. Specifically, it is "a system that provides specific information support to the decision-making process at each level of an organization" (Hurtubise, 1984, p. 28). A health information system first of all is a "system" (Helfenbein et al., 1987, p. 2). Like each system, it has an organized set of interrelating components which can be grouped under two entities: the information process, and the health information system management structure (see Fig. 2). Through the information process, raw data (inputs) are transformed into information in a "usable" form for management decision making (outputs). The information process can be broken down in the following components: (i) data collection, (ii) data transmission, (iii) data processing, (iv) data analysis, and (v) presentation of information for use in planning and managing the health services.

Monitoring and evaluating the process ensures that the right mixture of inputs produces the right type of outputs in a timely fashion. For example, the information needed is continuously changing with changing planning and management needs. This will in turn affect data collection and other components of the information process. A health information system can generate adequate and relevant information only insofar as each of the components of the information process has been adequately structured.

Fig. 2   *Components of a health information system*

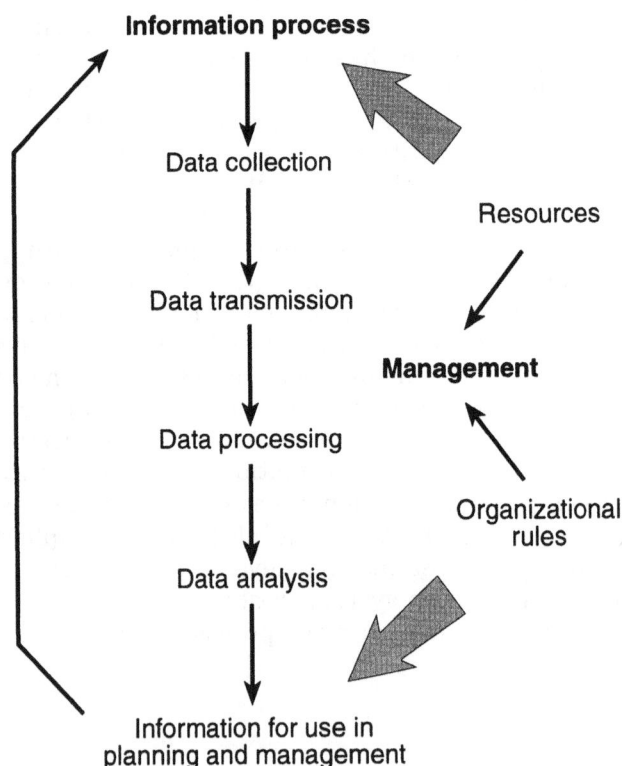

WHO 99362

The unfolding of this stepwise process in space and time is not necessarily the same in all situations. Sometimes data collected are used immediately and locally for a decision, with little processing or analysis. For example, by asking patients how well they responded to treatment (data collection), care providers can decide if follow-up visits are necessary (use of the information). Also, the decision-making process for daily management tasks often consists of a set of "routine procedures", where data are immediately linked to a series of actions. This is the case with standardized treatment guidelines, or with standard procedures for drug management. In other situations, each of the steps in the information-generating process takes place in a different location and at a different time. For example, data on the use of preventive services is collected at the time of the patient/client visits, aggregated every month and transmitted from the health facilities to the district, and processed at the provincial level. Each year, based on this data, coverage for preventive services is calculated and communicated to the district level for further analysis and action.

In order to make the information process efficient, a health information system management structure is required to ensure that resources are used in such a way that the information process produces high-quality information in a timely fashion. This structure can be further broken down into two components: (i) health information systems resources, and (ii) a set of organizational rules. Health information system resources include persons (e.g. planners, managers, statisticians, epidemiologists, data collectors); hardware (e.g. registers, telephones, computers); software (e.g. carbon paper, report forms, data-processing programs); and financial resources. Organizational rules (e.g. the use of diagnostic and treatment standards, definition of staff responsibilities, supply management procedures, computer maintenance procedures) ensure efficient use of health information system resources.

Thus designing or redesigning health information systems will need to address in a systematic manner each of these components of both the information process and the management structure. The ultimate objective is that health information systems provide specific information support to the decision-making process within the health system at large.

The relationship between the health information system and the health system at large

A health information system cannot exist by itself but is a functional entity within the framework of a comprehensive health system that offers integrated health services, including curative care, rehabilitative care, disease prevention, and health promotion services. The health information system structure should permit generation of the necessary information for rational decision making at each level of the health services system. This health system is composed of various levels between the centre and the periphery, each with different management functions, health services provision, and resource availability. Ideally, services and resources should be as available as possible to the periphery, to optimize access by the population. But there are limits to the degree of decentralization related to the provision of technical competence (technical limit); or to the efficient use of equipment (economic limit); or to the distribution of power (administrative limit). For example, it is neither possible nor desirable that every patient with a urinary infection be treated

Fig. 3   *Organizational model of the health services*

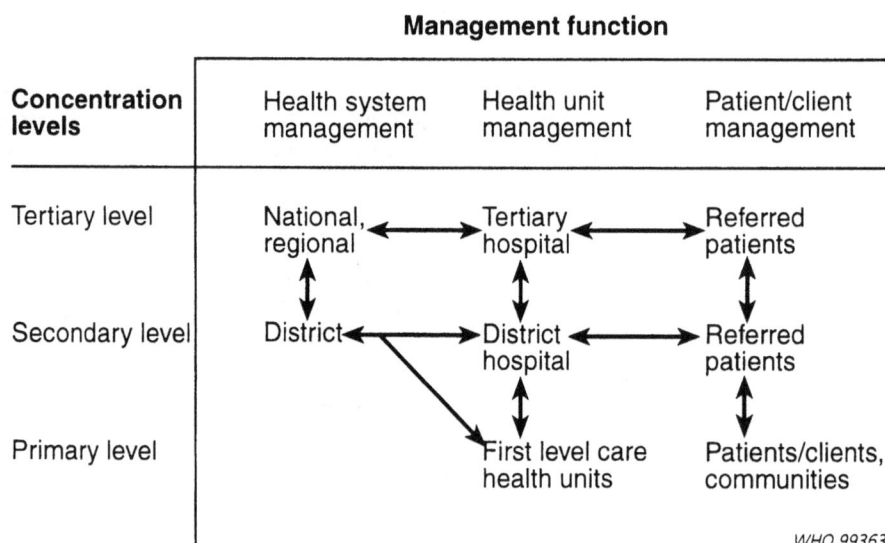

Management function

Concentration levels	Health system management	Health unit management	Patient/client management
Tertiary level	National, regional ⟷	Tertiary hospital ⟷	Referred patients
Secondary level	District ⟷	District hospital ⟷	Referred patients
Primary level		First level care health units	Patients/clients, communities

WHO 99363

by a urologist; or that each first-level care clinic has ultrasound equipment. We therefore call these levels "concentration levels". Classically, three concentration levels are described: the primary level, the secondary level, and the tertiary level. The primary level is the point of contact between the system and the population to whom health care is delivered. The other levels—the secondary or district level, and the tertiary level—provide specialized services as well as planning and management support. In many countries the tertiary level is further divided into regional (or provincial) and central levels.

Each of these levels has specific functions, implicating a series of specific decisions to be made, ultimately leading to improvement of the health of the population. From a management perspective, functions can be grouped in three types of management functions, related to (i) patient/client management, (ii) health unit management, and (iii) health system management (see Fig. 3). Patient/client and health unit management functions are directly related to the delivery of promotional, preventive, and curative health services to the population. They include all interactions between the health unit staff and communities in their catchment areas. The health system management functions consist in the provision of coordination and management support to the service delivery levels. Decisions to be made under each of these types of management functions are different. The management information systems literature would call the patient/client and health unit management decisions "operational", and the system management decisions "strategic planning" or "management control" decisions.

The organizational model of the health services described above and depicted in Fig. 3 will allow us to identify at each concentration level what the specific management functions are, who the information users are, and what decisions they have to make. This in turn will permit us, at each level, to define information needs and to develop or restructure data collection methods and instruments, data transmission and processing procedures, as well as appropriate feedback reports.

Patient/client management functions

The main patient/client management function is to provide quality care to patients and clients, curative as well as preventive and health-promotional, at the first level as well as at the referral level. A vast literature has been produced on how to define quality of care. An excellent semantic discussion is given in a World Bank Technical Paper by De Geyndt (1994). Quality of care assessment, according to the conceptual model of De Geyndt, should look at the inputs ("structure") of health care, at the process, and at the outcome. In the context of this book, we want to relate the provision of quality care to a series of decisions that care providers (and their supervisors) have to take at each level of the health services. How can an information system support these decisions in the most relevant and effective way? We prefer to focus on a process-oriented definition of quality care.

As explained before, quality care will be defined differently depending on the concentration level. Quality care at the first level is comprehensive, integrated, and continuous; it focuses on patients and clients in their immediate sociocultural environment (Public Health Research and Training Unit, 1980). Quality care at the referral level is much more dependent on the input of human and technical resources, and can therefore be defined in terms of technical excellence according to the "state of the art".

The user of information at the patient/client level is the care provider—the doctor, the health auxiliary, the midwife, but also the community health worker or the traditional birth attendant. A well-designed health information system can be a major tool in improving the quality of care delivered by care providers, by generating the information they need to make appropriate decisions, as in the following illustrations:

- The date, findings, and treatment prescribed during the last visit will help the care provider to make better decisions for a tuberculosis patient visiting a rural health centre (continuity of care).
- A child of 2 years is brought by his mother because of a skin rash and diarrhoea. Does the care provider have the necessary information support to know whether the child has already had measles or whether he was vaccinated (integration of care)?
- In order to decide what vaccine to administer to an 8-month-old child brought to the clinic, the health auxiliary needs to know what type of vaccines the child has already received and on what dates (continuity of care).
- The pathology results of a biopsy specimen of the cervix will assist the surgeon to decide whether to perform a hysterectomy.

Health unit management functions

The general management objective of a health unit is to provide health care to a defined population in the catchment area surrounding the health unit with a given amount of resources. Health units can be classified according to the level of concentration of resources: first-level care units, and referral-level care units. Management functions are specific for each type of health unit. They can be further subdivided into service delivery functions and administrative functions.

Service delivery functions are defined based on the health needs of the communities served by the health units. First level care units provide a package of general health care services. There is a great deal of variation in the setting of a first level care health unit, as shown by the various forms of such units: dispensary, clinic, health centre, basic health unit, rural health centre, sub-health centre, first aid post, community health post, and so on. These different facilities may also cover differences in functions. Until quite recently, most of these units provided only curative care, as indicated by the name "dispensary". In some instances, first-level care health units have been given specialized functions and activities: maternal and child health centres, tuberculosis centres, sexually transmitted disease clinics, family planning clinics. Often the availability of personnel determines the types of activities delivered at the first level. For example, if first-level care units are operated by a doctor, they probably can offer a wider range of services than if they are operated by a community-based health worker trained in 3 months. Also, material resources limitations can be at the origin of the range of services provided. For example, without refrigeration equipment, first-level care facilities cannot provide immunization services.

Since the conference in Alma Ata in 1978, most countries in the world have adopted the strategy of primary health care. This implies that a package of essential health care, including curative as well as preventive and promotional activities, should be provided to as large a segment of the population as possible. This package focuses on priority health problems in the community, for which simple and effective technologies exist, and which can be solved by general health care providers with essential equipment and drugs, taking into account the available resources in the country. The World Bank in its 1993 *World development report* suggests that, based on cost-effectiveness studies, the "minimum package" should include at least the following activities: prenatal and delivery care, family planning services, management of the sick child, treatment of tuberculosis, and case management of sexually transmitted diseases (World Bank, 1993). Most of these activities are housed in a first-level care unit.

At the referral level, hospitals and specialized outpatient clinics provide services and techniques for which the technical complexity and costs are not justified at first level care units. The district hospital is the first referral unit or secondary care unit. Provincial and national hospitals are mostly tertiary care units. Again, which specific services and techniques will be offered at what level will vary from country to country, or even from region to region. For example, in some countries, district hospitals do not offer ophthalmological surgery, while in other countries they do.

Table 3 provides a list of service delivery functions adopted by the Ministry of Health in Chad in 1989. In support of the service delivery functions, health units also have administrative functions, such as personnel management and training, financial management, drugs and supplies management, and information management. Obviously, such functions will increase in complexity with the size of facilities, from a first-level care unit staffed by a health auxiliary and a midwife, to a tertiary care hospital with hundreds of beds and staff.

Once functions and activities of the different types of health units in a given health services system have been clearly defined, we can easily identify the information needed for decision-making:

Table 3   *Service delivery functions in health units in Chad*

First level (dispensaries, infirmaries):
— to provide curative care services for the most common health problems
— to provide prenatal care services
— to organize under-5 clinics (including immunizations)
— to provide follow-up services for chronic diseases
— to organize nutritional rehabilitation clinics
— to provide family planning services
— to ensure communication with the population in the catchment area.

Secondary (or first referral) level (centres medicaux):
— to manage medical and surgical emergencies
— to provide X-ray and laboratory services
— to organize outpatient referral clinics
— to provide inpatient services (medicine, surgery, paediatrics, and gynaecology/obstetrics)
— to manage complicated deliveries.

Tertiary level (hôpitaux de préfecture, hôpital national):
In addition to the functions of secondary level,
— to provide all types of surgical interventions
— to provide specialized care.

Source: Translated and adapted from Unger (1989).

- A health centre is supposed to provide treatment to tuberculosis patients. The officer in charge would like to know how many patients out of those who started treatment in the health centre abandoned their treatment prematurely (dropout rate). This information can prompt the health officer to improve follow-up of tuberculosis patients.
- One of the functions of a health centre is to provide prenatal care to all pregnant women in the catchment area, and to refer those at risk for delivery to the district hospital. In the last few months, several women from surrounding villages are reported to have died in childbirth or shortly thereafter. The officer in charge and the midwife of the health centre would like to know how many women out of the total expected pregnancies in the catchment area of the health centre receive prenatal care. This information will guide the midwife in reorganizing prenatal care activities in a more effective way.
- A district hospital with 200 beds provides inpatient care to a population of 200,000. For about a year, beds have been constantly full, and patients are hospitalized on improvised floor beds. The superintendent would like to know the average length of stay of the patients in each department in order to decide whether more beds are needed, or whether alternative discharge procedures could solve the problem.
- A tertiary hospital functions with a given annual budget. Revenues come from government subsidies, from health insurance payments, and from user fees. In order to prepare an annual budget, the financial director of the hospital will need data of the previous year on revenues by source and on expenditures by cost centre.

Health systems management functions

The objective of health systems management is to coordinate and provide planning and management support to the service delivery levels. Some examples of generally accepted health systems management functions are:

— establishment of health policies and legislation;
— intersectoral coordination;
— strategic planning and programming;
— budgeting and financial resource allocation;
— organization of the system, including referral mechanisms;
— personnel development including continuing education;
— resource management, including finance, personnel, and information;
— distribution and management of equipment, supplies, and drugs;
— disease surveillance;
— protection of the environment;
— supervision of the health services.

Health system management functions vary for each concentration level. Their distribution from the periphery (classically the "health district" is the most peripheral health system unit) to the centre (regional and national levels) and, consequently, their decision-making power depends on the way the health system has been administratively organized in each country.

The main poles between which most national health systems can be situated are centralized and decentralized systems; government and private sector-managed systems; and horizontally managed health services systems and health services systems managed predominantly by vertical programmes. For example, budgeting and decisions on financial resource allocation will be made at the national level in a centralized health system; in other health systems, these functions have been delegated to the district level. In a country with a predominantly private sector-managed health system, most of the listed functions are performed by private institutions, whereas the government has only a regulatory role, setting policies and making legislation. In a health system managed mainly through vertically organized health programmes, programme managers have taken over responsibilities in resource management and supervision from the line managers. Table 4 lists management functions at central, regional, and district levels in a decentralized health services system as proposed by WHO (1988).

Again, based on the specific health system management functions at each concentration level, information needs can be rationally determined and data collection procedures developed to generate the required information. Health planners and managers can use a variety of information sources, but should be sure that the amount and nature of the data to be reported by the operational levels of the health services are reasonable to avoid burdening health care providers. Ideally, health services staff should only report data which are useful for patient/client management or for health unit management. All other information required at this level could be generated by data sources other than health unit-based reporting.

Essential public health management functions

More recently, as part of the "health for all" renewal effort and the discussions on the role of the state versus the private sector in health care provision, another group of management functions has been proposed— "essential public health functions". These functions have been defined as "a set of fundamental and indispensable activities carried out to protect the population's health and treat disease through means which are targeted at the environment and the community" (Sapirie, 1997). Typical

Table 4 *Health system management functions in a decentralized health service system*

The central level (Ministry of Health) is responsible for:
— health policy formulation, including policy on intersectoral activities;
— production of national health plans and regional and local planning guidelines;
— advisory role on allocation of resources, particularly capital funds;
— source of high level technical advice for specific programmes;
— control over purchasing pharmaceuticals and distribution of supplies;
— training and regulation of health personnel development;
— regulation of private profit and nonprofit health organizations;
— control of national health organizations and research institutes;
— liaison with international health organizations and aid agencies.

Regions and/or provinces are responsible for:
— regional health planning and programme monitoring;
— coordination of all regional health activities;
— employment and control of part or all of the health personnel;
— budgeting and auditing of health expenditure;
— approval and financing of large-scale capital projects;
— managerial and technical supervision of district health teams and district;
  heads of specific health programmes;
— provision of supplies and other logistical support.

Districts are given the following main functions:
— organizing and running the district hospital services;
— managing all other government health facilities;
— implementing all community-based health programmes;
— managing and controlling local health budgets;
— coordinating and supervising all government, nongovernment and private
  health services within the district;
— promoting active links with local government departments;
— promoting community participation in local health service planning;
— preparing an annual health plan;
— raising additional local funds;
— in-service training of health workers;
— supervising and controlling all community health workers in the district;
— collecting and compiling routine health information and forwarding it to regions and ministries
  of health.

Source: WHO (1988).

examples of such functions are disease surveillance and protection of the environment.

A working group on essential public health functions has further proposed to classify management functions according to three categories: personal health care, health system management, and public health (Sapirie, 1997). While the health system management category is very similar, the categories of this classification are difficult to compare with the one proposed earlier. As illustrated by the examples given in Box 1, this classification is particularly suited to ensure that during health system reform efforts essential public health functions are preserved somewhere in the system.

The design and implementation of an effective and efficient health information system are intimately linked with and have to fit into the organization of the health system for which it generates information. In this book, when discussing the different health information system elements, we will consider different organizational structures of health services systems, particularly when presenting country cases. Nevertheless, in a

---

Box 1   Essential public health and health system reform

A recent meeting on primary health care systems provided an opportunity to introduce the concept of essential public health and to attempt to create a map of the evolving concept of overall health systems in functional terms. There are some who view public health as falling within the broadened definition of primary health care. Without debating this point, an effort has been made to present the simplest possible view of the health system in terms of three categories of functions:

Health system management (health system maintenance and development)
This category would include such functions as health policy formulation; programme planning; resource mobilization and allocation; programme implementation, monitoring and evaluation; human resource development and management; management of health research.

Public health
These functions include maintenance of information about the health of the population, protection of the environment, prevention and control of disease, health promotion and education, health legislation and regulation, and specific public health services such as school health, occupational health, veterinary health services, and public health laboratories.

Personal health care
This category would include all personal health care services, whether public or private, possible organized in the traditional referral levels: primary, secondary, tertiary, and specialized care.

As health systems undergo reform processes, such a functional map can assist system designers in assuring that essential functions are preserved somewhere in the system. This does not belabour the question of where or what primary health care is, but instead attempts to depict specific, important health system functions.

Source: *Adapted from Sapirie (1997).*

---

more generic way we will base our approach for the development of health information systems on the model of a health services system as outlined above: a decentralized health system based on primary health care, with district level decision making and active involvement of the community, as put forward by WHO (1988).

Matching the health information system restructuring process with the health services system

Effective health information systems provide information support to the decision-making process at all levels of the health services. Thus health information systems should fit into the overall management structure of the health services system. The question then is, how, in a very practical way, can existing inadequate routine health information systems be transformed into effective management tools?

The health information system restructuring process itself is a challenging and complex undertaking, particularly in the context of government bureaucracies in developing countries (Sandiford, Annett & Cibulskis, 1992; de Kadt, 1989). Failures tend to be more common than successes. In addition to purely methodological factors, the actual political, sociocultural, and administrative context can influence the outcome of the reform process. In this chapter we focus particularly on the methodological aspects of health information system restructuring. An in-depth analysis of the impact of contextual factors on the health information system restructuring process is provided in Chapter 13.

The previously proposed health services model based on concentration levels with different patient/client, health unit, and system management functions as explained in previous paragraphs (see Fig. 3) is an excellent framework on which to build or rebuild health information systems. All along the health information system restructuring process, this model will provide conceptual guidance on the different steps of the process.

Health information system restructuring rarely involves a total overhaul of the system in a particular country or region. In fact, comprehensive restructuring efforts often fail. Rather, health information system restructuring should focus on the least functional aspects of the system, or be planned in connection with ongoing health system reforms. For example, reform of the financial management system of the health services requires particular health information system restructuring focused on financial information. Prior to any health information system restructuring process, an in-depth assessment is required to identify strengths and weaknesses of the existing system and to focus health information system restructuring on those areas that are the least functional or constitute particular country priorities.

In order to undertake a systematic assessment of the existing health information system, WHO proposes to categorize the health information system under five interrelated "subsystems":

— epidemiological surveillance for notifiable infectious diseases, certain environmental conditions, and risk factors;
— routine service reporting from the basic health services at community level, health centres, first referral hospitals, and tertiary hospitals;
— special programme reporting systems, such as tuberculosis control, maternal and child health, and school health;
— administrative systems, including health care financing systems, health personnel systems, drugs and logistic systems, financial management systems, health-training programmes, health research programmes, and health documentation management;
— vital registration systems for births, deaths, and migratory movements.

Chapter 5 provides a detailed methodological description of the initial health information system assessment.

The health information system restructuring process itself can be broken down into six steps addressing each of the health information system components presented earlier. The four initial steps deal with the development of the information-generating process: (i) identifying information needs and indicators, (ii) defining data sources and developing data collection instruments, (iii) developing data transmission and data-processing procedures, and (iv) ensuring use of the information. The two last steps involve setting up the health information system management structure necessary to ensure generation and use of the information: (v) planning for the required health information system resources and (vi) developing a set of organizational rules for health information system management. The approach we propose is to carefully match each of the health information system restructuring steps with the existing health services system. Within the chosen subsystem and for each of the health information system restructuring steps, particular attention needs to be given to ensure that the information can be made available and is used for decision making at the appropriate concentration level (from the periphery to the centre) and for the identified management functions (patient/client, health unit, and health system).

- *Step 1: Identifying information needs and feasible indicators.* The amount of effort and time needed for this initial step will depend upon the degree to which management functions have been defined at the time of health information system restructuring as part of the regular health services planning and programming activities. Therefore, initial health information system assessment should include a functional analysis of the health services, focusing on patient/client management, health unit management, and system management. Based on the results of this functional analysis, it may be necessary to first agree upon a clear set of management functions. For patient/client management, this could mean, for example, establishing standardized service procedures; or for system management, delineating functions between the district, regional, and national levels.
  With clearly defined management functions, identifying the information needed to make appropriate decisions at each management level will become relatively easy. The real challenge at this step is to set priorities and to select a limited number of feasible indicators, or variables that measure change, taking into account the available resources at each level, and without overburdening peripheral health workers with data collection. Most important, selected indicators have to be action-oriented and contribute directly to decision-making by care providers, as well as by health planners and managers. Chapter 4 will further detail this important step in the restructuring process.
- *Step 2: Defining data sources and developing data collection instruments for each of the indicators selected.* Most data for service delivery and resource management can be collected through the routine health information system. At the system management level, for policy setting and health planning indicators, data reported by health units can be complemented with data from other sources such as surveys or from other sectors. Data collection procedures need to be standardized and adapted to the technical skills of the health workers and the diagnostic equipment available. Data collection instruments should be designed to promote, to a maximum degree, immediate use of the information at the service delivery levels.
  Again, it will be important to make sure that the procedural interaction between different concentration levels and for different management functions is consistent and minimizes duplication. For example, standardized case definitions will ensure that epidemiological information at the primary level and at the referral levels is comparable. Or data reported through the monthly report forms should be easily retrievable from the patient/client record cards. Chapters 6 and 7 will

provide a detailed overview of routine and nonroutine data collection sources, methods, and instruments.

- *Step 3: Developing a data transmission and processing system.* The data transmission system should respect established management channels of the health services system and be responsive to the need for intensive information exchange between different concentration levels, between the community and the health services, and between first-level care and referral-level care institutions. Data processing mechanisms will also vary depending on management needs: for example, in a small health unit, data can be processed manually, whereas in big tertiary hospitals and for system management, computers will be required. Whatever the mechanics, data processing should generate information of acceptable quality for each management function and at all concentration levels (see Chapter 8).

- *Step 4: Ensuring use of the information generated.* Using information is the ultimate objective of each information system. The combined result of the first three steps of the health information system design process should be relevant and quality information. The most important step is to ensure that, based on appropriately designed feedback mechanisms and innovative approaches in data presentation, this information will be used to provide high-quality promotional, preventive, and curative services to patients, clients, and the community; in managing of first-level care centres as well as referral hospitals; in planning and managing the health services system from the district up to the national level; and in ensuring essential public health functions such as environmental protection and disease surveillance.

  The main challenge of this step is to convince decision-makers at central as well as at peripheral levels that quality information really can help them to make informed decisions for patients and clients, health units, and health system management, in other words, to create an "information culture". Succeeding in this endeavour, particularly at the peripheral levels, will also result in better quality of the data generated. Chapter 3 provides an in-depth discussion of potential strategies to improve information use.

- *Steps 5 and 6: Planning for health information system resources and developing a set of organizational rules for health information system management.* Health information system efficiency and sustainability will depend for a large part on the availability of human and physical resources and their organization into a well-designed management structure. This health information system management structure needs to be adapted to the physical and organizational realities of the health services system: organizational procedures; personnel planning and training; financial allocations; equipment procurement and maintenance; and stock management of printed and computer supplies.

  Again, the health services functions for patient/client management, for health unit management, and for system management should be the starting point for planning health information system resources and for developing organizational rules for health information system management. For example, training of health unit staff in data collection procedures should as much as possible be integrated with training in clinical procedures for patient/client management. Or, when designing a district level computerized system, the procedures for the production of feedback reports should be linked to the supervisory timetables of the district management team.

As was pointed out before, health information system restructuring does not necessarily address all concentration levels or all management functions. The initial health information system assessment will reveal the particular focus of restructuring. For example, if assessment of the epidemiological surveillance system shows that case finding is functioning in a satisfactory manner, restructuring can be limited to improving the transmission and processing of case information from the health unit to the national level. As an example, Table 5 gives a list of illustrative tasks for each step of the health information system restructuring process to ensure its fit with the health services system, focusing on the routine service reporting subsystem. The third and fourth columns indicate the link of the task with a particular concentration level or management function within the health services system.

Box 2 shows how practically the health information system restructuring process has been intimately linked to the existing health services

---

Box 2 Pakistan: design of a health management information system for first level care facilities

A general assessment of the existing health information system undertaken at the request of the Ministry of Health of Pakistan pointed out that the system did not provide adequate information for decision making, either to health managers for system planning and management, or to health workers for facility or patient management. The reasons were multiple:

- Overall health information system management was weak.
- Indicators did not always respond to specific information needs at different levels in the health system.
- Data collection in health facilities was poorly organized.
- Information flows were fragmented, because most national programmes had set up separate reporting systems and, often, separate supervisory systems.
- Data consolidation and processing, mostly done manually, were time-consuming and error-prone.
- Use of the information generated was greatly limited by the quality of the data collected, by the fragmented flow of information, and by the lack of feedback mechanisms.

After 20 years of "patching-up" interventions, the ministry felt that a more structured effort was necessary to transform the existing routine data collection system into a management tool. It wanted an information system that would provide all the necessary indicators for decision making at different management levels of the health services: the patient/client management level, the health unit management level, and the health system management level. A national workshop on health information systems was organized in May 1991 in Islamabad to decide on the content and process of restructuring the health information system. A general consensus was reached between federal and provincial health officials to transform the existing routine reporting system in government-managed first-level care facilities into a comprehensive and integrated health management information system (HMIS/FLCF). Priority was given to first-level care facilities because most priority health problems of mothers and children could be resolved at this level. Also, the quality of the information system in referral-level facilities was considered acceptable. Although the private for-profit sector provides a significant portion of curative care in Pakistan, it was felt that at least in an initial phase only government-managed institutions should be included. The United States Agency for International Development (USAID) and the United Nations Children's Fund (UNICEF) provided funding for technical assistance during the design phase and the initial start-up costs of the system.

The design phase followed a stepwise process, first revising the information-generating process based on the information needs for first-level care facilities, and then planning for the required resources to manage the information system. It used a consensus-building approach involving a wide range of future HMIS user groups. First the participants agreed on a standard comprehensive package of health care services and resource management activities that had to be performed in every first-level care facility. For each of these services and activities, essential indicators were defined. Relevant data collection instruments were revised or newly designed if necessary, with the help of experts. Then the participants agreed upon reporting procedures and data flows within the health services system. In addition, for the first time ever in Pakistan, participants decided to computerize the reports sent by the first-level care facilities, in an initial phase at the divisional level, and later on also at the district level. To this end, customized data processing software was developed. About a year later, after several months of field testing in a sample of health facilities, the Ministry of Health and the provincial health departments approved the newly designed HMIS/FLCF. The following are the main features of the system:

- HMIS/FLCF indicators were chosen based on the need for appropriate decision making related to first level care services and activities.
- The system called for determining catchment areas around each FLCF and collecting population data for all villages in each catchment area. This resulted in a population denominator that permitted calculation of coverage for preventive maternal and child health services in the targeted risk groups.
- Case definitions for the main health problems were standardized. To ensure uniformity and reliability of data, complete instructions on how to collect, record, and report data were provided to the care providers through a comprehensive instruction manual available in English and in Urdu.
- Data collection instruments were simplified and reduced to a strict minimum. For example, instead of 18 registers previously maintained by the FLCF staff for managing maternal and child health services, only 3 registers were needed under the new system to record preventive services for mothers and children.
- Only indicators needed for health system management were routinely reported through a single comprehensive monthly report. The report was designed in such a way that the health unit manager could directly use the aggregated information for better planning and management in the health facility in question. Also, whereas epidemic diseases were reported through the immediate report, the yearly report served to update demographic and infrastructural information.
- Feedback reports on the main health problems, on services performed, and on resources used were to be produced through simple customized database management software.
- A supervisory checklist was developed to assist district supervisors in assessing the quality of care given to patients and clients in the FLCFs and in providing supportive supervision to the FLCF staff.

HMIS/FLCF implementation started in 1993 through a massive inservice training programme for health managers and care providers. Although it is still too early to conclusively evaluate the system, the first results are encouraging. Care providers say that the new data collection instruments are easy to use and provide the information they need for daily management of their activities. HMIS/FLCF is also an invaluable tool in ongoing implementation of a decentralized district-managed health services system in Pakistan. District managers use the information in the recently established district level-planning process.

Table 5 *The health information system restructuring process of the routine services reporting system*

Restructuring steps	Fit with the health services system		
	Illustrative tasks	CL	MF
Step 1: Identifying information needs and indicators	• Identify information needs for follow-up of a pregnant woman in a primary level clinic	1	PC
	• Identify indicators to ensure efficient drug management in a referral hospital	2	HU
	• Identify indicators to monitor the quality of supervision by the district management team	2	HS
Step 2: Defining data sources and developing data collection instruments	• Develop an appropriate record form for follow-up of haemodialysis patient in a tertiary care hospital	3	PC
	• Develop a monthly reporting form for activities performed in a primary level clinic	1	HU
	• Define data sources for a situational analysis at the district level	2	HS
Step 3: Develop data transmission and data processing procedures	• Structure the information flow on pregnant women between the traditional birth attendant and midwife in the health centre	1	PC
	• Ensure that monthly report forms from health centres are entered in the district computer in a timely and accurate manner	2	HS
Step 4: Ensure the use of the information	• Develop user-friendly feedback formats for regional managers on the utilization of inpatient services in the region	3	HS
	• Train health auxiliaries in follow-up procedures for hypertensive patients using a standard record form	1	PC
Step 5: Plan for the required health information system resources	• Create positions of computer operators in cases where district-level data processing is computerized	2	HS
	• Submit revised recurrent cost budgets based on proposed new data collection procedures	3	HS
Step 6: Develop a set of organizational rules	• Develop standard case definitions	All	All
	• Change the job description of doctors in cases where health information system restructuring involves their active participation in data collection	1	HU
	• Develop an instruction manual for computer operators	2	HS

CL = concentration levels, 1 = primary level, 2 = secondary level, 3 = tertiary level, MF = management function, PC = patient/client, HU = health unit, HS = health system.

system framework during the design of an improved routine reporting system for first level care facilities in Pakistan in 1991–1992.

Conclusion

The proposed health information system restructuring approach will assist system developers in addressing the weaknesses of existing routine health information systems in developing countries in at least three ways. First, it is adaptive to the information needs of health services at different strategic planning and operational levels, with particular consideration of care providers. If the information system provides information directly useful for patient/client and health unit management, care providers will be motivated to improve the quality of the data collected for transmission to higher levels. Second, it permits the development of a health information system in support of the health services system in its entirety, rather than fragmented systems in support of separate disease-oriented vertical programmes. Such a comprehensive information system is much more effective in ensuring a continuous and bidirectional flow of information between health services levels. This exchange of information is the basis of patient referral and counter-referral systems, supervisory systems, management support systems such as drugs and supplies distribution systems, and the organization of essential public health functions such as disease surveillance. Finally, and most important, as a result of the improved information process and health information system management structure, more relevant and better quality information will be produced that is also more likely to be used in the decision-making process at all levels and for all management functions of the health system.

Using health information system development as a strategy to improve the general management environment, as mentioned in Chapter 1, makes the match of the information system with the existing or planned health services system even more imperative. For example, in Pakistan, building a population-based indicator such as maternal mortality into the newly restructured health management information system for first level care facilities motivated the health unit staff to seek more active community participation, a policy actively promoted by the national and provincial governments. Or the creation of a comprehensive monthly activity report combining previously separate report forms reinforced the effort to integrate the health services, a strategy that was part of the national health plan. Also, a well functioning *intra*sectoral health information system, established in a decentralized district health system with the active participation of the population, can be the starting point for the gradual development of an *inter*sectoral health information system, as proposed by de Kadt (1989).

References

De Geyndt W (1994). *Managing the quality of health care in developing countries.* Washington, DC, World Bank (World Bank Technical Paper, No. 258).

de Kadt E (1989). Making health policy management intersectorial: issues of information analysis and use in less developed countries. *Social science and medicine,* 29:503–514.

Foltz AM (1993). Modeling technology transfer in health information systems—learning from the experience of Chad. *International journal of technology assessment in health care,* 9:345–361.

Helfenbein S et al. (1987). *Technologies for management information systems in primary health care.* Geneva, World Federation of Public Health Associations (Issue Paper, Information for Action Series).

Hurtubise R (1984). *Managing information systems: concepts and tools.* West Hartfort, CT, Kumarian Press: 1–168.

Lippeveld TJ, Foltz A, Mahouri YM (1992). *Transforming health facility-based reporting systems into management information systems: lessons from the Chad experience.* Cambridge, MA, Harvard Institute of International Development: 1–27 (Development Discussion Papers, No. 430).

Public Health Research and Training Unit (1980). *Organisation des services de santé: résumé.* Material for an international course in health promotion. Antwerp, Institute for Tropical Medicine.

Sandiford P, Annett H, Cibulskis R (1992). What can information systems do for primary health care? An international perspective. *Social science and medicine,* 34:1077–1087.

Sapirie S, Essential Public Health Functions Working Group (1997). *Primary health care and essential public health functions: critical interactions.* Paper presented at the International Conference of the Council of International Organizations of Medical Sciences, Geneva, 12–14 March 1997.

Unger JP (1989). *Evaluation du système national d'information du secteur santé. [Evaluating a national information system for the health sector.]* N'Djamena, Ministry of Public Health: 1–25.

World Bank (1993). *World development report 1993: investing in health.* New York, Oxford University Press.

World Health Organization (1986). *Improving health care through decision-linked research: application in health systems and manpower development. Part II: Options for implementation.* Geneva, World Health Organization (unpublished document HMD/86.4.2; available on request from Evidence and Information for Policy, World Health Organization, 1211 Geneva 27, Switzerland).

World Health Organization (1988). *The challenge of implementation: district health systems for primary care.* Geneva, World Health Organization (unpublished document WHO/SHS/DHS/88.1; available on request from Evidence and Information for Policy, World Health Organization, 1211 Geneva 27, Switzerland).

3 Using information to make decisions

Rainer Sauerborn

The problem

As is stressed throughout this book, information is not an end in itself, but a means to better decisions in policy design, health planning, management, monitoring, and evaluation of programmes and services including patient care, thus improving overall health service performance and outcome.

The implicit assumptions underlying information systems are twofold: first, that good data, once available, will be transformed into useful information which, in turn, will influence decisions; second, that such information-based decisions will lead to a more effective and appropriate use of scarce resources through better procedures, programmes, and policies, the execution of which will lead to a new set of data which will then stimulate further decisions (Fig. 4), and so forth in a spiral fashion. This generic view of the relation between information and decisions is applicable to patient care, health unit, and system levels (Chapter 2).

Most would agree that information can only influence decisions if it is relevant, reliable, and available for the decision-maker in a timely fashion. Unfortunately, the availability of such high-quality information does not guarantee its appropriate use in the decision-making process. The literature abounds with anecdotal accounts of underutilization of data (Opit, 1987; de Kadt, 1989). Chambers (1994) described the scenario with a note of sarcasm: "Much of the material remains unprocessed, or, if processed, unanalyzed, or, if analyzed, not read, or, if read, not used or acted upon. Only a minuscule proportion, if any, of the findings affect policy and they are usually a few simple totals" (p. 53).

The purpose of this chapter, therefore, is to provide workers in the health system with strategies to enhance information use. To do this we first define the various uses and users of information. We then turn our attention to the broader issue of how policymakers, planners, and health care providers make decisions within organizations and the role of information in this process. The chapter concludes by exploring practical ways of enhancing the use of information.

Defining information use

We can distinguish a number of inappropriate uses of information such as nonuse, underuse, misuse, and premature use to overuse of information. However, for the purpose of this book, we focus on underuse and nonuse, since they constitute the greatest and most frequently found

Fig. 4   *Idealized relationship between data, decisions, resources, and programmes*

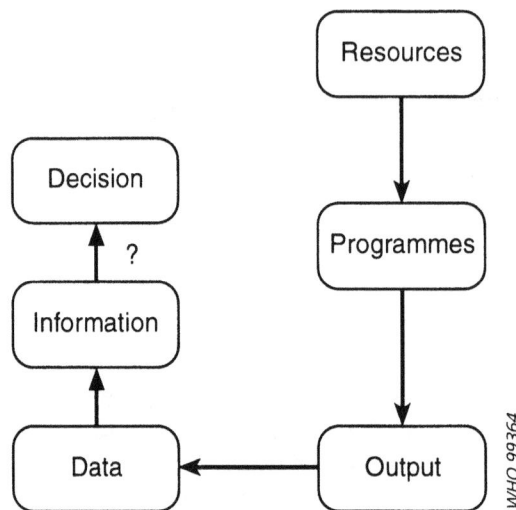

problems, both in our own experience and the published literature (Opit, 1987; Chambers, 1994; de Kadt, 1989; Campbell, Adjei & Heywood, 1996), as well as in the experience of many public health practitioners around the world.

Let us examine the left-hand side of Fig. 4, that is the transformation of data into decisions. As Einstein once noted, "Data do not speak for themselves." In fact, raw data are meaningless in and of themselves and need to undergo a series of cognitive transformations before they can influence decisions. Van Lohuizen (1986) proposed the cognitive model shown in Fig. 5.

As a first step in this knowledge-driven model of the decision-making process, data are turned into information through a process of selection and reduction. The use of indicators is a typical example (see chapter 4). Processing and analysing information with problem solving in mind leads to new knowledge. The interpretation of this knowledge, then, is guided by subjective judgement, rather than by objective, scientific rigour. As Weiss (1979) stated, the assumption here is that the "sheer fact that knowledge exists, presses it towards development and use".

Although this model is useful for delineating distinct steps which can be influenced separately, the model only incompletely reflects reality since it does not adequately address the political and social dimensions of decision making, which leads us to question how decisions are made, and what role information plays in this process.

How are decisions made?

Little is known about how decisions are made at the various levels of the health system. Most of what we know about how decisions are made comes from the analysis of the policy-making process, and most of those analyses are derived from sectors other than health. Assuming that the process of decision making is similar for policy making and for manage-

Fig. 5 *The knowledge-driven model of decision-making (modified after Van Lohuizen, 1986)*

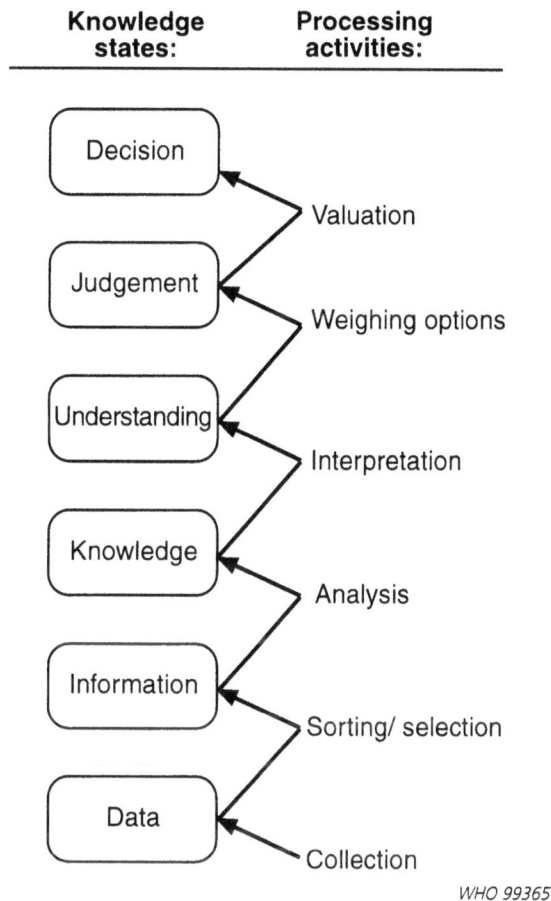

WHO 99365

ment, we give a brief overview of the factors involved in it. We then discuss how to extrapolate these findings to health information systems so that information can be optimally used throughout the health system.

The classical model of the policy-making process (Lasswell, 1975) identifies seven stages which follow each other over time in a linear and logical fashion, very much in the way a car is produced on an assembly line. These stages are shown in Fig. 6.

The conventional planning cycle or "planning spiral" (Green, 1992) as shown in Fig. 1 (see Chapter 1) is based on this model. The strength of this model lies in its emphasis on the process of decision-making, rather than on the individual decision-maker. Furthermore, the model stresses that there needs to be some sense of urgency and relevance for a problem to be put on the agenda and that this is not only done by the decision-makers themselves but by a wide variety of societal groups (community and special interest groups, the media, etc.). Once a problem is "on the agenda", several options for addressing it are generally developed and compared for their relative costs and benefits. The adoption of one of these options (the crucial decision-making step) in this model is influenced by a set of sociopolitical "pressure groups", such as political parties, special interest groups, and governments. The implementation

Fig. 6   *The classical model of the decision-making process (Lasswell, 1975)*

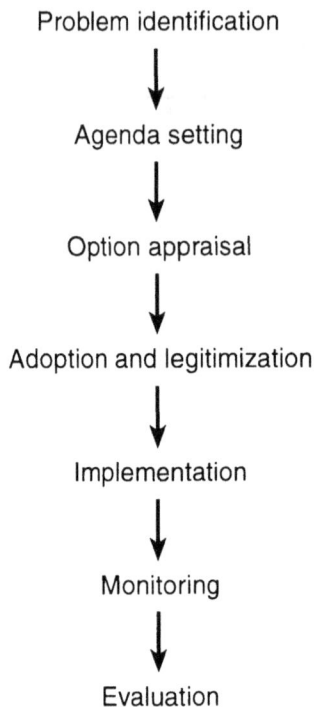

Problem identification

↓

Agenda setting

↓

Option appraisal

↓

Adoption and legitimization

↓

Implementation

↓

Monitoring

↓

Evaluation

WHO 99366

step is straightforward, followed by the final steps—monitoring, and evaluation—which may lead to the identification of new problems, making the linear process circular or, rather, spiral. In this model, information is but one of many inputs into the decision-making process (Fig. 7). We can understand how important it is that information be made available not only to decision-makers themselves but to the players influencing decision-makers, such as the media, donors, political parties, and so on.

Critics of Lasswell's linear decision-making model point out that in the real world decisions are not likely to be made in such a neat and logical way. Rather, phases overlap, and options are rarely compared methodologically. Proposing an iterative model of policy making, Grindle & Thomas (1991) acknowledge that a "policy reform process may be altered or reversed at any stage . . . by pressures and reactions of those who oppose it". They stress that there are a multitude of players with conflicting interests in the decision-making process and that decisions are made in an iterative rather than linear way.

Porter & Hicks (1995) emphasizes that problems, solutions, and political pressures converge in a window of opportunity that the prepared policy entrepreneur seizes. They suggest that in such a window of opportunity, there is a strong chance for information to influence the decision-making process.

How are these analyses of the policy-making process relevant to health information systems? We can draw several conclusions:

- The decision-making process is "messier" than the linear model suggests.

Fig. 7 *Political, noninformational factors influencing decision makers*

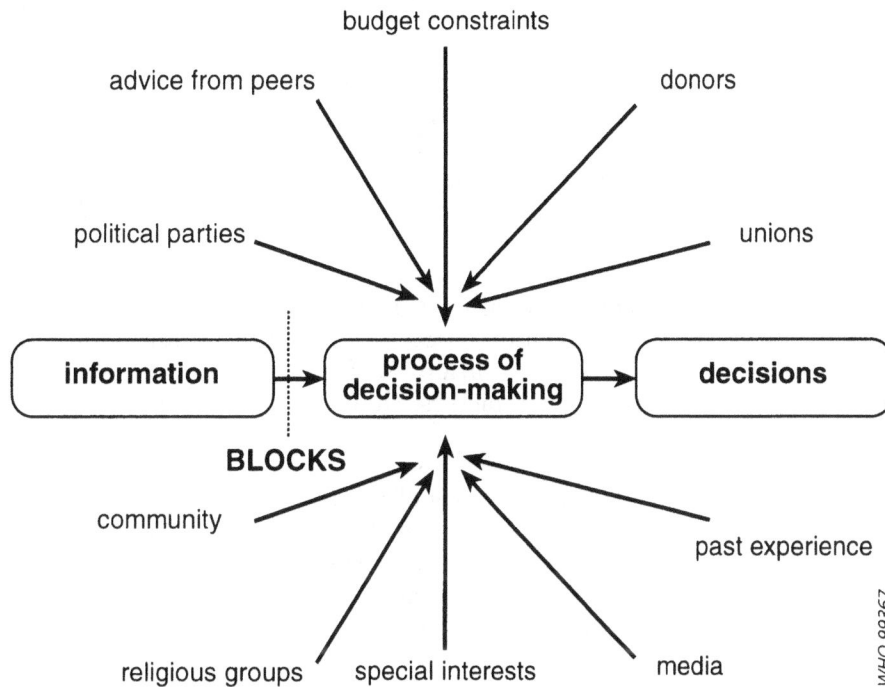

- The social and political dimensions of the decision-making process are critical, yet the knowledge-driven model (Fig. 5) does not acknowledge them. In this light, we can understand how it is crucial that "data people" be aware of the political environment in which decisions are made. For example, a physician's decision to start a campaign to foster the use of condoms in her catchment area commensurate with the standards of the national health plan is not only contingent on her knowledge of health information system indicators, such as low contraceptive prevalence rate, high fertility rate, and high estimates of maternal mortality rates, but also on the opinion of village heads, religious leaders, the local women's association, teachers, and the village council. She may have been warned by a colleague from a neighbouring health unit who experienced strong resistance to advertising condoms in his area and whose attempts to raise contraceptive use had failed.
- Advocacy and leadership are needed to put a problem on the agenda and to influence and "lobby" decisions. In order to foster the use of information, data people must leave behind the kind of political "abstention" that characterizes so many statistical departments at all levels of the health service pyramid all over the world. Rather, data people should become aware of the conflicting interests that influence decision-makers. They should consider it their task to communicate their information to all the main players (e.g. the media, political parties, donors, other ministries, etc.). Their role does not end with the delivery of a statistical yearbook; it only begins there. What is needed is for data people to engage in a continuous dialogue with decision-makers and those influencing them, and provide them with an arsenal of relevant and understandable information.

Ways to enhance the use of information in decision-making

Given the substantial—albeit rarely specified—resources that go into both health information systems and policy research, it is surprising that there is almost no empirical evidence to support the assumption that good information leads to improved decisions for health planning and policy. In fact, we could not identify a single empirical study of the actual use of information within a health system. We therefore must extrapolate again from the literature on the use of information derived from social science research for policy-making. In his seminal study of decision-making in private and public organizations (not in the health sector), Dunn (1980) examined the factors that enhanced or impeded the use of information. Modifying Dunn's classification, we can distinguish five broad factors that have been shown to be important in using information:

— characteristics of the data;
— characteristics of the problems and the decisions they require;
— organizational or structural characteristics;
— cultural differences between "data people" and "decision-makers";
— the communication between both.

We will now examine these five factors in greater detail.

Characteristics of the data

Ownership and relevance
Dunn notes that "research which conforms to the specification of the policy maker is more likely to be used." In order to ensure this conformity, we strongly advocate that a sense of ownership be fostered among all potential users of the information. From our experience (e.g. from Cameroon, see case study in Chapter 4, Box 9), potential users of a health information system can achieve a sense of ownership when they actively participate from its inception in all phases of the design. This includes identifying the data to collect, thus ensuring their relevance; choosing the indicators as well as determining the threshold values for actions and decisions; and defining what type of information should go to which users. This is the best way of ensuring that the information generated by a health information system is relevant to those who need it and thus more likely to be used in the decision-making process.

Validity and reliability
In addition, studies show that information tends to be used significantly more if decision-makers are convinced of its reliability and validity (Chapter 8). Potential users must be convinced that the data are of appropriate quality. For this reason, data quality is an important aspect to take into account not only at the start of the health information system, in the design phase, but throughout the operations of the health information system through regular checks on validity and reliability. Health information system designers often neglect to seek a consensus regarding what constitutes "appropriate" quality and what kind of checks should be applied. Users and producers of data should bear in mind their resource constraints and the trade-off between data quality and costs (Chapter 8).

Aggregation of data

Asked why they did not make more use of the information made available to them, decision-makers at the system level in Dunn's study frequently responded that they got too much detail with too little aggregation over time and space. From our own experience, those at the district or health centre level tend to deplore the fact that data are too aggregated and that they do not see how their specific district performs and compares with others. Tailoring the aggregation of the data to client needs is therefore a crucial part of the design of data feedback: different users need different outputs. As an example, Table 6 shows a part of the indicator definition achieved during the planning stage of the health information system in Cameroon. For each indicator, the different levels of aggregation are shown for each user in the right two columns. The task the indicator measures is the frequency of supervisory visits members of the district team pay to health centres. Although the rhythm of data collection is monthly, the reporting is not; at the systems level, only cumulative yearly data are shown by province.

It is essential that the detail of the original information remain available and can be recovered in the case of a special information request. For example, a supervisor from the Ministry of Health of Cameroon plans a visit to the provincial health team in Adamaoua Province. He notes that, overall, the average number of yearly supervisory visits to the health centres was below the national average in the preceding year. He now wants to see differences between health centre supervisory visits within the province. He incorporates health information system software that allows him to customize the aggregation of each indicator over time and space (see below).

Customizing information to users' needs

In a district-centred, primary health care approach, users should include the community, the local health facilities, the district and the central level, as well as the general public and the media. We would like to stress, along with Green (1992), that our list should include users of other sectors relevant to health, such as agriculture, education, housing, finance and planning, and so on. Table 7 maps the different types of information needs against the different types of users.

It is obvious that a health information system cannot and should not generate just one set of information for all users. Rather, we should make sure that the health information system is highly selective in tailoring the type and aggregation of information communicated to each of them. Table 7 provides an example of the types of information important for different users.

Timeliness of feedback

Listening to decision-makers, we are very likely to hear that one of the strongest impediments to proper use of information is the fact that it often arrives much too late, so that decisions must be made in its absence. We hear the same complaint regarding delay of feedback from those who produce the information. Chapters 6 and 8 deal with strategies to speed up data collection, transport of data, and data analysis.

Characteristics of the required decisions

Decision-makers use information more extensively in tackling short-term problems than in tackling long-term ones. In general, the clearer

Table 6   *Decision-oriented indicators: defining who gets what data in which aggregation (the example of the health information system in Cameroon)*

Task		Problem	Indicator		Data source aggregation	Rhythm		Decision			
Level	Description		Numerator	Denominator		Collect	Report	User	Cut-off	Type	
1	2	3	4	5	6	7	8	9	10	11	
District	Monthly supervision visits to each health centre (HC)	Supervision intervals exceed 1 month	No. of HCs with >3 months since last supervision	Total no. of HCs in district	Supervisory sheet/ district	Monthly	1 month	District team leader	>25% of HCs	Review logistics and motivation; revise supervision plan	
					Supervisory sheet/ district		6 months	Provincial team leader	>25% of districts	Logistics, motivation? Include in next district supervision; review supervisory plan	
					Supervisory sheet/ province		1 year	MOH	Province with >25% districts	Review resource allocation (personnel, fuel, transport)	

MOH = Ministry of Health.

Table 7 *Types of users and their different information needs. The number of crosses in each category is meant to reflect the relevance of information for the potential user*

Type of information needed	User				
	Community	Facility/ district	Central/ MOH	Other sectors	General public/ media
Demographic data	++++	+++	++++	++++	++++
Social and economic data	++	++	++++	++++	++++
Health care coverage	++++	++++	++++	+	++++
Health status	++++	++++	++++	++++	++++
Quality of care	++++	++++	++++	+	++++
Building/equipment	+	++++	++++	+	+
Personnel	++	++++	++++	+	+
Financial information	+++	++++	++++	+	++++

Shaded: Users that are often forgotten in health information system design.
Note: Facility/district and Ministry of Health (MOH) information needs differ mainly in the aggregation of data, not in the type of data.

and more formalized the decision, the more likely information will be used for that decision, provided that the information is available and aggregated for ease of use by the decision-maker. Since decisions for which the health information system is designed are often highly specific and foreseeable, we should expect these rules derived from research into the decision-making process in policy formulation to work in favour of information use in the health sector. We remind the reader of the need to define precisely the types of decisions for which a given indicator will be used (Chapter 4). In many instances, the type of decision prompted by the value of an indicator can be defined, as in the health information system in Cameroon (see Table 6, column 11). However, this only makes sense under two conditions: first, the decisions need to be very strongly linked to one indicator alone; and second, there needs to be a consensus among users that the specified action makes sense. In no way do we wish to advocate a health information system that replaces judgement with predefined computer algorithms, though these can help.

Conversely, decision-makers are likely to rely on input other than information when they face high-risk decisions which may cause conflict. Such decisions are more likely to occur at the systems level when new policies are formulated. The more routine decisions are and the less conflict they engender, the more likely they are to be based on information. This is not to say that we should accept these tendencies. On the contrary, we should insist that crucial and conflict-laden decisions be based to a large extent on the rational use of information. This requires active and timely promotion or brokering of the information to those facing hard decisions.

Characteristics of organizations

Dunn (1980) found that private organizations with profit incentives use information for decisions substantially more often than public ones. Nothing is known, however, about whether this finding can be extrapolated to the health sector. A plausible but unsubstantiated explanation is that public organizations are not under as much pressure to perform as private ones. From industry we know that information is used as a means to develop and monitor good quality.

Particularly in developing countries, the incidence of information-based decision making is particularly low in the health sector compared with other sectors and industries (Rodrigues & Israel, 1995). When the incentive to perform and to monitor quality is low, the use of information can be expected to be equally low. Conversely, we argue that offering incentives for performance, such as annual premium payments for reaching specific targets (Sauerborn, Bodart & Owona, 1995), promotes the use of information. Research on the link between institutional set-up, performance orientation, and information use in the health sector is clearly welcome.

Clearly established procedures to incorporate information in the planning process also have the potential to stimulate the use of information. In Cameroon, provincial budget plans were accepted by the Ministry of Health only when they incorporated data on past performance from the health information system.

Knowledge generated from inside the organization itself is used more frequently for decision-making than knowledge from an outside source, researcher, or evaluator. Applied to health information systems, there should therefore be a strong tendency to use information as long as the system was designed and agreed upon "from inside" rather than imposed by outside forces.

Cultural differences between data people and action people

Several authors have stressed that the psychology or the "culture" of people who use information ("action people") is quite different from those who collect, collate, analyse, and report information ("data people"). Health information system managers and staff would be included in the latter group. Ukwu (1995) went so far as to speak of "mutual disdain and distrust". Table 8 identifies a number of areas in which these two crucial players in a health information system may differ.

Of course, these distinctions are idealized and are less likely to be found the lower one goes in the health system pyramid. In fact, the health care practitioner at the health unit level is at the same time provider and user of information and data, and decision-maker.

Lack of attention to these cultural differences may lead to poor adaptation of the health information system to the information needs of decision makers (during the design phase) and to poor communication of information from data people to decision-makers (during operation of the health information system). This, in turn, is likely to block use of information.

Data people must leave their restricted realm of forms, computers, and reports and feel responsible for how they use data. Moreover, they need to become information promoters and lobbyists, interested in and committed to fostering change through information. The better data people understand the needs and constraints of decision makers, the more data will be used. Conversely, the more decision-makers know what data they need and communicate these needs to data people, the more useful

Table 8 *Different characteristics of the users (action people) and the providers of data (data people)*

Characteristics	Action people	Data people
Incentives/main objective	Reelection, good standing with supervisors, change	Publication (researcher); detailed report (health information system)
Time horizon	Short: weeks or days, works under strong time pressure	Long: months, years
Main interest in looking at data	Relative values, comparing: • current state with performance objective • two regions • time trends	Absolute values and totals
Cost orientation	Strong, always want to know what an action costs	Weak, frequently not interested in costs
Language	Action-oriented, managerial jargon	Precise, academic jargon
Communication style	Short memos, executive summaries, business meetings	Full reports, written publications, conferences
Training	Administration, economics, management, medicine	Statistics, informatics, medicine
Familiarity with data	Limited	Excellent
Familiarity with substance	Excellent	Limited
Computer literacy	Limited	Excellent

the data will become for them. How can we promote such mutual understanding?

One way is to clearly specify how to use what data for which types of decisions. As an example, the Ministry of Health of Pakistan developed a specific instruction manual for first-level care workers, explaining the meaning and use of each indicator in the health information system. Health workers found it particularly effective in fostering use of information.

Another way of promoting understanding is through training. Data people should receive short courses on the main substantive issues, the decisions that need to be made, and their time frames, whereas decision-makers need to learn more about data collection problems, data quality, transmission, and analysis. Both should receive explicit training in the use of information for decision making. Such training is only effective if clear ideas and procedures for information use are in place, as we stressed in the preceding paragraph.

A third way to foster cooperation is to facilitate teamwork between action people and data people from the start, that is the design and implementation of the health information system. When the flow of information starts, there should be regular meetings comprising both groups to discuss the implications of the information for decision making and how information can be improved for that purpose. It is essential that this communication not be relegated to written reports alone. This leads us to the next factor that influences the use of data: from the design phase to the feedback phase, good communication is likely to increase mutual understanding of constraints.

Finally, incentives—pecuniary and nonpecuniary—for proper use of information in management and planning should be offered (i) to those involved in health information systems in an effort to improve the quality and completeness of data and (ii) to decision-makers at all levels for the actual use of information.

Communication

The way information is communicated is a critical pathway (bottleneck) for the use of information. It can be improved by attention both to the process of communication and to its products.

Communication process within a health team

We fully concur with Green's (1992) point that verbal and personal briefings on the main results are much more likely to stimulate the use of information than written reports alone. As an example, such verbal feedback can take the form of regular half-day staff meetings at the district or central level, or informal meetings at the community level. Every effort should be made to create a culture of regular dialogue and exchange between data people and action people. Finally, in the primary health care spirit of intersectoral cooperation, we should seek to communicate relevant information beyond the health system (see above "advocacy") to the media, funding agencies, as well as education and agriculture ministries, to name just a few (see Table 7).

Feedback process

The feedback process has been stressed above. Speed of feedback is of paramount importance to motivate health practitioners or managers at the periphery to use information. Modern technology such as the Internet can help speed up feedback and allow interactive communication regarding its interpretation.

Communication products

Many health information systems produce endless tables as their main form of data presentation. While precise and detailed, these tables rarely help decision-makers find the most crucial information in a short time. Written reports should be customized according to major issues (e.g. policy issues, efficiency, budgetary advocacy) and to the time pressure of decision-makers: they should be short (not more than 10 pages, including a 1-page executive summary), and tentative conclusions keyed to major issues should be spelled out for discussion. The full report should act as a backup rather than as the main document for communication, and as something to which the interested decision-maker can refer for further detail. Wherever possible, different options for action should be specified, together with their likely consequences and costs. Ukwu's (1995) suggestion to hire professional writers to rewrite research results for decision-makers could also prove helpful for health information system reports.

The information should be related to a meaningful population denominator. For example, it is more useful for decision-makers to report the percentage of all children in a given area aged 1 year that have been fully immunized instead of the total number of children immunized.

The art of creating a useful feedback report lies in the use of meaningful comparisons rather than absolute figures. Such comparisons include:

- Time comparison. Trends comparing past and present information.
- Geographical comparison. Between health units and districts (position of performance of health centre X with the mean of all health

Fig. 8 *Graphical display of health facility performance*

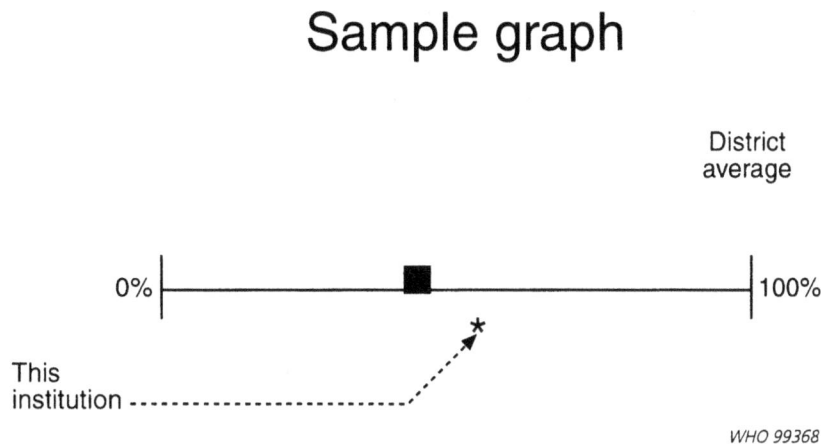

Sample graph

District
average

0% ├────────────■──────────────┤ 100%

*

This
institution ----------------------------´

WHO 99368

Source: Pakistan Child Survival Project, 1994.

centres). A link to a geographic information system is particularly useful. A more in-depth discussion of geographic information systems and their tremendous potential for increasing information use is provided in Chapter 12.

- Comparison of actual performance versus mean performance. Fig. 8 shows in graphical format where a given health unit stands with regard to the mean.
- Comparison of actual versus planned performance. Wherever possible, the current value of an indicator should be put in relation to the objective set for this indicator. As an example, "20% of planned supervisory visits were carried out" makes more sense to a decision-maker than "34 supervisory visits were carried out". Unfortunately, much of the output of health information systems is based on total values, such as the total number of new cases per month, the total number of children under 1 year fully immunized, and so on. Such information is meaningless for the decision-maker who needs to decide whether there is a deficit in performance and hence a need for action (e.g. check cold chain, vaccine availability, work motivation, or equipment; examine cases of immunizable diseases, review reasons for population non-compliance with immunization schemes). Performance charts are action-oriented because they relate current to planned performance. As Fig. 9 shows, such graphs visually depict any gap that requires decisions. For a health centre in Cameroon, the chart displays the monthly cumulative number of new outpatients seen (lower line). The upper straight line shows the performance objective set by the health centre team in conjunction with their district supervisor. The endpoint of the straight line is the performance target the health facility team had set out to achieve at the end of the year. The origin of the straight line is the actual number of monthly outpatient visits at the beginning of the year. By linking both points we assume a linear progression, which is certainly a simplification, but a reasonable one.
- Comparisons between population subgroups. For example in terms of health status, health care utilization, and risk factors.

Fig. 9 *Performance Chart: actual number of outpatients seen compared with performance targets (Beka Gotto health area, Adamoua Province, Cameroon)*

Number of new cases of curative consultations

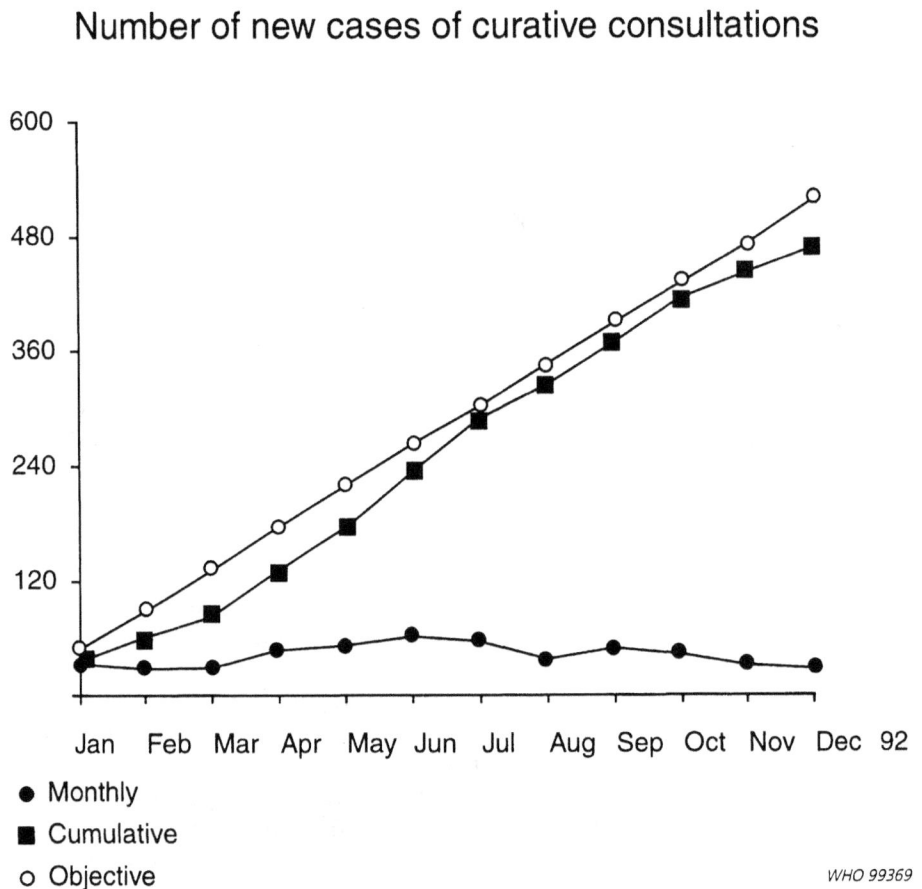

● Monthly
■ Cumulative
○ Objective

WHO 99369

Source: Cameroon Provincial Health Information System.

Outlook and sketch of a research agenda

We have pointed to many gaps in the empirical evidence with regard to the decision-making process in health care planning and provision, and the relative importance of using information within this process. We strongly advocate that operational research be commissioned that sheds more light into these areas. Illustrative examples of areas for further research include:

— the use of information for a series of purposes, such as budgeting, establishing annual work plans, supervision, infrastructure, and personnel planning;
— the relationship between the format in which information is displayed (maps, action-oriented graphs) and its use in health planning;
— the relationship between training to use information and actual use of information;
— the relationship between various ways of disseminating and using information;

— the effectiveness of broadening the target audience of information from the decision-maker to political groups that influence the decision-making process (see Fig. 7);
— analyses of cost-effectiveness of information for decision-making.

Conclusion

The objective of a health information system is not to produce information but to use it. While many factors other than information influence the decision-making process, we have shown that the potential for using information is rarely achieved. We identified a number of deficiencies in the data and their presentation, and most important, in how information is communicated and "lobbied" to those who make and influence decisions. We have shown ways to address these deficiencies and enhance the use of information for health planning. More research use is urgently needed on how health information systems function and on the extent to which the strategies outlined in this chapter actually enhance information.

References

Bertrand WE (1988). Information as a primary health care intervention: the impact of new technology on improving health for all. In: Wilson RG et al., eds. *Management information systems and microcomputers in primary health care.* Geneva, Aga Khan Foundation: 21–26.

Campbell B, Adjei S, Heywood A (1996). *From data to decision making in health—the evolution of a health management information system.* Amsterdam, Royal Tropical Institute: 1–96.

Chambers R (1994). *Rural development: putting the last first.* New York, Longman.

de Kadt E (1989). Making health policy management intersectorial: issues of information analysis and use in less developed countries. *Social science and medicine,* 29:503–514.

Dunn WN (1980). The two-communities metaphor and models of knowledge use: an exploratory case survey. *Knowledge,* 1:515–536.

Green A (1992). *An introduction to health planning in developing countries.* Oxford, Oxford University Press.

Grindle MS, Thomas JW (1991). *Public choices and policy change, the political economy of reform in developing countries.* Baltimore, MD, Johns Hopkins University Press.

Lasswell HD (1975). Research policy analysis: the intelligence and appraisal functions. In: Greenstein FI, Polsby NW, eds. *Handbook of political science.* Reading, MA, Addison-Wesley.

Opit LJ (1987). How should information on health care be generated and used? *World health forum,* 8:409–417.

Pakistan Child Survival Project Team (1994). *Extension period, final report.* Islamabad, Pakistan Child Survival Project.

Porter RW, Hicks I (1995). *Knowledge utilization and the process of policy formation: towazrd a framework for Africa.* Washington, DC, United States Agency for International Development.

Rodrigues RJ, Israel K (1995). *Conceptual framework and guidelines for the establishment of district-based information systems.* Barbados, Pan American Health Organization, Office of the Caribbean Program Coordination (document PAHO/CPC/3.1/95.1).

Sauerborn R, Bodart C, Owona R (1995). Recovery of recurrent health service costs through provincial health funds in Cameroon. *Social science and medicine*, 40:1731–1739.

Ukwu IU (1995). *Health research and health policy in Nigeria.* Enugu, Institute for Development Studies, University of Nigeria.

Van Lohuizen CW, Kochen M (1986). Introduction: mapping knowledge in policy-making. *Knowledge*, 8(1):3–11.

Weiss CH (1979). The many meanings of research utilization. *Public administration review*, 39:426–431.

4 Identifying information needs and indicators

Claude Bodart and Laura Shrestha

Introduction

Chapter 2 suggests that the design and implementation of an effective and efficient health information system are intimately linked and must fit into the organization of the health system for which it generates information. In the same chapter, it is argued that the development of a rationally structured routine information system can potentially contribute to the overall improvement of the management capabilities of the health services.

In this chapter, we look at ways health planners and health system professionals can achieve these goals by determining information needs and indicators—that is variables that describe a given situation and thus can be used to measure change—based on a functional analysis of health services, focusing on patient/client management, health unit management, and system management. Restructuring any health information system means first of all identifying strengths and weaknesses of the existing system to focus on the least functional areas.

Some information can be used directly to make decisions. For example, the stock level of a specific drug item can easily trigger a decision about the urgency of ordering the drug. However, in most instances, the direct use of raw data in this fashion is not feasible. Therefore, selecting appropriate indicators allows health system professionals to transform crude information into a form that is more suited for decision making.

Until recently, information needs were primarily at the national level, for example statistical reports which focused primarily on measuring facility-based diseases. With increased financial constraints in the health care sector and a greater concern for decentralization and democracy, there has been a move towards more information access across the spectrum of health care management. Recent trends have shown that defining information needs must be based on consensus building among all the actors involved in collecting the data and using the information produced. Both consumer and provider concerns must be heeded.

Just as information must reflect the needs of consumers and planners alike, so, too, should an information system be customized to meet specific needs for specific circumstances (Helfenbein et al., 1987). It is essential that a country develop its own indicators, even though specialized UN agencies, bilateral donor organizations, and nongovernmental organizations have proposed sets of indicators for the health sector. Specifying individualized indicators will ensure ownership of the end product, result in an adequate set of indicators tailored to local needs, and contribute to the development of institutional capacity of the country. The search for uniformity in the definition and methods of collecting the data advocated in the international fora should not undermine the importance of each country developing its own set of relevant indicators. Our intention is not to present long lists of indicators by levels of care or programmes—although many examples can be found throughout the chapter—but instead to describe a methodology for defining information needs and indicators.

A general framework for defining information needs and indicators

The proposed framework for defining information needs and indicators, described below, is based on the same premise as the more general health services framework presented in Chapter 2: information in support of the decision-making process at all levels of the health services.

- *Step 1: Perform a functional analysis at each management level of the health services system.* Defining information needs starts with an analysis of functions of the different management levels of the health system. This functional analysis should focus on priority health problems, national goals and strategies, essential health services for the prevention and management of priority problems, critical health resources for carrying out the essential services, and important management processes needed to plan, monitor, and control the services and resources. It includes both individual care and essential public health functions. While it is preferable that a complete analysis of all health system functions take place, this may be unrealistic within a modest time period. Even without a complete functional analysis, it is possible for national working groups to confirm priority health problems and the services and resources that must be directed towards their prevention and control within reasonably brief group processes conducted at various levels in the health system (policy, central programme management, regional or district).
- *Step 2: Identify information needs and select feasible indicators.* Once priority services and resources have been defined, it becomes possible to identify the relevant information to monitor the functioning of the system. Based on the information needs so defined, appropriate indicators can be developed. It is important to set priorities at this stage to select a limited number of indicators. This requires judgement calls on their validity; their specificity and sensitivity; the required resources to collect the data; and the importance of the decisions to be made based on these indicators (relevance). Finally, indicators will only be retained after defining a number of characteristics to enable their operationalization. Operationalizing indicators requires defining the sources of the data; determining the frequency of collection and processing of the indicator; determining appropriate levels of aggregation; setting levels of thresholds and target; and determining possible actions if a threshold is reached.

Needless to say, what counts in defining appropriate information and indicators is not only the methodology described here but also the extent to which the information needs of the actors involved are taken into account (health care providers, health consumers, data collectors, and users). Defining information needs according to this framework will help in developing a health information system that will be proactive, dynamic, and action-oriented, as suggested by Finau (1994).

The process described in this chapter is not meant to be applied in a rigid way. The intent is rather to provide a guideline that can help define appropriate "action-led" information needs and essential indicators, that is limiting the quantity of information and indicators though ensuring that they are well balanced as a set; improving the quality of data; and defining indicators that are operationally feasible and meet national needs. It is an iterative process, meaning that at any step one can return to previous steps to revise them. The process described can be used either to identify a new list of indicators or to revise an existing one. The benefits of revising an existing list of indicators must, however, be weighed against its costs in terms of lost opportunities to measure trends over time.[1]

The remainder of this chapter presents and discusses each of the steps involved in defining appropriate information and indicators.

Performing a functional analysis at each management level of the health services system

Routine health information systems should support three types of management functions (patient/client management, health unit management, and health system management) that are required at various levels of the health system (district, regional, and national).

In a broader context of health care reform, many countries have adopted a decentralized approach where the health district becomes the operational unit of the health system. Unfortunately, in most countries, information systems have not followed the pace of decentralization and therefore are not suited to the information needs of local health professionals. Table 9 summarizes the main functions at the different management and health system levels.

Identifying information needs

Information required for action for the three types of management functions is specified below.

Patient/client management

Although quantities of clinical data are collected about patients during each episode of illness, only the most relevant to patient management should be kept and filed. For details, see Box 3.

---

[1] For instance, in the United States, in efforts to measure the prevalence of disability in the population, a question about health conditions that limit or prevent the use of public transportation was introduced in the 1980 decennial census. Recognizing that the query addressed only a limited fraction of the disability experience of Americans, the question was dropped in the 1990 census and replaced by two questions which addressed the individual's ability to perform activities of daily living. While these questions better captured the prevalence of disability in the United States, the opportunity to measure trends in "public transportation" disability were lost (see Shrestha & Rosenwaike, 1996).

Table 9 *Main functions at national, regional, and district level in a decentralized health system*

	Management functions		
	System management	Health unit management	Patient/client management
District level	• Plan development and routine activities of the health district • Evaluate the annual workplan • Manage all district resources (financial, human resources, equipment, etc.) • Organize promotive activities in the district • Manage the health information system • Provide feedback to and supervise health facilities in the district • Integrate specialized programmes in the health system of the district • Identify the needs for and carry out operations research • Rationalize health care to improve its efficiency, quality, and acceptability • Promote intrasectoral (private sector, NGOs) and intersectorial collaboration	Health Centre • Service delivery — first level curative care — antenatal care — under-5 care — immunization — chronic patient care — nutritional activities — family planning — outreach activities • Resource management — management activities (drugs, finances, transportation, personnel, etc.) • Community participation — community dialogue Hospital • Services delivery — referral curative care — emergency surgery — dentistry — diagnostic activities (X-ray and laboratory) — hospitalization (paediatrics, surgery, medicine, obstetrics) — high-risk pregnancies and deliveries • Resource management — management activities	Health Centre • Provide quality curative and preventive care to individual patient/client Hospital • Provide quality secondary care for referred patients
Regional level	• Regional planning and coordination of health activities • District supervision, monitoring, and evaluation • Feedback on the districts on consolidated and analysed data • Budgeting and auditing • Logistical support for districts • Financing and monitoring of capital investment	Hospital • Service delivery — specialized surgery and internal medicine — some specialties (ophthalmology, etc.) — specialized diagnostic tests • Resource management — management activities	Hospital • Provide quality tertiary care for referred patients
National level	• Policy formulation • National planning for resource allocation • Regulatory role • Coordination between private and public sector and liaison with international agencies • Training and regulation of personnel development	Hospital • Service delivery — all types of specialized care — teaching activities — clinical research • Resource management — management activities	Hospital • Provide quality tertiary care for referred patients

NGOs = nongovernmental organizations.

The nucleus of information gathering in the health centre is the information kept on individual clients. Most information derived from this level will be used for decision-making concerning the individual patient or client. Information on patients and clients at this level is important

---

Box 3 Examples of important information needs for patient/client management

- *Identifiers:* name, address, sex, age, information on other family members, socioeconomic status of the family
- *Follow-up on risk episodes:* vaccination status, follow-up information on other risk episodes (antenatal care, under-5 consultations)
- *For women:* number and ages of children, information on contraception, illnesses during pregnancies, and post-partum
- *Information on important episodes of illnesses*[2] (especially of chronic illnesses, human immunodeficiency virus (HIV) infection, perinatal problems for infants, and childhood diseases)
- *Information on risk factors and allergies.*

---

because it improves the quality of care provided to the client (see Box 4), and determines the quality of the data used at subsequent levels of the system.

Health unit management

At the health unit management level, two distinct types of information are recommended: the aggregated data from the patient/client level and the internal management data from the health unit. The exact requirements for information will depend on the type of facility (hospital, health centre, etc.) and the nature of the services provided.

Where possible, it is recommended that service delivery data be combined with data on the characteristics of the defined catchment population, to see whether service use is adequately meeting the needs of the population. Data on community characteristics are also helpful, but may require special studies.

Internal management data from the health unit provide an indication of how particular facilities work. This latter category addresses whether facilities have the resources, both tangible and intangible, that are required to carry out the mission of the unit (Bulatao, 1995). It includes such things as adequate infrastructure and equipment, effective logistics, clear and sensible decision-making procedures, trained and dedicated staff, the research and evaluation capacity required, and so on. It also considers whether the capital and resources are being used efficiently.

The type of data needed for decision-making at the health unit management level depends on the degree of decentralization of management. Box 5 illustrates the types of information that are required.

---

[2] The definition of important episodes of illnesses will differ depending on the local epidemiological profile (most episodes of malaria are considered insignificant in hyperendemic areas), the management capacity of data of the providers, and the local culture.

Box 4   How does the information system promote quality care?

Major characteristics of quality of care are continuity, integration, comprehensiveness, and rational care. All four characteristics can be promoted through the information system:

- *Continuity* of care can only be achieved through an effective information system in the health unit that will increase client compliance with curative and preventive care. Carefully designed cards can help the staff to be aware of follow-up appointments. When patients do not keep their appointments, staff need to remind them. Reminders can take several forms: home visits, telephone calls, or written reminders. Relevant individual information on each patient is usually kept on a card or a more sophisticated medium, and the appointments database is regularly updated. In this way, continuity of care greatly improves the effectiveness of care.
- *Integration* of curative and preventive care is achieved primarily with the help of the individual information kept on each patient. Each patient-provider contact is used to deliver curative as well as preventive care according to client needs and acceptability. Integration leads primarily to more efficient use of scarce resources. Standard diagnostic and treatment guidelines can be developed in a way that maximizes every provider-patient contact in terms of curative and preventive care.
- To ensure *comprehensiveness* in the delivery of care, the care provider needs to be informed about the patient's household and socioeconomic milieu. This can be achieved through household records filled out during a census of the population living in the catchment area of the health unit as discussed in Chapter 5. This census will generate useful information on the community and will initiate a dialogue between the community and the health care providers. At the same time, it produces demographic data that will be useful in generating information on use and coverage needed at the health unit and system management levels. In urban settings or developed countries where catchment areas are more difficult to define due to competition among providers, comprehensiveness can be promoted for a catchment population. A typical example is the case of health maintenance organizations in the United States, which deliver a package of activities to a defined population recruited through voluntary membership.
- *Rational* care at the patient/client level can be promoted by the use of standard diagnostic and treatment guidelines. Proper use of these guides can improve classification of health problems and monitoring of patient health status and therefore they are part of the information system. Their capacity to improve care depends on the quality or validity of the guidelines themselves, as well as implementation in day-to-day practice. Constraints on the effectiveness of the guidelines are numerous and result generally in poor use of these tools. It is suggested that economic incentives might be more effective in changing the provider's behaviour than clinical guidelines (Feder, 1996). There is a need for further research on appropriate incentives (economic, regulatory, etc.) for compliance with standard diagnostic and treatment guidelines.

Box 5 Examples of important information needs for health unit management

Data on use and coverage of curative and preventive services:

— absolute number of clients receiving particular services (e.g. acceptors of family planning, prenatal care visits, measles vaccination
— proportion of the population at risk that receives a service (family planning users as a proportion of all fertile women in union in a catchment area)
— aggregated data on continuity of care (number of pregnant women who return for a second prenatal visit, after having had a first visit at the health facility)
— aggregated data on referral (number of referred cases of high-risk pregnancy registered at a facility which provides essential obstetric services)
— measurements of actual and perceived quality of care
— estimates of community access (such as the absolute number and proportion of population in a catchment area with or without relatively easy access to services)
— data on population catchment area (population size, population age and sex distribution, population at risk of particular ailments, vital statistics on births and deaths).

Resource management data, to gauge how facilities are functioning:

— human resources (e.g. the ratio of health personnel to 1000 inhabitants; estimates of the number of service and fieldworker personnel who are theoretically supposed to deliver services who have or have not received requisite training)
— material resources, including infrastructure, medial equipment, and so on (such as an inventory of vehicles [both in and out of service], and assessment of future requirements)
— pharmaceuticals, vaccines, and contraceptive management
— availability of a logistics information system which provides estimates of availability and future needs for services
— maintenance
— financial management (mobilization, cost, accounting)
— unit costs (per episode), which is important for planning and for pricing (fee-for-service and reimbursement schemes).

Health system management

Information needs at the system management level (national, regional, and district) will vary according to the level of decentralization of the health system. At the national level, information needs must guide policy formulation and strategic planning. At the regional level, information needs are geared towards the technical and logistic support of districts and strategic mid-term planning. Information needs at the district level must primarily satisfy operational needs to measure the functionality of the district health system. As shown in Box 6, the information needed for health system management often has to come from outside the health services, for example from the community, or from other sectors. It will therefore require data from sources other than the routine health information system. This issue is further discussed in Chapters 6 and 7.

Box 6 Examples of information needs at health system management level

Community profiles:

— epidemiological profile
— demographic and socioeconomic profiles (household income and expenditures, willingness and ability to pay, mother's literacy, etc.)
— environmental profile of the community.

Aggregated data on functioning of health services:

— data from health unit level on use and coverage of curative and preventive services.

Aggregated management data:

— data on management of services (planning, supervision, information activities, quality of care, community involvement)
— data on referral between health care levels.

Macrofinancial data:

— financial resources by source: public sector, medical insurance, out-of-pocket, foreign aid
— health expenditures by level of the health system, in rural and urban areas, in the public and the private sector, and for minorities
— technical efficiency (use of financial means for cost-effective interventions).

Resource distribution:

— geographical distribution of health infrastructure (and services actually delivered), equipment, and human resources by type.

Legal and regulatory framework:

— legal and regulatory documents.

Information from other sectors:

— education, agriculture, transportation, banking, justice, women's affairs, and so on.

Defining and classifying essential indicators

Defining indicators

As seen in Box 7, the literature provides numerous definitions of the term "indicator". At the outset of this chapter, we explained that an indicator is a variable that evaluates status and permits measurement of changes over time. An indicator does not always describe the situation in its entirety, but sometimes only gives an indication of what the situation might be and acts as a proxy. For example, the incidence of diarrhoea

---

Box 7 Some definitions of the term "indicator"

- Indicators are variables that help to measure changes, directly or indirectly (WHO, 1981).
- Indicators are "an indirect measure of an event or condition". For example, a baby's weight for age is an indicator of the baby's nutritional status (Wilson & Sapanuchart, 1993).
- An indicator is "a statistic of direct normative interest which facilitates concise, comprehensive, and balanced judgments about conditions of major aspects of a society" (Department of Health, Education, and Welfare, 1969).
- "Indicators are variables that indicate or show a given situation, and thus can be used to measure change" (Green, 1992).

---

determined from data collected in a health centre represents only a fraction of the cases of diarrhoea that occur in the community.

Indicators should lead as much as possible to action. In most instances, however, the information provided by the indicator will need to be complemented by further investigation, such as a supervisory visit to collect more qualitative data, special studies, or operations research, before it leads to action.

Indicators are quantitative measurements, and generally include a numerator and a denominator.[3] The numerator is a count of the events that are being measured. The most common denominator is the size of the target population at risk of the event (under 5, pregnant women, newborn, etc.). Indicators which include a denominator are useful for monitoring change over time and comparing areas. At the health centre and sometimes at the district level, the indicator might be more meaningful when presented as an event (numerator only) rather than as a proportion or a rate especially for rare but important events such as a case of haemorrhagic fever or meningitis, a maternal death in a health centre, or the number of health units with a stockout in measles vaccines.

At least four types of indicators can be identified:

- *Count indicators* simply measure the number of events without a denominator:

  Count indicator = number of newly detected cases of tuberculosis

- *Proportion indicators*, whose resultant values are typically expressed as a percentage, are indicators for which the numerator is contained in the denominator:

$$\text{Proportion indicator} = \frac{\text{number of health centres without ivermectin}}{\text{total number of health centres}}$$

- *Rate indicators* measure the frequency of an event during a specified time, usually expressed per 1000 or 100,000 population, k. The rate

---

[3] Some indicators, however, measure only the number of events, and have only a numerator.

is the basic measure of disease occurrence because it is the measure that most clearly expresses probability or risk of disease in a defined population over a specified period of time (Mausner & Kramer, 1985):

$$\text{Rate indicator} = \frac{\text{number of cases of malaria in children under 5}}{\text{mid-year population of children under 5}} \times k$$

- *Ratio indicators* are indicators for which the numerator is not included in the denominator:

$$\text{Ratio indicator} = \frac{\text{number of male AIDS deaths}}{\text{number of female AIDS deaths}}$$

Is it not always possible or relevant to provide quantitative information for decision-making. For example, the quality of the interpersonal communication between a nurse and his or her patients is best measured by direct observation of the nurse's interaction with a patient. This type of information will be collected during supervisory visits and characterized by measurement on a categorical scale, that is a nominal or ordinal scale.

Index (or composite indicators) is a term reserved for more complex, multidimensional measures composed of an aggregation of indicators. Indices are usually developed in research circles and are of limited practical use.[4] Recent efforts to measure the burden of disease using disability-adjusted life years (DALYs) are an example of the search for a global index of health (World Bank, 1993). DALYs represent the present value of future disability-free years that are lost as the result of premature deaths or cases of disability occurring in a particular year. It is the preference attached to the value of years of life by age and the trade-off between a year of ill-health and a year of death that makes it difficult to establish the appropriateness of this index. Murnaghan (1981) suggests that it makes more sense to concentrate on more generic measures as indicators since they are simpler to construct, interpret, and use, are more versatile in their applications, and less vulnerable to cross-cultural differences.

Classifying indicators

The proliferation of indicators calls for a rational system for classifying them. Various ways of classifying indicators have been proposed, depending on how they are used. It is sometimes difficult to prescribe a clear-cut typology because the categorization is not always conceptually clear: for example, the incidence of diarrhoea cases with dehydration in the catchment area could be an impact indicator for a control of diarrhoeal disease programme. However, the number of dehydrated children with diarrhoea seen at the health centre can also be a process or output indicator to calculate the number of oral rehydration salt packets required each quarter. Three common types of classification of indicators are briefly described.

---

[4] However, there are instances where indices might be of practical use. The "family planning program effort score" has proven to be highly used and respected in the area of family planning. See Parker & Ross (1991).

The input, process, output, and outcome spectrum of indicators and its attributes (see Annex 1)
A common typology distinguishes five classes of indicators: input, process, output, and outcome and determinant[5]. This classification system is based on a logical framework in which inputs eventually lead to outcomes:

- Input indicators refer to resources needed to carry out the activities.
- Process indicators monitor activities that are carried out.
- Output indicators measure results of activities, including coverage, knowledge, attitude, and behavioural changes that result from the activities.
- Outcome indicators determine developmental long-term effects, including changes in the health status of the population.
- Determinant indicators refer to conditions that contribute to or are precursors of disease such as human behavioural factors or unhealthy environmental conditions.

The following example illustrates this continuum:

Immunization equipment, vaccines, and trained staff (input) can progressively be applied to vaccination activities (process). This, in turn, raises the immunization coverage (output) and consequently reduces morbidity and mortality from preventable diseases (outcome).

Table 10 shows that the need for different classes of indicators varies with the type of management and, hence, the functions at that level. Health system management mainly uses outcome indicators; health unit and patient/client management depend more on input, process, and output indicators. Each of the four classes of indicators targets specific attributes. These attributes can be defined as the major concerns of a health system such as equity, efficiency, effectiveness, accessibility, coverage, costs, sustainability, and so on. Ideally, the health information system indicators should target major attributes of the health system to end up with a well-balanced set of indicators which will provide complete but concise information on important aspects of the health system. Annex 1 provides an example of such a balanced list.

Programme indicators
Indicators can also be classified by programmes or activities (e.g. family planning, reproductive health, and nutrition). In some cases, this typology is not advisable as it may lead to a verticalization of activities and an increase in the number of indicators. However, special programmes like the Expanded Programme on Immunization, Control of Diarrhoeal Diseases, Acute Respiratory Infections, Tuberculosis, and Maternal and Child Health and Family Planning need not undermine primary health care, and in many countries may lead to enhanced service coverage and quality within integrated services at the community and health centre level (Sapirie & Orzeszyna, 1995).

Within programmes, indicators are usually categorized according to input, process, output, and outcome.

---

[5] Determinants of health are increasingly considered as a distinct class of indicators, although some authors tend to include them in one of two classes: input or outcome.

Table 10 *Link between functions, management level, and indicator categories*

Indicator categories				
Mission/functions	Type of management	Input	Process and output	Outcome
Policy (evaluation)	Health system	++	+	++++
Planning (monitoring and evaluation)	Health system	+++	++	+++
Implementation (monitoring)	Health unit and patient/client	++++	++++	++

Indicator use increases from + to ++++.

Monitoring and evaluation indicators

Indicators can also commonly be grouped into monitoring and evaluation indicators. There are at least two interpretations of this type of grouping. Monitoring indicators can be interpreted as those measuring project input and process, whereas evaluation indicators measure project output and impact. For others, these groups relate more to the frequency of measurement of the indicators. Monitoring means the regular measurement of indicators over time, whereas evaluation refers to a measurement that occurs at the end of a project or programme. When referring to frequency of measurement, an indicator can be either a monitoring or an evaluating indicator.

Selecting essential indicators

Identifying characteristics of "good" indicators for action

Choosing appropriate indicators requires a high degree of judgement and consensus building among potential users and other parties interested in the information generated. In fact, lists of indicators usually become too inflated, and it is therefore advisable to follow the old adage: keep it straightforward and simple (KISS). Drawing from our own experience and recommendations of a WHO Expert Committee (1994), the questions in Box 8 can help standardize the selection process and reduce the number of selected indicators.

What is the indicator supposed to measure?

Defining what an indicator is supposed to measure is not always an easy task, because it must be unambiguous to all health staff. Does it really measure what it intends to measure? The following examples illustrate the difficulty in validating certain indicators:

- The number of meetings held by the local health committee is used in many programmes as a proxy for measuring community involvement. Does it really measure community involvement? In many cases it measures the passivity of the community representatives who merely attend without any real involvement.
- What does the caesarean section rate in a hospital measure? Is it the quality of care provided in the maternity ward of the hospital? Or, rather, the effectiveness of the referral system between health centres and hospital? Or the greed of the hospital obstetrician who might

---

Box 8   Helpful questions in selecting indicators

While judgement and intuition are crucial in defining and selecting indicators, the following questions can help standardize the selection process.

* What is the indicator supposed to measure (validity)?
* What will be the cost of measuring the data?
* What is the relative importance of the subject matter to be addressed and the decision to be made based on the indicator (relevance)?
* Does the indicator actually capture changes that occur in the situation under study (specificity)?
* Is the change shown by the indicator a true change in the situation under study (sensitivity)?

Once selected, one needs to ask whether the indicator contributes to a balanced set of essential indicators. For instance, we do not want too many indicators targeting inputs to the exclusion of outputs. Alternatively, we do not want 10 indicators to measure characteristics of tuberculosis if no indicators for malaria are suggested in countries where both diseases are important. See Annex 1 (page 253) for details on balancing sets of indicators.

---

suggest caesarean sections for women who physically do not require the procedure?

* What does an increase in the incidence rate of pulmonary tuberculosis mean? Is it merely a reflection of improved diagnostic procedures and motivation of personnel? Or does it indicate a true increase in the number of cases of tuberculosis due to an extension of acquired immunodeficiency syndrome (AIDS)?

What will be the cost of measuring the data to arrive at the numerator and denominator of the indicator?

This refers to the complexity of the data collection methods discussed in Chapters 6 and 7. Nevertheless, implications for resources (financial, human, equipment, etc.) have to be discussed at this point because they are a vital part of the decision to keep or reject an indicator. For some indicators, the costs involved in collecting data are high, and the decision to reject them is easy to make. For others, the appropriate decision is less clear because the costs have to be weighed against the benefits of collecting the data. Consider the following examples:

* Measuring infant mortality on a routine basis at the level of a health district is not feasible in most developing countries. It requires collecting data from every infant death in the community over a long period of time. Reaching the level of organization required for this purpose would be extremely costly. Therefore, infant mortality will almost never be part of an appropriate list of indicators for the district level if measured from facility records.
* The choice of the appropriate data collection method for calculating immunization coverage is less clear-cut. Two options are commonly used at the district level: the routine information system and the cluster sampling method. Since cluster sampling is a nonroutine

method, its full cost must be calculated. For the routine system information method, only the marginal cost of adding the information on immunization needs to be taken into account. In addition, the routine information system provides data on a regular basis (monthly or quarterly) and allows for better management; cluster sampling instead provides more reliable and accurate data. Clearly, the choice of the method requires careful deliberation. If resources are available, both methods could be combined to check the quality of the data provided by the routine information system, as explained in Chapter 8.

- Measurements of maternal mortality also tend to be very expensive. In many countries, and usually in those locations that lack vital registration systems, only a percentage of maternal deaths will occur in health facilities. In such circumstances, it is useful to compare data from the facilities with information on deaths in the community. Maternal mortality can be measured by incorporating questions on pregnancy and deaths into large-scale household surveys. The disadvantage of such approaches is that they require very large sample sizes, which result in extremely expensive and time-consuming efforts.

A common issue is the level of accuracy required for an indicator. Accuracy represents the distance between the true and the measured value of the indicator. The level of accuracy required depends on the importance of the decision to be made. If a decision has important consequences, accuracy should be higher. Usually, higher accuracy implies higher costs (Green, 1992). Box 9 gives an example of a trade-off between accuracy and cost (see also Annex 2).

What is the relative importance of the decision to be made based on the indicator?
The importance is primarily defined by (i) the relative importance of the subject matter to be addressed by the indicator, which should address the priority health problems, their determinants, and the critical health services response to these problems; and (ii) the usefulness of the indicator to the staff recording the data. An indicator is useful if decisions based on the measurements contribute to improvement of the staff's work and, hence, the effectiveness and efficiency of the health system.

For example, in the Democratic Republic of the Congo, health centres were asked to report the number of cases of gastritis on a monthly basis. There is neither a specific diagnostic test nor any known "epidemic" of gastritis. Reporting the number of gastritis incidents does not lead to any rational decisions, since there are no effective treatments. Hence, the information obtained is not immediately or potentially useful to the staff.

The collection of useless disease data is not limited to gastritis. For instance, there is a growing controversy among public health professionals concerning the importance of routinely collecting long lists of diseases in developing countries for the purpose of compiling an epidemiological profile of the diseases. Henderson (1978) describes this data as "a laundry list of most diseases known to mankind". Unger and Dujardin (1992) argue that the need for epidemiological information for health service planning is relatively low. Unfortunately, this remains one of the most time-consuming tasks for health care providers.

What diseases merit collection and reporting by the health services? Table 11 classifies diseases according to their informative value for

Box 9   Trade-off between accuracy and cost

The denominator of many indicators is demographic data on a population at risk. Common examples are number of infants, under-5 population, women of child-bearing age, adolescents, and so on.

Demographic data can be collected in several ways involving different costs. The census is the most thorough method but also the most costly, and new data are generally available only every 10 years. In developing countries, most administrations collect demographic data on births, deaths, and migrants, although few developing countries have complete vital registration systems. Traditional and political authorities usually keep some sort of account of their constituencies. The quality of data, however, is questionable.

In 1989, the Ministry of Health of Cameroon decided to organize a systematic household registration in every catchment area of district health facilities. The demographic data from the registration were to be used as a denominator for many indicators. After the first experiences with the registration, the government realized that the costs were disproportionate to the benefits and that updating the data could not be assured.

From there, Cameroon decided to rely on more easily available data from the administration and from traditional leaders in spite of the lack of accuracy of this source of information. Total population figures were broken down according to national estimates of the crude birth rate and so on in order to derive the size of the different risk groups.

For monitoring activities, the manager compares measurements between health centres of a district and over time for the same health centre. A systematic error in determining the denominator will not change the assessment of the performance of a health centre and will not lead to important variations in the allocation of resources within the district.

Table 11   *Classification of diseases according to their pathology and informative value for health service management*

Types of pathology	Examples	Group
• Universal diseases showing variations that are not likely to justify special resources	— tuberculosis, diarrhoea, acute respiratory infections	1
• Diseases with geographical variations, whose frequency alters resource allocations:		
— deficiency diseases	— iodine deficiency, acute malnutrition	2
— endemic infectious diseases	— trypanosomiasis, schistosomiasis, onchocerciasis, leprosy	3
• Diseases with important chronological variations, justifying changes in the resource allocations:		
— regular cycles	— epidemic malaria, seasonal cycles	4
— epidemics	— cholera, yellow fever, typhoid, meningococcal meningitis, HIV/AIDS	5

Source: Adapted from Unger & Dujardin (1992).

health service management (resource allocation). Diseases of group 1 can be monitored routinely in all first-level care facilities. Diseases of groups 2 and 3 should be monitored in certain types of health centres or within a specialized programme because their geographical variations alters resource allocation. Diseases of groups 4 and 5 with important chronological variations need epidemiological surveillance but should be the responsibility of specialized services for cost and quality reasons.

Indicators and specificity

Another characteristic of a good indicator is its specificity: the indicator should reflect changes only in the phenomenon concerned. For example, infant mortality is not a specific indicator of the effectiveness of health care because infant mortality is influenced by many other determinants, including the socioeconomic conditions of the household and the caregiving of the mother.

Indicators and sensitivity

An indicator is sensitive when small changes in programme effectiveness are reflected in variations in its values. Sensitivity is a matter of degree and often implies quantification. For instance, one would expect that "the percentage of infants who receive appropriate vaccinations" would be a sensitive indicator, since its value changes easily after targeted information, education, and communication campaigns to encourage women to bring their infants to facilities for immunization. An example of an insensitive indicator is whether or not the government officially supports family planning or abortion; this changes rarely, though when it does it can mark a milestone (Bulatao, 1995). The maternal mortality rate would also be an insensitive indicator to measure whether large investments in improving the training of providers in emergency caesarean section improved maternal outcomes for women, if an operating theatre and appropriate supplies and medications were not available.

Finally, the appropriateness of an indicator is a judgement call based on the responses to the different questions raised above. For example, the importance of the decision to be made might offset the high cost involved in collecting the data needed to compute the indicator. On the other hand, a cost that is too high might lead to the decision to drop an indicator even if the decision to be made is of great importance. This process will greatly limit the number of indicators by eliminating those that are difficult to measure, of poor validity, or that lead to less important decisions.

Boxes 10 and 11 illustrate the selection of essential indicators with examples from Cameroon and Georgia. Although the objectives were the same, the processes followed were quite different. In Cameroon, a bottom-up approach to the selection of indicators was emphasized, which encouraged participation and consensus building among a large group of users. Although the selection process was time-consuming, the ultimate result was that a wide range of actors accepted the new indicators because they had contributed to their definition. In Georgia, in contrast, the process, although more efficient in terms of time spent to select essential indicators, might suffer from insufficient ownership. These two case studies show that there is a trade-off between time spent on selecting indicators (efficiency) and the number of potential users that are involved (ownership). We think that countries should be prepared to allocate enough time to the selection of indicators to guarantee ownership of the design of the information system, although we recognize that the experience of

---

Box 10   Definition and selection of national indicators: a participatory approach in Cameroon

In 1991, the Ministry of Health of Cameroon decided to completely overhaul its health information system after an assessment revealed major deficiencies in the information system in place. The ministry wanted this exercise to be as participative as possible. Potential users (health units, district, provincial, national level, and community representatives) and other resource persons were selected, including representatives of the private sector, other ministries (social affairs, finance, and planning) and donor agencies. The methodology adopted was to list all the functions and activities at every level of the health system, and then to define information needs and indicators. Reflecting the fact that Cameroon's priorities were managerial rather than clinical or epidemiological, the system was called the health management information system (HMIS).

After debating for 2 years during workshops and "long" meetings, a list of 255 indicators was prepared, weaknesses in the information system were identified, and solutions for reforming the system were developed and tested. Most participants in the indicator selection process realized that the list needed to be drastically reduced. Programme directors were very hard to convince when it came to reducing the number of indicators related to their programmes. Epidemiologists were even less flexible and were not ready to admit that some indicators were intellectually captivating but operationally difficult to measure. At times the debates became quite emotional.

Objective selection criteria with measurement scales were defined in order to rank the indicators, such as validity of the indicator, difficulty and cost in collecting the data, and importance of the decision. Quite often people's opinions diverged on the rating. After one more year, the rank list of indicators was available. The ministry decided then, quite arbitrarily, that the HMIS would include the 50 first indicators appearing on the new list. The other indicators were kept "on standby" until a need for their use arose.

Although this participative process was somewhat inefficient, it was nonetheless successful in engaging all of the actors involved. Through the many months of discussion and debate, the enthusiasm and emotions of many of the participants were piqued. As a result, health professionals from the health centre level up to the central ministry felt that they had contributed to defining the national indicators.

Cameroon is an extreme case in terms of time allocated to this selection process.

Figure 10 illustrates the process that was used in Cameroon to select an indicator measuring the stock level of drugs in a health centre to prevent decapitalization. Three indicators were initially proposed for this purpose. The third indicator was considered the most appropriate when applying the different characteristics of "good" indicators. The context in which the indicator is used is important to understand the selection process. During supervision, when district officers check how well the health centres are performing in terms of drug management, they need a reliable summary indicator. Some health districts include up to 25 primary health centres, and the drug system is not yet computerized at

Box 11   The experience of selecting essential health indicators in Georgia

In its efforts to revise and strengthen its health information system in support of overall health reform, the Ministry of Health of Georgia undertook a process to define essential health indicators. This was done at several levels of the health system in the following way:

The initial step was to convene a group of managers and staff of priority health programmes, including staff from the regional and municipal levels. This group identified the key measures of each priority health problem, the critical services for preventing and managing the health problem, and the essential health resources required for providing the critical health services. On this basis they were able to propose a list of essential indicators felt to be feasible for monitoring within their programmes with routine data obtained from their services.

Immediately following the programme indicator selection, a group of Ministry of Health decision makers met to review the results and add indicators to monitor progress in health sector reform, for example the proportion of hospitals that had implemented fee-for-service procedures.

The next step was to take the process to the municipality and rayon (district) level. Facility and service managers were assembled in one region to propose indicators for monitoring priority health problems, services, and resources from their service-oriented point of view. The product was again a set of indicators which was based on the information needs for service-oriented action and the availability of data at that level.

The results of these three processes were then studied by a health information working group located in the new health management centre. Priority health problems were reconfirmed, and the consolidated list of indicators reviewed to ensure that relevant indicators were defined for all priority health problems, services, and critical resources. In addition, the working group considered activities suggested by the previous workshops for improving the health data system and developed a plan of action for assessing and strengthening the information system comprising four streams of activities:

— assessing and strengthening the disease surveillance system;
— assessing and standardizing clinical diagnostic, treatment, and recording procedures;
— enhancing central programme and local level health-planning procedures, while updating the essential health indicators;
— strengthening computerized health databases and report generation.

The set of essential indicators will continue to be reviewed and updated, and will be used to assist the health information system review and design tasks as the plan of action is carried out.

Source: Sapirie & Orzeszyna (1995).

Fig. 10   *Selection process of an indicator for stock management*

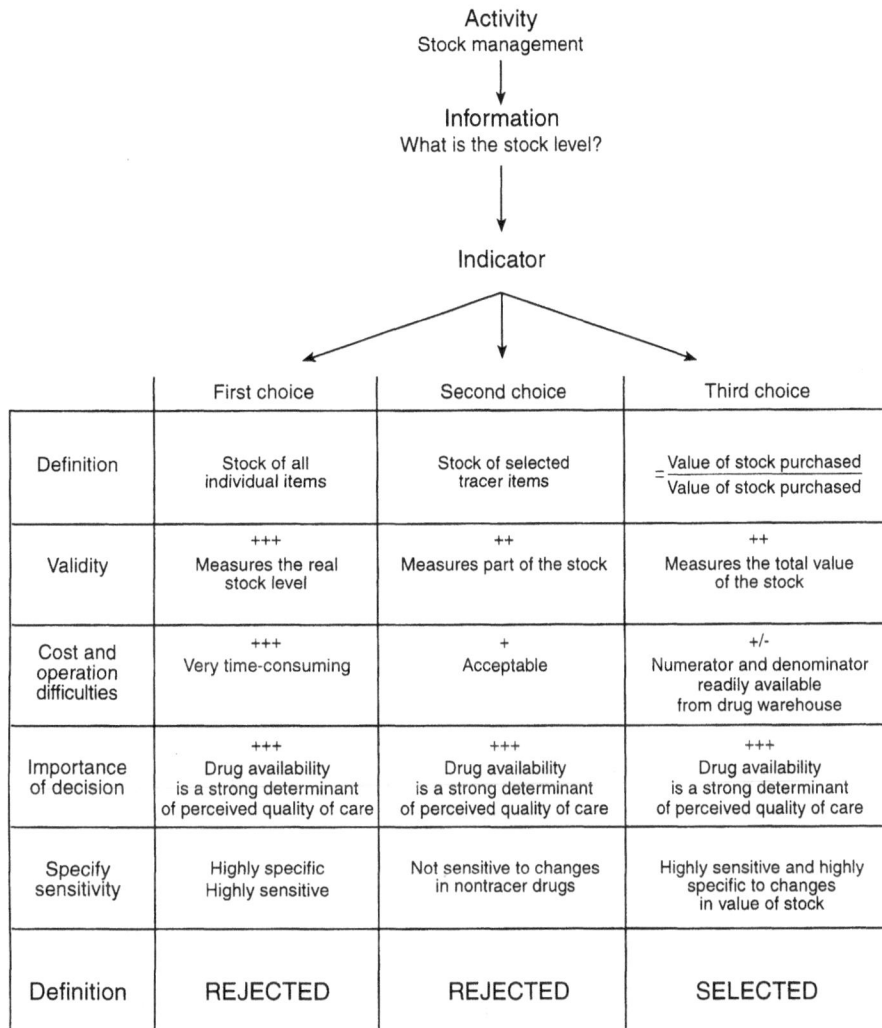

Activity
Stock management

↓

Information
What is the stock level?

↓

Indicator

	First choice	Second choice	Third choice
Definition	Stock of all individual items	Stock of selected tracer items	$=\dfrac{\text{Value of stock purchased}}{\text{Value of stock purchased}}$
Validity	+++ Measures the real stock level	++ Measures part of the stock	++ Measures the total value of the stock
Cost and operation difficulties	+++ Very time-consuming	+ Acceptable	+/- Numerator and denominator readily available from drug warehouse
Importance of decision	+++ Drug availability is a strong determinant of perceived quality of care	+++ Drug availability is a strong determinant of perceived quality of care	+++ Drug availability is a strong determinant of perceived quality of care
Specify sensitivity	Highly specific Highly sensitive	Not sensitive to changes in nontracer drugs	Highly sensitive and highly specific to changes in value of stock
Definition	**REJECTED**	**REJECTED**	**SELECTED**

WHO 99370

the district level. Of primary concern to the district manager is the stock level, that is, is there depletion or excess storage of drugs at the health centre level? Going through the individual stock cards of each of the health centres would be extremely time-consuming (since each health centre handles about 70 items) and would not provide a global picture of the general stock level. In contrast, at the district warehouse information on the amounts of drug purchased and drugs actually sold at the health centres (distributed) is readily available. Amounts of stock purchased at the district warehouse should roughly be equal to the amount of drugs used (sold) at the health centre in order to maintain the same level of stock, provided the same price list is applied.

Operationalizing the indicator

Once an indicator has been considered appropriate, it needs to be further defined in order to make it operational. At this stage, previously selected indicators can be rejected because they are not easy to operationalize. This step is central to the development of the health information system because it has many implications for the design of health information systems, for example data collection instruments, data flow and

---

Box 12 Helpful questions for operationalizing an indicator

The following questions will be helpful for operationalizing indicators:

- What are the sources of the data (numerator and denominator)?
- At what frequency should the numerator and denominator be collected?
- At what frequency should the indicator be processed and analysed?
- Who will actually make use of the indicator (determining the level of aggregation over time and space)?
- What is the target (objective) of the indicator that needs to be achieved?
- What is the threshold, the minimum or maximum value, of the indicator that should trigger an action?
- What will be the nature of the action (decision) once the indicator reaches the threshold?

---

processing, and decisions to be made. Asking the questions listed in Box 12 can help operationalize the indicators. How health planners and managers employ these questions is discussed below and is illustrated by the examples from Cameroon (Table 12).

What are the sources of the data (numerator and denominator)?

Answering this question will help decide who will be responsible for data collection and what the data collection method will be, as developed in Chapters 6 and 7. For example, for measles immunization coverage, the data of the numerator (number of children under age 1 year immunized) will be collected from each individual operational card, and the denominator (total number of children under the age of 1) will come from the last local household survey or census in the health centre catchment area. Specifying the source of the numerator and denominator will constitute a basis for designing data collection forms. Additionally, it provides information about the need for coordination when numerator and denominator have different sources. This will also be very helpful in designing software for and computerizing the information system (see Chapter 11).

At what frequency should the numerator and denominator be collected?

The urgency of the decision to be made or the speed of changes of the measured variable determines the frequency of data collection. Financial and stock indicators usually require close monitoring, and therefore these data are usually collected more frequently, that is on a monthly basis in a health centre in developing countries. In modern industry, stock management is quasi-instantaneous, managers being able to get information whenever they ask for it. In contrast, the ratio of nurses to population changes only slowly over time. Thus, an annual collection of data will suffice.

At what frequency should the indicator be processed and analysed?

For some indicators, the frequency of data collection differs from the frequency at which the data need to be processed in order to produce an

Table 12 *Operationalizing indicators (examples from Cameroon)*

Sources of the data?	Frequency of collection?	Frequency of processing indicator?	Level of aggregation?	Target?	Thresholds and actions?
Indicator for health centre: Measles immunization coverage for children under 1 year of age					
• Numerator: operational cards of each individual child for immunizations • Denominator: census data for denominator	Monthly	Every 6 months	• Health centre catchment area • Health district • Province	• 50–60% depending on health centre • 50% • 50%	• 40%: strategic meeting with community leaders and media campaign • 35%: ad hoc supervision visits of the health centre • 40%: emphasis on vaccination activities during quarterly supervision of districts
Indicator for district hospital: Rate of caesarean sections					
• Numerator: surgery registry for caesarean sections • Denominator: maternity registry for births	Monthly	Annually	• District hospital	• 5%	• 2%: review of newborn deaths at maternity, checking on references from health centres
Indicator for health district management level: Proportion of patients exempted from payment of fee for service					
• Numerator: exemptions from accounting records • Denominator: curative consultation from health centre and hospital outpatient department	Monthly	Annually	• Health centre and district hospital • District management level	• Less than 5% • Less than 5%	• 5% and above: tighter control of exemptions • 8% and above: ad hoc inspection and review exemption policy and financing if necessary

indicator. An indicator such as measles immunization coverage can be processed every 6 months or on an annual basis. Analysing vaccination data too frequently—say on a monthly basis—is inadequate because coverage can be influenced by external factors, for example the illness of a nurse or bad weather, which decrease attendance at the health centre. On the other hand, waiting a long time to collect the raw data required to process the indicator on vaccination coverage places a burden on health centre personnel that can greatly jeopardize the quality of the data.

Who will actually use the indicator?
Answering this question will determine the level of aggregation over time and space needed for decision-making. The indicator should first be analysed and used by the staff collecting and reporting the data. No data that do not have a use at the recording level should be requested from a service level to be reported to higher levels. Some of the indicators will be channelled vertically to a higher level of the health system (central ministries, aid agencies) or horizontally to the community (see Chapter 8). Determining what level data need to be reported to is important because it influences the level of aggregation of the indicators over space and time. For instance, the central ministry of health might choose to aggregate information on couple-year of protection for family planning activities either by regions or health districts over a period of 6 months or a year depending on their information needs.

What is the target (objective) of the indicator that needs to be achieved?

Determining a target for an indicator is another helpful mechanism to ensure use of information, because the gap between actual measurement and the target will help in making decisions. Targets should be set by the immediate supervisor in agreement with the persons in charge of carrying out the activities. It will depend on local resources available and should take into account national objectives. For example, in the Adamaoua and South Provinces of Cameroon, tetanus immunization coverage for pregnant women was drawn on a wall chart on a monthly basis. Each month, the actual results were compared with the objective. This helped health staff and community members to analyse the gap between the two lines and to make appropriate decisions to increase attendance by pregnant women.

What is the threshold, that is the maximum or minimum value, of the indicator that should trigger action?

When appropriate or feasible, determining a threshold for an indicator helps in making decisions. There can be more than one threshold per indicator according to the level of the health system. Health staff should determine reasonable thresholds according to local needs and resources available. For example, the threshold for antenatal care coverage can hardly be the same in both rural and urban areas in a poor developing country. These thresholds need to be fine-tuned over time and should be "negotiated" between supervisor and supervisee.

What will be the nature of the action taken based on the measurement of the indicator?

Information systems tend to become ends in themselves. They are not useful until actions are taken based on the information provided by the system. Actions will vary according to the information provided. Consider the following example from the Health District of Bandundu, Democratic Republic of the Congo. In this district, health centre nurses had decided on the following actions according to the level of measles coverage in their catchment areas (it was assumed that vaccine was available): (i) less than 55% coverage: sensitization of all community leaders in order to organize promotional activities in the community; (ii) less than 35% coverage: same as previously and, in addition, household visits in the community by the health centre staff.

To illustrate the above steps in operationalizing indicators, Table 12 shows three examples from Cameroon. WHO (1996) recently published a list of "operationalized" indicators for system management. The list contains 57 indicators, 22 related to infants and children, 10 addressing issues specific to the health of women, and the rest concerned with general population issues.

Summary

This chapter examined how health planners and health system professionals can improve the management capabilities of health services by determining information needs and monitoring indicators. A general framework for defining information needs and indicators was developed and illustrated at the beginning of the chapter. The remaining part was devoted to presenting and discussing each of the steps involved in defining appropriate information and indicators. Finally, a detailed discussion which highlighted how to define, classify, select, and operationalize indicators was presented. The common typology distinguishing four classes of indicators (from inputs to outcomes) was illustrated.

Routine health information systems should support three types of management functions: patient/client management, health unit management, and health system management at various levels of the health system. A well-designed information system starts with functional analysis, as well as with procedures for identifying information needs and indicators, at each management level.

References

Bulatao RA (1995). *Key indicators for family planning projects.* Washington, DC, World Bank (World Bank Technical Paper, No. 297).

De Geyndt W (1994). *Managing the quality of health care in developing countries.* Washington, DC, World Bank (World Bank Technical Paper, No. 258).

DHEW (1969). *Towards a social report.* Washington, DC, Department of Health, Education, and Welfare.

Donabedian A (1980). *Exploration in quality: assessment and monitoring.* Vol. 1: *The definition of quality and approaches to its assessment.* Ann Arbor, MI, Health Administration Press, School of Public Health, University of Michigan.

Donabedian A (1988). The quality of care: how can it be assessed? *Journal of the American Medical Association,* 260:1743–1748.

Finau SA (1994). National health information systems in the Pacific Islands: in search of a future. *Health policy and planning,* 9:161–170.

Feder G (1996). *How can clinical guidelines improve the quality of care in general practice?* The East London Collaborative Clinical Guidelines Project. Paper presented at the 13th International Conference of the International Society for Quality in Health Care, Jerusalem.

Green A (1992). *An introduction to health planning in developing countries.* Oxford, Oxford University Press.

Helfenbein S et al. (1987). *Technologies for management information systems in primary health care.* Geneva, World Federation of Public Health Associations (Issue Paper, Information for Action Series).

Henderson DA (1978). Surveillance of smallpox. *International journal of epidemiology,* 5:19–28.

Mausner JS, Kramer S (1985). *Epidemiology: an introductory text,* 2nd ed. Philadelphia, PA, WB Saunders.

Murnaghan JH (1981). Health indicators and information systems for the year 2000. *Annual review of public health,* 2:299–361.

Parker MW, Ross JA (1991). Family planning programs: efforts and results, 1982–1989. *Studies in family planning,* 22:350–367.

Sapirie S, Orzeszyna S (1995). *Selecting and defining national health indicators.* Geneva, World Health Organization.

Shrestha LB, Rosenwaike I (1996). Can data from the decennial census measure trends in mobility limitation among the aged? *Gerontologist,* 36:106–109.

Unger JP, Dujardin B (1992). Epidemiology's contribution to health service management and planning in developing countries: a missing link. *Bulletin of the World Health Organization,* 70:487–497.

Wilson R, Sapanuchart T, eds. (1993). *Primary health care management advancement program.* Geneva, Aga Khan Foundation.

World Bank (1993). *World development report 1993: investing in health.* New York, Oxford University Press.

World Health Organization (1981). *Managerial process for national health development.* Geneva, World Health Organization: 57–60 (Health for All Series, No. 5).

World Health Organization (1994). *Information support for new public health action at the district level: report of a WHO Expert Committee.* Geneva, World Health Organization: 1–31 (WHO Technical Report Series, No. 845).

World Health Organization (1996). *Catalogue of health indicators.* Geneva, World Health Organization (unpublished document WHO/HST/SCI/96.8; available on request from Department of Organization of Health Services Delivery, World Health Organization, 1211 Geneva 27, Switzerland).

Assessing health information systems

Steve Sapirie

Introduction

This chapter addresses health information system assessment as an essential component in the early stages of developing a health information system (see Box 13). The intention is to provide guidelines for conducting focused assessments capable of yielding useful findings rapidly. Health care workers and managers should undertake such assessments both as an early step to strengthen the health information system at national and regional levels, and periodically to evaluate success in improving generation and use of data. While the literature is replete with statements on the need for information for management of health services and descriptions of the different "information systems", there are no references which either document the need for assessing the health information system or present the steps involved to implement such an assessment.

If it is believed that information is indispensable for effective management and development of health services and that, furthermore, it has to be meaningful, reliable, accurate, and timely (Hartshorne & Carstens, 1990; Sandiford, Annett & Cibulskis, 1992), then health system managers should be "keeping an eye" on the information system and its performance. They should monitor and evaluate staff performance in generating, using, and reporting data the same way they monitor disease control programmes, including the periodic assessment of information use for action taking in patient/client, community, health unit, and system management levels.

Managers should base their decision for health information system improvement on concern about real problems in health care delivery rather than deciding to improve the health information system as an end in itself. They should look for innovative approaches for managing information in order to monitor output, coverage, quality, and efficiency of the health system in a way that will identify the population groups with the greatest need and the least access (Taylor, 1984). Thus, health information system assessment should embrace the principle of equity in health care delivery.

Assessment as a step in the development and implementation of the health information system

Previous chapters have presented the framework and principles for the design and restructuring of the health information system (Chapter 2), how information can be used to improve decision-making at all levels of

---

Box 13   What is health information system assessment?

The assessment of a health information system is essentially a measurement of the performance of selected components or subsystems of the information system to support health care delivery and management of the health services system at various levels. Specifically, these components are assessed in terms of:

— data generation;
— data management (storing, processing, communicating, and sharing);
— data analysis and reporting;
— data use.

---

the health services system (Chapter 3), as well as the concept of essential health indicators (Chapter 4). This chapter assumes that health information system assessment will be carried out as an early step in a strategy for strengthening the health information system. It often takes place immediately after selecting or confirming essential health indicators. Such assessments help in planning further developing and restructuring of the health information system. They are facilitated when the health information system is oriented towards the generation, analysis, and reporting of data for monitoring essential health indicators which have been selected for all priority health problems and programmes, service performance (coverage and quality), and resource availability and use. If essential health indicators have not been identified prior to the health information system assessment, it is recommended that this be done before designing and undertaking the assessment. The data required for such indicators thus become the vehicles for assessing the current performance of the health information system. The problems discovered with the data and their use then become the subject for subsequent steps in strengthening the health information system.

A framework for assessing the health information system

In this chapter, we present an approach to health information system assessment which has been developed by WHO and used in a number of countries. It encourages the selection of subsystems and domains for assessment because normally it is not possible to assess all health information subsystems in one study. The assessment does not have to be nationwide but could, for example, focus on one region. The approach provides a comprehensive review of the health information system from different perspectives (e.g. use of information, resources in support of the subsystem, managerial support, outputs, and organizational aspects).

When discussing the assessment of the health information system, it is recommended that the system be thought of as a set of interrelated subsystems, as defined in Box 14. This general categorization includes the following basic subsystems: epidemiological (health or disease) surveillance, routine service recording and reporting, special health programme information (maternal and child health and family planning, tuberculosis control, etc.), administrative information systems, and the vital registration (birth and death) system. Even though vital registration does

---

Box 14 Common subsystems of health information systems

In most countries, the following subsystems of health information can be found:

— *epidemiological surveillance* for notifiable infectious diseases, certain environmental conditions, and risk factors;
— *routine service reporting* from the basic health services at community level, health centres, dispensaries, first-level hospitals, referral hospitals, and special and tertiary hospitals;
— *special programme reporting* systems such as tuberculosis control, leprosy control, malaria control, maternal and child health and family planning, Expanded Programme on Immunization, and AIDS prevention;
— *administrative systems*, including health programme budget management, health financing systems, health personnel systems, health supply and logistic systems, health training programmes, health research management, health documentation management, and managing external resources for health;
— *vital registration*: births, deaths, and migration.

---

not administratively belong to the health sector, it is included among the five general health information system subsystems because of its importance as a source of data for population estimation and health impact. It is also included because of the role the health services can play in strengthening the registration of births and deaths. Obviously, subsystems of the health information system will vary from country to country, and need to be defined specifically for the country at the outset of an assessment. Rarely are all subsystems assessed at the same time; instead, attention is focused on those subsystems which are felt to be most critical for providing the data to monitor essential health indicators.

In addition, managers can choose to focus on all health information system components (as defined in Chapter 2) for the assessment, or to select only a few. For the purpose of such assessments, health information system components have been categorized as follows:

— *data input*: validity and completeness of data recording and collection, including surveillance, routine case and activity data, surveys, data emerging from administrative processes, and registration data;
— *data analysis, transmission, and reporting*: efficiency, completeness, and quality of data analysis, processing, and presentation, at all levels of the health system, in order to produce actionable information;
— *use of information*: decisions and actions taken for patient/client, community, health unit, programme, and executive management;
— *information systems resources*: availability, sufficiency, and use of critical resources to support: the health information system budget; staff with necessary training and expertise; facilities such as space for record storage, records, and formats; and necessary equipment for data communication, storage, analysis, and document preparation (faxes, computers, printers, photocopy machines, etc.);

Table 13   *Health information system assessment framework*

Possible components of health information system assessment					
Health information subsystems	Data input Recording and collection	Data analysis Transmission and reporting	Use of information Decision and action	Information system resources Finance, staff, facilities, computers	Information system management Coordination and networking
Epidemiological surveillance					
Service reporting, e.g.: Community level Health centres First-level hospitals Referral/special hospitals					
Programme reporting, e.g.: Malaria Immunization Maternal and child health and family planning Tuberculosis control					
Administration, e.g.: Budget Personnel Training Supplies Facilities Research management Document management External resources					
Vital registration					

— *information systems management*: organization and coordination mechanisms for assuring that data and information are properly defined, standardized, produced, maintained, shared, and reported.

Table 13 displays the overall health information system conceptual framework which can be used to select the subsystems and domains to be assessed. This format can also be useful for recording the issues to be addressed during the assessment. Decision-makers and designers of the assessment usually identify such issues at the time the terms of reference of the assessment are formulated.

Reasons for health information system assessment

The decision to undertake a health information system assessment should be made by the managers of the health service system, or programmes supported by the health information system and their subsystems. Such a decision must be motivated by a need for action to improve service performance and by a commitment to use the findings for taking appropriate corrective action both within the services and in regard to the information system. The decision should be based on the intent to improve, for example, the quality of data, its timeliness, and its use for decision-making at all levels of the health system, but especially at service delivery levels in managing cases and community health.

The role of a health information system has been described in the previous chapters. The objectives of an assessment of a health information system may therefore be stated as:

— to determine the performance of one or more subsystems of the health information system in terms of the generation, use, and reporting of data needed for essential indicators and databases. These indicators and databases are essential in managing the delivery of priority health services and support systems, and monitoring the health situation;
— to identify problems of the information system and propose activities for their resolution; and, as a by-product,
— to provide first-time participants in the health information system assessment process with the capabilities to undertake similar assessments in the future.

It is important that the staff who use the health data and manage the subsystems carry out the assessment process, rather than outside "experts". It is also important that the assessment be focused and rapidly completed, with the results used immediately for taking corrective measures to strengthen the system.

Managers begin a health information system assessment with a decision on the broad topics and issues to be addressed, and clarification of how the results will be used for decision-making and action to strengthen the system. The process of identifying the issues starts with specification of the general and specific objectives of the assessment. On the basis of these objectives, a series of issues to be addressed in the assessment are then identified, which become the subject of the assessment.

To achieve its specific objectives, the assessment should focus on a few major issues confronting the health services and the health information system. Issues of concern should be expressed as specifically as possible so that managers can select the appropriate service levels and data sources for assessment, formulate the most relevant ways to measure the problem (sensitive and valid indicators), and determine the most appropriate methods to conduct the assessment.

Basic steps of health information system assessment

This approach proposes that the following steps be undertaken within a health information system assessment:

— formulate the terms of reference for the assessment (which includes the objectives and constraints of the assessment);
— assemble and review relevant existing information;
— confirm the services and service issues to be studied;
— identify the indicators of health information system performance and the sources of data for each;
— design and test the assessment tools and formats;
— prepare for field data collection;
— conduct the assessment (data collection);

— analyse the results and prepare the assessment report;
— formulate recommendations and prepare a follow-up plan of action.

Formulating the terms of reference for the assessment

The terms of reference are intended to specify the purposes of the assessment and the conditions under which it must be completed. The terms of reference document defines the objectives, the main issues to be addressed, the specific information subsystems and/or domains to receive the most attention, the staff and resources being made available, the nature of the assessment report and when it is due, and the expectations regarding the next steps. In particular, health planners and managers should identify the current issues and problems pertaining to health data and information under examination.

The terms of reference are best formulated through discussions among the senior managers who are calling for the assessment. These managers are usually highly motivated by the need to improve the health information system and therefore committed to using the results of the assessment. Table 13, which presents the common health information system subsystems and possible health information system components for assessment, has proven useful in identifying issues and setting the limits of the assessment. Initial issues pertaining to each subsystem being assessed may be entered in the table under the relevant assessment component.

Box 15 provides a list of questions which can be used as a guide for formulating the terms of reference.

Box 15 Terms of reference for health information system assessment

- Who has asked for the assessment? (Indicate the institution or office which has requested the assessment and to which the results should be delivered.)
- Why is the assessment being requested? (Indicate how the findings will be used; the nature of the decisions or actions to be taken on the basis of the results.)
- When must the assessment findings be available?
- Who will participate in the assessment, and what special perspectives and skills will they provide?
- How will the costs of the assessment be met?
- What health services, public health functions, and information subsystems will be the subject of the assessment?
- What national health objectives, targets, and priority services are relevant to the chosen subjects and should be used as a basis for assessing adequacy of data generation and information use?
- What health indicators defined for monitoring and evaluating the services or public health functions should be selected for review during this assessment?
- Are there any levels of the health service or the health system which should receive special attention during the assessment?
- Are there any assessment components which should receive special attention (input, processing, reporting, data use, resources, information management)?
- What are the issues of current concern which must be addressed during the assessment?

Assembling and reviewing existing information

A health information system assessment should be undertaken with knowledge of existing information about the system, its management, operation, and use. Background information should, therefore, be assembled and reviewed. Such documents should provide descriptive information on the health system and organization in the country, on the health information system, and specifically on the subsystems targeted for assessment as mentioned in the terms of reference. The relevant documents could be:

— descriptions and diagrams of the structure of the health service and information system;
— documents presenting priority health problems, health development and programme objectives and targets, and indicators for monitoring and evaluation;
— reports of recent surveys and evaluations;
— routine data flow charts;
— current routine and ad hoc reports;
— lists of existing information support staff (statisticians, epidemiologists, statistical clerks) and extent of specialized and general computer literacy;
— lists of computers in various offices, institutions, and service facilities;
— descriptions of existing or planned projects for developing components of the health information system, including externally supported projects.

Confirming the services and service issues to be studied

The goal of a health information system assessment is to resolve health information system problems in order to improve health services, planning and decision-making at each level of the national health system. The terms of reference for the assessment may initially specify service and information issues to be given attention during the assessment. However, new issues will be identified in the process of reviewing existing documentation and information. All the health information system issues (i.e. problems with the current management and use of health information) should be causally related to health and health service problems. Annex 3 gives examples of issues which were identified in one country when assessing epidemiological surveillance and routine reporting systems.

As service and information issues are identified, it becomes clear which types and levels of health services will need to be studied and therefore visited during field data collection. Generally, several levels of health services need to be included in the visits, such as district hospital outpatient departments, health centres, maternal and child health centres, dispensaries, village health workers, and offices of disease control programmes.

Identifying the indicators of health information system performance and the sources of data

The key question which should be answered by a health information system assessment is whether the information system is capable of providing the data and summarizing information needed for health care and public health action. A health information system assessment is expected to determine the existence and magnitude of initially perceived problems as well as additional problems discovered during the course of the assessment. Each issue or problem is measured in terms of indicator(s) which define the magnitude of the problem.

If the health information system assessment has been preceded by the selection of "essential health indicators", then the assessment can focus on whether the data for the essential health indicators exist and are being appropriately used.

Health information system performance indicators can later be used to monitor how the information system's support to the health care system is progressing. They can also be used in the evaluation of the information system development effort to judge to what degree the information system is being used to monitor and manage the services. (Note: health information system performance indicators should not be confused with "essential health indicators" used to monitor health problems, services, and resources.)

At the operational level, at least three types of indicators for assessing a health information system, or its subsystem, can be identified. These are health information system indicators of data input (completeness and validity), data analysis and use (action taking), and the suitability of information outputs or products (quality, completeness, timeliness, etc.). All indicators should be simple, easily interpretable, sensitive, specific, valid, objective, ethical, and useful for monitoring and evaluating the health information system. In practice, health information system performance indicators have often been stated in terms of those types listed in Box 16.

Table 14 provides examples of health service issues with corresponding health information system issues and indicators. As each indicator is formulated, it should also be noted where the data for the indicator can be found, for example from records maintained in health centres, or by

---

Box 16   Types of health information system performance indicators

- *Staff knowledge*: target groups, service targets, calculation of coverage, occurrence and trends of diseases and deaths, case definitions, use of treatment guidelines
- *Recording performance*: case diagnosis, cause of death, consistency of registers and records, completeness of registers
- *Reporting performance*: timeliness of report submission, data consistency (between registers and reports), submission of disease notifications
- *Reporting feedback*: response to reports from higher levels and to lower levels
- *Availability of materials*: guidelines, records and forms, wall charts
- *Performance monitoring*: coverage with targeted services, knowledge of unserved populations or areas of low coverage
- *Supplies management*: recording vaccine use, age and temperature, monitoring drugs supplies

Table 14 *Health information system issues and indicators*

Common health service issues	Corresponding health information system issues	Examples of information system indicators
• Problems in providing critical supplies continuously	• Lack of accurate and timely stock inventory reports	• Proportion of health facilities submitting regularly their stock inventories and requisitions.
• Inadequate detection and control of communicable diseases	• Failure to receive reports of notifiable communicable diseases from government services	• Percentage of government health units submitting disease notifications as required
• Inadequate planning and scheduling of critical activities and services at facility and district level	• Certain facility types or service levels not regularly submitting routine operational plans and monitoring reports	• Percentage of district health offices and health centres which have routinely submitted their quarterly operational plans and implementation reports
• Inadequate attention is given to finding and serving high-risk and underserved populations	• Patient and clinic records fail to identify high-risk patients, families, and communities	• Percentage of dispensaries and health centres able to identify in their catchment areas high-risk pregnancies, malnourished children, defaulters in tuberculosis treatment, and families and communities in greatest need of service attention and follow-up
• Inadequate health protection and services provided to poor populations	• Lack of up-to-date population data which identifies less advantaged population groups	• Proportion of health facilities with service area population data broken down into key demographic and social categories
• Inadequate action by health staff at facility and district level to monitor and correct deficiencies in service coverage and quality	• Staff at facility and district level do not maintain records and present data in a manner which enable monitoring of coverage and quality	• Proportion of health facilities with up-to-date service charts and graphs of important indicators of service coverage and quality
• High staff turnover	• Lack of clear job descriptions and career development opportunities	• Percentage of facilities with up-to-date job descriptions and training records for all staff

interviewing staff to determine their ability and practice in using the subject data. Table 15 gives examples of health information system issues, indicators for measuring health information system performance, and the sources of data for measuring the indicators.

Designing and testing assessment tools and formats

Some key questions must be answered in the course of preparing the data collection methods and tools:

What data are needed for each indicator (i.e. for exploring each issue)? Where must the data be obtained?
The types of data to be collected for the health information system assessment are determined by the indicators. These data are, however, likely to come from a variety of sources: official government documents, stock inventories, by observation, through staff interviews, and so on.

How will the data be collected?
Appropriate instruments (questionnaires and data collection formats) should be designed in such a way that all field teams will easily and consistently elicit and record the required information during visits to selected facilities and offices.

Table 15   *Selected health information system issues, indicators, and data sources*

Issue	Assessment indicator	Data source
• Lack of complete and reliable information on immunization	• Percentage of health centres with complete and reliable information on EPI coverage in their area • Percentage of health centres using the data in the EPI quarterly report for planning the next quarter's EPI activities	• Observation, at the health facility, of the presence of: — EPI tables and graphs; — the EPI quarterly reports; — EPI activity schedule • Interview health workers on their knowledge of the coverage/targets (hospitals/health centres)
• Lack of use of clinic register data for monitoring child health	• Percentage of facilities following the established procedures for identification and follow-up of EPI defaulters and malnourished children • Percentage of facilities establishing a list of EPI defaulters	• Review of the child registers • Interview health workers on defaulter identification and follow-up • Check for list of EPI defaulters
• Lack of information on the level of vaccine use and wastage	• Number of health centres with vaccine stock books correctly maintained	• Review of the completeness of vaccine stock books (dates of receipt and expiration), quantity received, issued/used, wastage
• Lack of information on maternal mortality in spite of the existence of a notification system	• Proportion of maternal deaths known by health centre staff • Proportion of maternal deaths notified	• Review and comparison of the information recorded in the monthly report and the number of maternal death reports submitted through the civil registration system
• Absence of data on antenatal care coverage	• Proportion of facilities following the procedure for identification of antenatal cases • Proportion of health centres establishing a list of antenatal care defaulters based on the antenatal care register	• Review of ANC registers • Interview health workers to determine knowledge of ANC coverage calculation • Review of records and interviews to determine action taken on ANC defaulters
• Lack of information on the performance of community health workers	• Proportion of health centres visiting community health workers at least monthly • Number of health centres recording information from village health workers registers	• Interview health workers on the periodicity of their visits with village health workers • Review village health workers' information extracted from their registers

EPI = Expanded Programme on Immunization; ANC = antenatal care.

Data collection methods which are commonly used in health information system assessments include:

— reviewing and extracting records;
— checking equipment and supplies;
— observing and recording consultations;
— interviewing staff;
— holding focus group discussions with staff and clients.

A number of different data collection methods and instruments may be needed for a single health information system assessment to be able to obtain the necessary information from the different sources.

Testing data collection instruments

After the working group has designed the various instruments, it is important that they be tested in typical facilities of the types to be visited in the actual sample. Difficulties in wording and formatting of questions will be found and the instruments modified as necessary.

How will the resulting data be analysed and presented (including the design of tables)?

Data requirements and indicators needed for studying each issue can be summarized in a table indicating facility types and levels of service to be studied, and how the data will be collected. Data summary tables should also be prepared in advance to show how each indicator will be computed, and how the anticipated results will be presented.

This systematic approach to planning an assessment of a health information system extends to the preparation of the tools to be used for collecting the data by whatever method. Going through the issue-information matrix systematically formulating questions to be asked or information to be collected through observation assures coverage of all issues and minimizes collection of redundant data.

Examples of health information system assessment questions and their formatting in field questionnaires are given in Annex 4.

Preparing for the assessment

The success of a health information system assessment depends to a large extent on how well the exercise is planned. The planning process should cover not only the content of the assessment but also the timing and resources. The following is a checklist of what should be carefully planned:

— the timetable of the assessment activities;
— securing the support of the specific staff needed for the assessment (by name and office) in order to adequately perform the assessment tasks in the field;
— preparing and procuring the material (forms and supplies) and equipment (computers and calculators) for data collection, analysis, and report preparation;
— arranging transport and accommodations, and communicating with the facilities;
— ensuring necessary financial support (budget);
— training the field teams in the use of the questionnaires.

Two important questions to be answered when arranging for the conduct of the field work are these:

How many (and what type of) facilities and/or people should be targeted for data collection to ensure validity of the measurement of the indicators?

Practical attention has to be paid to the sampling procedures to be followed, and the sample sizes. Planners may need to stratify the sampling if service and health information system performance are likely to be different in the different strata or regions. For example, it may be necessary to look at the assessment results for the government and non-government sectors separately. Ultimately, the total size of the sample of facilities and offices is determined by the time and resources available. The data collection for most health information system assessments is planned to be conducted within 4 to 7 days with the use of three to five teams visiting different provinces or regions.

Who should be in the teams visiting or contacting the various facilities to collect the various types of data?

It is necessary to determine the level of expertise needed for carrying out the various types of observation and data collection, and the training (content and duration) necessary for the people who will be collecting the data. Some of the team members should be health service staff experienced in clinic and programme management. Others may be statisticians or epidemiologists.

Conducting the assessment (field data collection)

The quality of the assessment and the validity of the results can be compromised by errors during the data collection process. This often results from misunderstanding the questions to be asked, lack of motivation of the data collection team, poor supervision, and so on. It is therefore extremely important that experienced people who are acceptable and respected by the data collectors monitor the data collection stage of the assessment. The supervisors should continually check whether the procedures and guidelines are being followed by all the people involved in collecting the data. They should monitor the supplies (data collection tools) to ensure that fieldwork can be undertaken without interruption and delays, and that time allocated for data collection is sufficient, and is efficiently used.

Data management in the field and in the central office of the assessment team is equally important. Strong and efficient supervision is needed if the data collection effort is to be effective. It is important to monitor whether the procedures for data handling are properly followed, for example whether data are checked for completeness and correctness as soon as they are received. A means for maintaining the data safely should be provided.

The level and degree of sophistication to be used in analysing the assessment data depend on the demands of the assessment terms of reference, the available technical expertise, other support resources, and the characteristics of the data to be analysed. Basic analysis of the data should result in computation of the quantitative assessment indicators (normally the proportion of facilities visited with a certain condition) or description of the qualitative indicators. Since, during the course of data collection, extensive interaction with health workers and observation of activities take place, a considerable amount of information which may not have been foreseen, both quantitative and qualitative, often becomes available. That information should be taken into account during the data analysis and report-writing stages.

The depth and detail of the analysis depend on the assessment objectives and the nature of the performance indicators of the proposed health information system. It is advisable to have a plan of how the data are to be analysed according to the indicators and the desired tabular presentation in the various assessment domains. Use of a computer for assessment data handling, analysis, and report preparation is often appropriate.

Analysing the results and preparing the assessment report

The report of the assessment exercise should be seen as a rapid and practical means of communicating the findings and recommendations of the action to be taken to all those involved in the health care system. The report should therefore communicate rather than simply be a record of the activities undertaken during the assessment. It should be brief, readable, and understandable by those for whom it is intended.

The report should be prepared in line with the terms of reference and fulfil the objectives of the assessment. The report should normally provide a detailed description of the adequacy of data generation, management, and use in support of the critical service tasks and functions highlighted for attention during the assessment, and a plan of action. Detailed presentation of the performance indicators of the health information system is important, but clear descriptions and qualitative assessment are also crucial.

Examples of data presentation resulting from a health information system assessment appear in Annex 5.

The plan of follow-up

Normally, health information system assessment teams are also asked to formulate recommendations on how to resolve deficiencies found in the health information system. This step includes preparing an implementation plan that recommends actions and proposes steps, including how to monitor implementation of activities, and evaluate, after a reasonable time, the effect of the changes on performance of the health information system. The recommendations should be practical and aim at improved service performance, not just better data recording and reporting. Table 16 lists common health information system deficiencies and the types of activities which are sometimes suggested for their resolution.

Changes of registers and records should be undertaken only after other efforts to strengthen and make better use of existing information have been made. When changes in records are necessary, they should be made primarily for the purpose of enhancing service performance while simultaneously reducing the amount of data to be recorded and reported. Implementing the recommendations should not require extensive resources or staff time at the expense of regular activities.

The process of preparing a plan of action should involve extensive consultation with the people who will be implementing it. A brainstorming process to elicit corrective actions may be a very useful way of embracing the views of the people who are likely to be involved in implementing the plan of action. The plan of action should be endorsed at the highest level to ensure its rapid acceptance, appropriate allocation of resources, and effective implementation. A health information system steering committee should be established to oversee the plan's implementation. Further strategies on the health information system restructuring process are developed in Chapter 13.

Conclusion

The process described in this chapter has been carried out in a number of countries which have recently embarked on a practical strategy for strengthening their health information systems. The assessments appear very similar to evaluations of primary health care or specific

Table 16 *Possible responses to common health information system problems*

Problem	Possible action
Problems associated with service level case diagnosis, recording, and data use	• Assess the current diagnostic and recording performance of selected types of clinical work at different service levels. • Produce standardized treatment and recording guidelines. • Review and revise clinical registers, records, and report formats as necessary to capture data essential for sound case management. • Prepare standard national case definitions for infectious and reportable diseases. • Conduct in-service training in diagnostic skills for important health problems currently being improperly diagnosed. • Conduct "district team problem-solving" including analysis of assigned health problems, followed by the design and implementation of local solutions to these problems, and the monitoring and evaluation of the implementation and effect of the solutions (reduces health problems while enhancing district level data use).
Communications problems	• Strengthen the health sector communications ability with fax or electronic mail to facilitate the feeding of disease data to designated offices for data entry and analysis at regional and national levels. • Produce a monthly health (epidemiology and service performance) report and distribute it throughout the services as a form of information feedback to reporting units. • Begin a process of rapid evaluation of priority services (e.g. maternal health, communicable disease control) involving staff from several service levels.
Data analysis problems (in the services and at programme management level)	• Provide training in basic data analysis techniques to programme managers and surveillance staff. • Develop database and data analysis packages for use at regional or provincial health offices or disease surveillance and control units. • At the central level, review and revise the organization of databases and data analysis in order to reduce redundancies, facilitate the sharing of data across programmes, and respond better to user requirements for planning and monitoring. • Obtain standard statistical computer packages and distribute to regional centres in support of statistical analysis training.
Problems in reporting	• Strengthen legislation and regulations requiring medical practitioners to report infectious diseases. • Develop and maintain practical disease and programme databases for managing the data flowing from service levels, and to support the preparation of required reports. • Develop a monthly public health report which summarizes all infectious disease reports from around the country along with data on certain critical services and articles on especially effective case detection and outbreak control. • Develop a comprehensive annual health report which provides a complete qualitative and narrative assessment of the health situation and service performance in the country, based on essential health indicators. Distribute to service staff and programme managers, senior decision makers and politicians, the public, nongovernmental organizations and international agencies.

health programmes, and indeed involve assessing the way staff work in their clinical and community workplace.

However, the emphasis throughout the design and conduct of such health information system assessments is to confirm the availability, use, and utility of data required for selected health indicators that have been identified as essential for managing cases, health units, and priority programmes. One of the types of indicators used frequently for such assessment is the knowledge of staff about important health conditions and services. This gives evidence that the staff are analysing their data and using them to redirect their attention to unserved populations.

Experience has shown that as such assessments are undertaken, the study teams, with the involvement of staff in the facilities they are visiting, generate many ideas for improving the way data are recorded, analysed, and used. Not all these ideas are ultimately deemed worthy of implementation, but there are many fresh ideas from which to develop a practical plan for improving the health information system.

The findings of past assessments point to weaknesses in programme planning and management which can be addressed simultaneously in the recommendations and plan of action. For example, at the central level, it has been found that staff often cannot describe their programme's performance in relation to its objectives and targets. Many times they are unaware of the indicators their programme is supposed to be using for monitoring progress and evaluating health impact. Clarifying programme objectives, targets, and indicators can become an important step in improving both programme management and performance while enhancing the use of routine data.

References

Hartshorne JE, Carstens IL (1990). Role of information systems in public health services. *Journal of the Dental Association of South Africa*, 45:313–317.

Sandiford P, Annett H, Cibulskis R (1992). What can information systems do for primary health care? An international perspective. *Social science and medicine*, 34:1077–1087.

Taylor CE (1984). *The uses of health systems research*. Geneva, World Health Organization (WHO Public Health Papers, No. 78).

Theo Lippeveld

Use of routine versus nonroutine data collection methods

In the previous chapter, we discussed the choice of appropriate indicators for decision-making at all levels of the health services. The next question is how to collect the data to generate this information. Data can be collected through a variety of methods. We have found it useful to classify these methods into two groups: routine methods and nonroutine methods. Routine health unit-managed data collection is the most classic form of routine data collection. Data are collected based on patient/client encounters, in the health facility, or through outreach. Routine data collection can also be managed directly by the community (see Chapter 9; Reynolds, Bryant & Inam, 1988; O'Neill, 1993). Civil registration is another form of routine data collection. Nonroutine methods of health data collection include surveys, quantitative and qualitative rapid assessment methods, and other special studies.

No single data source can provide all the information required for planning and managing the health services. A national health information system in support of the health services will always use a combination of data collection methods. The main reason is the nature and use of the information for which data need to be collected. Routine health unit data collection is particularly geared towards data based on the health care services provided in the facility and provides information on the health of the people who use the regular health service (Woodall, 1988; Anderson et al., 1989; Claquin, Reynolds & Marsh, 1993). This can be a problem in countries where access to or use of the health services is low.

For more comprehensive understanding of health problems in low-access communities, other methods of data collection need to be used, such as population-based sample surveys (Anderson et al., 1989), or, as we discuss below, health unit data collection needs to be expanded to include community data. Mortality data can be obtained from hospitals and civil registration systems, but often need to be generated through other methods such as prospective studies of communities (Garenne & Cantrelle, 1989) or retrospective demographic surveys.

The particular function for which the information will be used and the related type of indicator often determine which data collection method will be most appropriate (see Table 17). Information for ongoing programme monitoring is easier and more efficiently obtained through routine data collection, whereas information for the purpose of an impact evaluation will probably need to be generated through nonroutine methods such as longitudinal studies or through sample surveys. Researchers mostly use nonroutine methods of data collection to gener-

Table 17 *Indicators and data collection methods*

Data collection methods	Indicator category				
	Input (health resources)	Process (health activities)	Output (health services provided)	Outcome (health status)	
				Morbidity	Fertility and mortality
Routine health unit data collection	+++	+++	+++	+	+
Routine community data collection	–	++	++	++	++
Civil registration	–	–	–	–	+++
Nonroutine methods	+	+	+	+++	+++

ate their information (WHO, 1990). Other nonroutine methods include rapid assessment methods, developed in the last decade for the collection of data for use at various levels (Anker, 1991) or for information on attitudes, behaviour, and opinions for use in programme planning and management (Scrimshaw & Gleason, 1992).

Available routine or survey data sets are often not sufficient to understand underlying causes of problems, particularly at the district and local levels. Informal investigations (Rodrigues and Israel, 1995) and "soft" information obtained through meetings with individuals and groups (Green, 1992) can be important sources of information to answer such questions. Finally, information from other sectors such as education, agriculture, and economics can contribute in major ways to improved decision-making, particularly for health policy formulation and planning of primary health care-based health services (de Kadt, 1989).

The choice of appropriate data collection methods is also linked to certain characteristics of the method itself, such as its complexity and cost (Klaucke et al., 1988; Thacker, Parrish & Trowbridge, 1988). Certain data collection methods such as national sample surveys and large-scale prospective mortality studies are very resource-intensive, requiring highly trained staff and equipment. Without external financial and technical assistance, most developing countries cannot afford to rely on such data collection methods for generating information.

But, as explained in detail in Chapter 4, whatever data collection method is chosen, the data collected should fulfil a particular information need. Routine health unit-based data collection can become very expensive if it takes time and effort away from care providers trying to deal with the multiple health problems in their communities. As eloquently stated by Van Lerberghe, Mercenier & Van Balen, (1987): "The normal functioning of the health service has to be recognized as a constraint to data collection, a constraint which is mandatory if relevance is to be ensured."

This chapter provides an overview of routine data collection methods. We first present different types of methods. Then, we describe the features of appropriate data collection instruments for use at different levels of the health services system. Finally, we discuss specific design and implementation issues when restructuring routine data collection methods. Where appropriate, the chapter illustrates the various methods with practical examples, models of data collection instruments, and case studies. An overview of nonroutine methods will be presented in Chapter 7.

Types of routine data collection methods

We classify routine health data collection methods according to three sources: health unit data collection, community data collection, and civil registration. As will be discussed later, there are substantial overlaps between these three types of methods: many health information systems combine health unit and community data collection; and both methods can include some form of vital events registration. Most discussions on this topic come down to the question of who uses the system (Reynolds, Bryant & Inam, 1988; O'Neill, 1993).

Health unit data collection

The most common type of routine health data collection is health unit-based. Data are recorded by the regular health staff within the facility while performing their daily health care activities. Routine health unit-based data collection is the most obvious way of collecting data for patient/client and health unit management (Van Lerberghe, Mercenier & Van Balen, 1987), for monitoring resources used and services provided, and for disease surveillance (Claquin, Reynolds & Marsh, 1993). Yet it is also the most criticized (Nordberg, 1988; Anderson et al., 1989; WHO, 1994b). Several problems with existing health information systems, as described in Chapter 1, are associated with this type of data collection: the quality of the data collected is poor; too much of the health care providers' time is spent collecting data; and the aggregated data are not representative of the population at large in countries with low utilization rates of the health services. But we do not share the pessimism of authors such as Anderson et al. (1989) who consider these problems nearly insurmountable: "The repetitive nature of the data registration processes, in the absence of prompt use of the data to improve heath, tends to result in reduced accuracy and quality over time ... Schemes to deal with deteriorating quality of data with repetition rest with various supervisory processes, often implying quite elaborate and time-consuming bureaucratic procedures."

On the contrary, this book demonstrates that health information systems based on routine data collection in health facilities not only can be transformed into helpful planning and management tools for the health services but can become the trigger for sustained improvement of the management environment in government health services (Lippeveld, Foltz & Mahouri, 1992). Later in this chapter we will discuss more particularly how data collection procedures can be improved as part of the restructuring process of routine health information systems.

One way of dealing with the problem of quality of data for use at higher levels is to use sentinel sites to report more complex data in addition to universal health unit-based data reporting. Sentinel site reporting is in fact a subtype of health unit-based data collection, whereby the staff of a selected number of facilities (mostly big hospitals) receive special training and supervision to collect and report data on a set of usually more complex diseases or activities. The resulting information is more complete and more accurate (Kirsch, 1988). This type of reporting is particularly useful in disease surveillance when health units in remote rural areas lack sufficiently trained staff and diagnostic equipment to accurately diagnose the diseases under surveillance. In Chad, one of the criteria for selection as a sentinel site was the availability of laboratory services. Sentinel sites reported on diseases for which a laboratory diagnosis was required (Lippeveld, Foltz & Mahouri, 1992). Box 17 gives a summary on the local area monitoring system, an example of a sentinel site reporting system (Kirsch, 1988).

The problem of the lack of representativeness of the information generated by health unit-based data collection can be addressed by expanding the system with some form of community-based data collection. For example, information on activities from community health workers or other outreach workers can be reported to the health unit; or in some cases, community members help to collect data from households (Claquin, Reynolds & Marsh, 1993). This has been done to a varying degree in different countries and projects, as will be demonstrated below.

Another common flaw of routine health unit data collection procedures is their organization into separate programme-specific data collection systems. An example of this "vertical" approach to information systems was the routine data collection set-up in the government services in Pakistan before restructuring. Each national programme (Expanded Program on Immunization, Control of Diarrhoeal Diseases, Malaria Control, Maternal and Child Health, Tuberculosis Control) had a separate set of data collection instruments handled by separate staff, and supervised by programme-specific supervisors (Frere, 1987; Lippeveld, Foltz & Mahouri, 1992). These categorical systems often are very well structured: external technical staff help develop action-oriented indicators; health care providers are well-trained and supervised, and use standardized sets of instructions; and reporting regularity is high, ensuring quality of data.

Many lessons can be learned from these programme-specific information systems regarding improving the quality of data collection (WHO, 1994b) which should be taken into account when restructuring routine systems. Unfortunately, the information generated pertains only to the activities of the basic health services covered by these programmes. This set-up is obviously very resource-intensive, and is in general possible only with external donor funding. In a government-funded district health system operated by polyvalent staff, such a data collection system becomes quickly and severely "overloaded". Also, some concern exists about the reliability of data collected by the same staff who are in charge of programme planning and management (WHO, 1994b). For example, coverage estimates obtained from routine Expanded Programme on Immunization statistics in Guatemala were consistently higher than those obtained by independent surveys (Goldman & Pebley, 1994).

WHO (1994b) states that "significant efforts are currently being made by some programmes to integrate data collection ... into the routine system". Our experiences in health information system development in Cameroon, Chad, and Pakistan show that it takes serious and sustained efforts to convince vertical programme managers of the well-founded basis of integrated data collection. Magnani (1990) describes how "the national-level programs at the Department of Health [in the Philippines] have been reluctant to relinquish control over what data is to be collected in the information system and how." These experiences provide the rationale for using a potentially time-consuming but rewarding

Box 17   Local area monitoring

Routine surveillance of the incidence of vaccine-preventable diseases has not proved sensitive enough to demonstrate the impact of the Expanded Programme on Immunization (EPI) in many countries. In order to document progress since the start of the EPI in 1979, data are needed for several years prior to that. In most developing countries these can be found only in major cities or large hospitals. Therefore a system of sentinel surveillance, the Local Area Monitoring Project is being set up in selected institutions in the major cities of the developing world.

The goal is to include the major city of each of the 25 largest developing countries, with a total population of 115 million. These 25 countries together account for 85% of all births in the developing world. In some cases the city was selected because it had an excellent municipal reporting system. For example, the Istanbul Health Office collects data from 169 hospitals, primary health centres, maternal and child health clinics and other institutions, and provides compiled municipal figures within 6 weeks. The trend of measles cases seen at the Children's Hospital exactly matches the trend for the city as a whole, indicating that for measles, at least, the Children's Hospital is an excellent sentinel site representative of the whole city. Manila has a hospital to which all cases of infectious disease are routinely referred, which is also a good sentinel site. In Rangoon it has been necessary to survey four hospitals, and in Jakarta seven, to cover all the target diseases.

By the first half of 1987, 12 years of retrospective data from 5–12 cities (depending on the disease) had been collected. Reporting was most complete for poliomyelitis and measles (76–80% of cities reporting), least complete for tetanus and neonatal tetanus (20–28%).

An attempt was made to assess the quality of the data from each sentinel site by reviewing the records for continuity, and comparing the number of cases of infectious disease with those expected or those found from other surveys. If the site was a hospital, the size of the population served had to be calculated in order to compute incidence rates, or else the total city population was used as a proxy. In order to compensate for variations between cities in the incidence rates, and to give each city equal weight in the analysis, the average of each city's percentage change from baseline (1974–1978) was used.

Judging from this, for the cities concerned, there has been a 62% reduction in the incidence of reported poliomyelitis by 1985, a 61% reduction for neonatal tetanus, 59% for diphtheria, 39% for measles, 35% for pertussis, and a decrease fluctuating between 0% and 24% for tuberculosis. Measles immunization was added late to many country immunization programmes; therefore, the decrease in incidence began later than for the other diseases. BCG (Calmette-Guérin bacillus) vaccine has its greatest effect on the severe childhood forms of tuberculosis, but the sentinel institutions do not usually report separately childhood, miliary or meningeal disease, hence the lack of a demonstrable trend. For the other target diseases, sentinel-site surveillance is proving to be a useful method for measuring programme impact.

Source: Kirsch (1988).

consensus-building approach during the design phase of a health information system reform effort.

Community data collection (see also Chapter 9)

The primary health care strategy promoted by WHO and adopted by most governments in the world calls for a reorganization of the traditional health services system, adapting health care delivery to the needs and limitations at the community level, and involving the community in the planning and management of local health services (Kleczkowski, Elling & Smith, 1981). This includes restructuring of health information systems not only to give health care managers and providers a better understanding of community needs but to also increase community involvement in the generation and use of information.

Based on these principles, ministries of health and nongovernmental organizations have expanded the classic health unit data collection methods with community routine and nonroutine data collection methods. Community nonroutine methods will be discussed in Chapter 7. As for routine data collection in the community, an important distinction to be made is whether it is part of a health information system primarily managed and used by the health services system or by the community itself. Most community data collection systems are managed by health care professionals at the district or health unit level, as an extension of the routine health unit information system. O'Neill (1993), in a study on community information systems, found that out of nine projects, seven were managed directly by health care professionals.

Community data collection can be used for a number of purposes:

— to monitor activities performed in the community by health unit staff or by community health workers (in most countries where such activities take place);
— to obtain more representative data on the health status and living environment of the communities served, including data on births and deaths in the community, agricultural and meteorological data, data on education, and so on (Kark & Berggren, 1981; Garenne & Cantrelle, 1989; Brown, 1990; de Kadt, 1989; Amonoo-Larston et al., 1994);
— to assist in planning for health services that are more accessible to the community (Taylor et al., 1983).

Community data collection systems managed by the community members themselves are rather uncommon, although the rationale for such systems is obvious: if communities need to be involved in planning and management of primary health care services, they will need information to carry out such functions and to make appropriate decisions (Reynolds, Bryant & Inam, 1988). What is less obvious is how to develop such systems and how to link them to health unit-based systems. Although in most communities human resources are available with experience in information management (merchants, teachers, etc.), they need assistance from professional health staff in determining the exact nature of community participation and related information needs for decision-making. Often the health professionals (from district or health unit level) themselves are not well trained to provide such assistance.

Examples of community-managed data collection systems in Thailand (in collaboration with the government) and in Bangladesh, Kenya, and Pakistan (in collaboration with the Aga Khan Health Network) are given by Reynolds, Bryant & Inam (1988) in their excellent overview article. Other data collection systems managed by the community are mentioned by Taylor (1992) and by O'Neill (1993). A transitional form between health unit-managed and community-managed data collection is described by Van Lerberghe, Mercenier & Van Balen (1987). In Kasongo (Democratic Republic of the Congo), a household registration system was set up to improve coverage and continuity of care. In order to avoid substantial time inputs from the paramedical staff at the eventual expense of the quality of care, it was decided that a clerk, paid by the community, would administer the data collection. A more in-depth discussion on the development of community-managed health information systems is provided in Chapter 9.

Civil registration systems

Civil registration systems are also a form of routine data collection related to health. In developed countries, these systems, in combination with census data, are the main source of mortality data. In developing countries, they often do not exist, and if so, they function poorly, so that the data are not useful for decision making (de Kadt, 1989; Helfenbein et al., 1987). In some countries in Asia and Africa, colonial administrators developed well-functioning systems, but mostly with authoritarian methods and substantial financial resources. After independence they gradually stopped functioning (Garenne & Parvez, 1991). Most developing countries therefore have to rely on other data collection methods for demographic estimates. Often indicators such as infant and child mortality rates are obtained through costly national surveys. Cause-specific mortality rates, maternal mortality ratios, and geographical breakdowns of mortality data are generally not available for strategic and programme planning.

Although a detailed discussion on the set-up and organization of civil registration and vital statistics systems falls outside the scope of this book[1], it should be mentioned that the development or restructuring of civil registration systems is a complex task. Often it is not very clear who should take administrative responsibility for the system, since data on births and deaths are crucial not only to the health sector but to most development sectors. In Pakistan, for example, debate is still ongoing as to whether the system should be administered by the Federal Bureau of Statistics, the Ministry of Interior, the Ministry of Local Bodies, or the Ministry of Health (Garenne and Parvez, 1991). In addition, substantial resources in terms of staffing, equipment, and supplies are needed to maintain the registration systems at an acceptable functional level. As Shahidullah (1995) writes: "No real hope can be expressed that most developing countries, whose economies are already burdened for many reasons, will soon afford the cost of maintaining and operating these systems."

Alternative methods for obtaining vital statistics are retrospective sample surveys and prospective follow-up studies of communities. The latter method is particularly promising and is further described under

---

[1] We refer the reader to the *Handbook of vital statistics and methods*, published by the United Nations (1991).

the nonroutine methods (see Chapter 7). In countries where regular population censuses are organized, governments can obtain information on fertility and mortality by adding specific questions to the census forms. Also, as part of the routine health information system, care providers and managers of the basic health services can organize data collection on births and deaths. Obviously, the community needs to be actively involved in this activity. Finally, care providers and managers can also obtain mortality data through indirect techniques such as Brass methods for infant mortality, or the sisterhood method for maternal mortality (Graham, Brass & Snow, 1989).

Data collection instruments

The quality and ultimate use of the data collected through routine information systems will depend substantially on the relevance, simplicity and layout of the data collection instruments. In the following section we will present an overview of various types of data collection instruments. Based on existing instruments, the literature, and our field experiences, we will discuss form design issues, operational advantages and disadvantages, and use of these instruments. Based on the health information system design framework presented in Chapter 2, and constantly keeping in mind future use of the information generated through these instruments, we have classified them according to the three types of management functions of the health services: data collection instruments for patient/client management, health unit management, and system management.

Data collection instruments for patient/client management

Data collection instruments for patient/client management can be anything from a simple piece of paper, to a fancy coloured plasticized card, a health booklet, or an electronic file. Their main purpose is to record data that will assist care providers in health services delivery to individuals or to communities at large, at the facility itself, or through outreach activities in the community.

Types
Medical records are data collection instruments to record data related to the management of the health status of an individual patient or client. Their content and format can vary as a function of the particular service provided: acute curative care; follow-up of chronic diseases; preventive follow-up for risk episodes such as a child under 5 or a pregnancy; or inpatient care in a hospital setting.

Other types of data collection instruments for individual patients or clients are laboratory forms (requests or results), forms for other specialized technical services such as X-ray and ultrasound exams, or referral forms to ensure communication between the first level and the referral level. In Bangladesh, household records were designed to record data during household visits (Helfenbein et al., 1987).

For preventive care activities, most countries use individual cards for follow-up of children under 5, pregnancies, or family planning services. A maternal and child health card used in Pakistan, for example, provides comprehensive data on the pregnancy of the mother as well as on the child from birth up to 3 years of age. We refer the reader to more detailed descriptions and prescriptions of child follow-up data collection instruments (Nabarro, 1987; Tremlett, Lovell & Morley, 1987; Helfenbein et al., 1987) and of maternal records (Helfenbein et al., 1987; WHO, 1994a).

Family registration records are particularly helpful in generating information for comprehensive and continuous care to patients and clients as members of a family. They permit "a more collective dimension to the individual contact; for example, the recruitment of children for the under-fives programme when a mother comes to the antenatal clinic; or the identification of specific family or social problems" (Van Lerberghe, Mercenier & Van Balen, 1987). As discussed further, by enumerating all members of the community in the catchment area, they provide the denominator for a series of health unit management indicators such as coverage of services. Although such records can be initiated in a simple way, to keep the records up to date can be quite cumbersome and time-consuming for the health unit staff. Most examples of well-functioning family registration were part of research projects such as Kasongo (Van Lerberghe, Mercenier & Van Balen, 1987), Khanna (Wyon & Gordon, 1971), Narangwal (Taylor, 1983), Matlab, or managed by a nongovernmental organization (e.g. Save the Children). Family registration is part of the national primary health care system in Costa Rica. In order to alleviate the problem of data collecting being too time-consuming, the Kasongo community hired a clerk (Van Lerberghe, Mercenier & Van Balen, 1987; see Box 18).

Content
What should be recorded on data collection instruments for patient/client management? Again, this depends first of all on the information the care provider needs in order to make appropriate decisions. For acute episodes of illness at the first level, simple diagnostic and treatment notes will suffice. Recorded on a simple form given to the patient, or kept at the facility on a medical record form, these notes act as a memory aid to the care provider if the patient returns. For significant health episodes (such as a pregnancy, a child under 5, or a chronic disease), more extensive data are necessary, permitting identification of risk factors and organization of continuity of care. Hospital medical records can contain detailed data on initial status upon admission, laboratory results, current diagnosis and treatment schedules, and follow-up notes on a daily and even hourly basis, depending on the condition of the patient. The hospital inpatient record in Kasongo permits staff to summarize the information at the top of the record, not only by describing the patient status at discharge (cured, improved, etc.), but also evaluating whether the hospitalization was justified (Kasongo Project Team, 1982). Referral forms should have at least two parts: one part filled in by the first level care provider who is referring the patient, and another part for the consultant at the referral level to communicate results on treatment provided and follow-up needed back to the first level.

The comprehensive nature of first-level care calls for a data collection instrument on which summary information on a patient or client can be kept, for example a health booklet retained by the patient, the summary card in Kasongo (see Box 18), or the maternal and child health card in Pakistan. A child growth chart should also contain data on immunization, or on acute episodes of illness such as diarrhoea which can influence the nutritional status of the child (Tremlett, Lovell & Morley, 1987), or on hospitalizations.

**Box 18 Family registration in Kasongo
(Democratic Republic of the Congo)**

In 1971, the Kasongo public health project was given overall responsibility for health care in the Kasongo area to about 200,000 inhabitants. Its major goal is to obtain satisfactory coverage of the target population with integrated and continuous care. Planning is based on a compromise between the health service's assessment of needs and the expressed demands of the population. The medical service is based on a two-tier structure consisting of a decentralized network of health centres responsible for providing individual primary health care, and a reference level in the form of the town hospital. Each health centre covers about 10,000 inhabitants. It is run by a team of one auxiliary nurse, one medicosocial aide, one orderly, and one clerk, whose salary is supported by the community, and who is responsible for the major part of the paperwork.

The health centre is the place where information is kept on individual members of the community for care provided in the health centre as well as in the hospital. The instrument is the household record. The file of household records is established during a census conducted by the health centre. It is further updated as families move into the area and come to register themselves. However, it is not the establishment of an exhaustive file of household records that prompted these censuses. The main reason was to establish contact with the population in order to give them sufficient information to permit participatory discussion about the health centre system, and for the nurse to get to know the population and its problems.

In a household record, summary cards for each individual client are filed according to a geographical classification. Summary cards contain information on episodes considered significant to the patient's health in the longer term: high-risk periods (children under 5, pregnant women, couples under contraceptive control); and certain chronic conditions (e.g. tuberculosis, hypertension). As such, household records permit a more collective dimension to the individual contact, for example the recruitment of children for the under-5 programme when a mother comes to the antenatal clinic, or the identification of specific family or social problems.

In addition to its usefulness for patient/client management, family registration also contributes to health unit management. Based on a census, the file of household records makes it possible to relate all data to population figures; for example, vaccination or antenatal care workload data can be transformed into information on coverage. The census data, which are regularly updated by recording vital events and by validity checks every few years, are sufficiently reliable for routine decision making, even if they might not be accurate enough for detailed epidemiological or demographic analysis. The geographical classification of the household records allows for a spatial dimension to the population-related figures.

Source: Adapted from Van Lerberghe, Mercenier & Van Balen, (1987).

One way of assisting paramedical staff in making the right decisions is to organize the record forms in an action-oriented manner. For example, if a certain risk factor during pregnancy is identified, what action will be taken on an immediate basis, or in the long term? Options can be given on the prenatal record form.

Table 18   *Patient-retained cards: what are the pros and cons?*

Some advantages of patient-retained records	Some problems with patient-retained records
• The time necessary to retrieve records in the facility can be used instead for service. • Patients have a personal health database they can present if they go to other units for service. • Village health workers can determine patients' follow-up health needs (immunizations, family planning) during home visits. • Certain community-based health surveys are more easily conducted. • Patient-retained records can be used for patient education and to stimulate patients' responsibility for their own health care. • Especially in large outpatient units (such as in hospitals), it has been found that more records are lost by the clinic than by the patients. • Hospital discharge information can be integrated into the patient-retained card, thus providing information for follow-up outpatient care.	• Patients lose cards, or forget to take them with them when they visit the health facility. • The records get wet and deteriorate quickly. • Confusion arises when the colour or the form of the record is changed. • Follow-up of chronic patients is more difficult, because there is no paper trace in the health facility.

Source: Adapted from Stinson (1983).

Record filing: patient-retained versus health unit-retained

A heavily debated issue is, who should keep the patient/client record, the recipient or the care provider? (Stinson, 1983; Helfenbein et al., 1987; Wyatt, 1994a). The concept of patient-retained cards was introduced mainly with the growth charts showing the "road to health" to mothers in a particularly intelligible manner (Helfenbein et al., 1987). Patient- or client-retained records are good vehicles to stimulate more involvement in decision-making related to patients' and clients' own health. But opponents maintain that too many patients lose their cards. Also, they make follow-up of patients and clients by the health unit more complicated. There are probably no final answers. Two consulting reports quoted by Stinson (1983) illustrate the debate very clearly (see Table 18).

Perhaps the best solution is to combine both systems. For example, in Pakistan follow-up of tuberculosis patients was ensured through a facility-retained card to identify missed appointments, but patients themselves kept a small card with a registration number so that the health unit could easily find the card. The patient card also contained a brief case history, in case patients changed the location of treatment.

For efficient patient/client follow-up, the "tickler file system" is particularly well suited. This simple and appropriate technology consists of two file holders which can accommodate the size of the record forms, for example two hanging file drawers or, very simply, two wooden boxes. One box, the "days box", is divided into 31 slots. The other box, the "months box", is divided in 12 slots. Tickler files are particularly useful for chronic episodes of illness such as hypertension or tuberculosis, and for preventive risk episodes. At the end of a visit, the record card is filed in the "day slot" or "month slot" (if the appointment is in a different month) of the next appointment. Remaining record forms at the end of the day are missed appointments for which follow-up procedures can be instituted. At the end of the month, all records in the next "month slot" are transferred to the "day slots". Fig. 11 shows how the tickler file system in Kasongo was linked with the family registration system.

Fig. 11   *Tickler file system for continuity of care in Kasongo, Democratic Republic of the Congo*

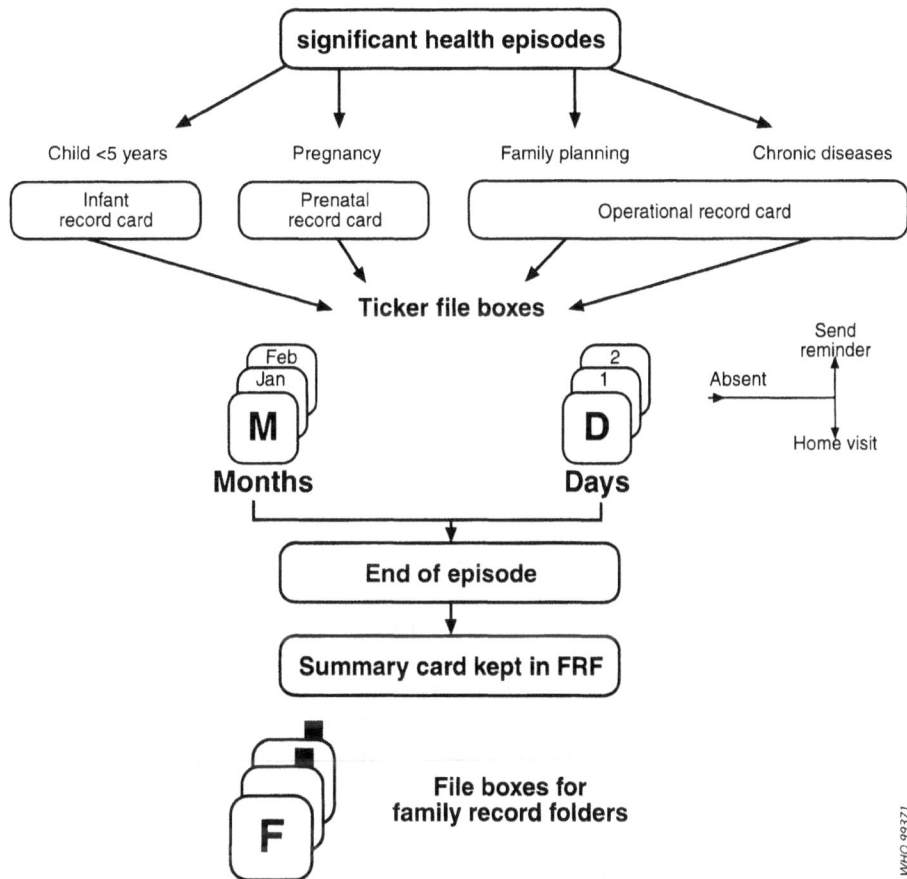

Layout

The layout of the record form is important for patient/client data collection instruments, particularly if the instruments are kept by the patients or clients themselves. For example, data items in medical records should be arranged in a logical order to guide care providers during clinical examinations. Disease- or problem-focused checklists are often pre-printed on the record forms. This not only reduces the time needed to fill them in, but makes them also more legible.

Forms are rarely self-explanatory; often abbreviations are used to save space, or terms and procedures are given without definition. If possible, abbreviations should be explained somewhere on the form itself, or instructions could be given on the reverse side of the form. If not, instruction manuals should be readily available, and health staff trained in using the forms.

Multicoloured record forms are more attractive than black-and-white forms, but are obviously more expensive. In Pakistan, a red band was added to the referral form. The idea was that patients referred by first-level care facilities would be more easily recognized by health staff in the hospitals who could save these patients from queuing again. Colours are particularly well suited for patient-retained records. UNICEF and other organizations issued growth-monitoring charts on which the "road to health" was coloured green above the 80th percentile line, yellow between the 80th and 60th percentiles, and red under the 60th percentile. Although this made the card very attractive, it drew too much attention away from the more important dynamic nutritional follow-up: Is the child gaining or losing weight between visits? So later the colours were removed. Tremlett, Lovell & Morley (1987) also advise using the right colours in each cultural setting. For example, in developed countries, red indicates danger, whereas green signifies "no problems". Yet in some other countries, red is the colour for health.

In countries with more than one national language or with a multitude of local languages, the language used on the record form can be an important issue for patient-retained cards or in settings with minimally trained health staff. In Pakistan, for example, health managers decided to print most patient cards in Urdu.

For the same reason, the use of pictorial elements can improve understanding of the form by illiterate health workers or by patients and clients. A vast number of such pictorial cards have been produced and are used all over the world (see an example in Annex 6, page 263). A good discussion on pictorial forms is provided by Helfenbein et al. (1987). One of their conclusions is that the production of a relevant, intelligible, and culturally acceptable pictorial record form is not an easy task, and extensive field testing is required. In Pakistan, a mother-retained maternal and child health card originally had many more pictures. Although during the field testing phase villagers had understood and accepted all the pictures, the health services managers themselves, to whom the card was shown for final approval, decided to remove several pictures because they feared that they would be considered "obscene" by most of the husbands.

Finally, partial or complete computerization of health information systems makes its own special demands on form design (Helfenbein et al., 1987). For example, if the data from patient/client forms need to be entered in the computer, the layout should permit easy data entry.

Production form
Particularly for patient/client records, the size and material can be determining factors in their effectiveness. Although larger growth charts can contain more information, they are more easily damaged (Tremlett, Lovell & Morley, 1987). Mothers often fold them to put them away. It is therefore advisable to prefold them to avoid early damage. The material is very important. The general rule is that the thicker the form, the longer it lasts, but also, the more expensive it is to produce. The thickness of each form will thus be a compromise between longevity and cost. Certain record forms, like patient tickets for acute curative care, can be made out of cheap paper. Patient-retained follow-up record cards should be made out of cardboard or plasticized paper. This last material, although more expensive, eliminates the necessity of providing a small, protective plastic bag for maternal and child health records (Tremlett, Lovell & Morley, 1987).

Electronic patient records
In developed countries and in some higher-income developing countries, more and more hospitals and even first-level care facilities use computerized data collection systems for patients and clients. According to Wyatt (1994a), electronic patient records are the best approximation of what he describes as the "ideal" patient record form. For a good description of computerized clinical data systems, we refer the reader to the

series of articles by Wyatt (1994a, 1994b and 1995). In most developing countries, the use of computer technology at the patient/client level cannot be considered "appropriate". The problem is not with the technical complexity of computerized clinical data systems. On a pilot basis, they have already been successfully implemented in rural settings in developing countries (Murthy & Patel, 1988). Rather, the problem lies in the prevailing organizational environment of the health services (Foltz, 1993). Two main impediments are the lack of trained staff and of hardware and software maintenance capacity at the health unit level. Another factor is obviously cost. Computerization of clinical data systems in developing countries will therefore remain a marginal phenomenon in the next decades. The first obvious candidates for implementation of such systems are tertiary care hospitals in major urban settings.

Data collection instruments for health unit management

Types

At the health unit management level, data are collected to permit health unit staff to make operational decisions. These decisions can be categorized into two main groups: (i) service delivery management decisions and (ii) resource management decisions. Similarly, we have also divided data collection instruments into two groups:

- Service delivery records
  The main purpose of service delivery records is to gather information for planning and management of the main services provided. For example, data from prenatal care registers after aggregation will permit calculations of coverage in combination with population data. Or curative care registers can be used for determining the geographical origin of the patients. They can be used for fixed as well as for outreach activities (Helfenbein et al., 1987). In some countries, service records are also considered legal documents.
  In addition, service records often constitute the main database for system management data. Data from these records are aggregated into reports to be transmitted to higher levels. Or supervisors use them to check on quality of care. For example, in Chad, supervisors checked on appropriate use of drugs by verifying the treatments prescribed in the curative care register. Sometimes service delivery records are used for both health unit and patient/client management. In Pakistan, maternal and child health cards are retained by patients. To check on missed appointments, health staff put a square sign in the column of the month of the next visit in the child care register (see Annex 7, page 264).
- Resource management records
  Resource management records gather data for management of different resources: personnel, equipment, supplies, transport, drugs and vaccines, and finances. Again, only data necessary to make the appropriate planning and management decisions are necessary. The data from these records are also mostly aggregated at certain time periods for reporting to higher levels.

As pointed out by Van Lerberghe, Mercenier & Van Balen (1987), merely recording data on service delivery and resource management records does not guarantee their use for health unit management. In fact, the data need to be aggregated from the different registers and presented in a summary form to make them easier to interpret and use for decision making. Our experience has shown that report forms provide the most

101

efficient format for these purposes. In addition to serving as a vehicle for reporting raw data to higher hierarchical levels, this form can be transformed into a summary record for health unit management. We will further elaborate on this when we discuss reporting data.

Production form
The most common form of service record is the register in which patients or clients are recorded by name and certain demographic characteristics, such as age and sex. Then a number of columns permit the registration of data for service indicators, such as date of visit, diagnosis, nutritional status, and so on. Registration by name takes time. If the data are collected only for aggregation purposes, it is often simpler just to use tally sheets (see Annex 8). Tally sheets can also be combined with registers. For example, in Pakistan, where data on health problems were recorded in the curative care register, a tally sheet (in the form of an "abstract register") was used to aggregate the data in the monthly report. The daily clinical treatment record presented by Husein et al. (1993) is another proposal for effectively recording daily curative care data.

Registers can also be used for inpatient registration. Particularly effective and easy to use is the hospital daily attendance sheet used in Chad (see figure, Annex 9). This sheet, combined with daily information on patient movements in the ward, permits quick calculation of the average bed occupancy and length of stay.

One way of directly linking data collection and use of the information is data collection instruments in the form of wall posters. For example, weight and height wall charts are used for nutritional follow-up of children under 5. In Pakistan, data collected on population in the catchment area were recorded on the population chart and posted on the wall in all first level care facilities (see Annex 10).

Layout
For health unit management data collection instruments, a rationalized and simple layout is more important than the presentation. The layout can have a major impact on the accuracy of the data. Columns in registers and open spaces on tally sheets should have sufficient space to record the required data. The headings of the columns should clearly indicate what data item needs to be filled in. Service delivery records can also have pictorial elements for illiterate health workers (Helfenbein et al., 1987). Checklists are easier to fill in, more legible, and quicker to aggregate. A good example is age registration. If age data will be analysed by age category, it is more effective to have age checked off in separate age category columns in the register instead of filling in an open-ended age column. The order of the data on the record forms and registers should take into account the sequence of procedures health workers will perform.

Size and material of the data collection instruments are also important. Large registers permit more data collection per page but are often not very handy on small desks in a rural health facility. Registers used for long periods should be made from sturdy materials to prevent the register from becoming a heap of loose folded pages. In countries where paper is a relatively rare commodity in rural areas, numbering the pages of a register can prevent too many pages ending up as wrapping paper.

Computerization of health unit data collection

The same arguments used for electronic patient records are valid for computerization of health unit management records because they are intimately linked to each other. Prior to the decision to computerize large health units such as tertiary care hospitals, careful study is required to ensure the availability of adequate resources such as trained staff and hardware and software maintenance facilities. Also, it is advisable to plan for an incremental implementation scheme. For example, physical resource management systems such as inventory control could be computerized in a first stage. Computerization of service delivery records would be done simultaneously with the introduction of electronic medical records.

Data collection instruments for system management

Types and content

As part of a routine health unit-based information system, information for system management can be generated from two sources: the health units, through reporting of aggregated data, and through primary data collection. By primary data, we mean data collected directly by the staff located at the system level, such as district supervisors and regional or national staff. We therefore will discuss separately report forms originating from health units and data collection instruments for system management.

- Health unit report forms
  In routine health unit-based information systems, most of the information needed for system management is collected by the health units and then reported to higher levels on report forms. The content of these reports, their actual number, and their frequency depend on the information needs of the health planners and managers and on the organizational set-up of the health services. Data reported mainly pertain to the health status of the population, services provided, and resources used. In order to ensure future use of the information, only data that contribute to the decision-making process at higher levels should be reported. This principle also applies to the frequency of reporting. If data on drug consumption are analysed once a year to establish standard drug supply packages for the health units, reporting once a year is sufficient.
  As described earlier, the routine reporting system often has become fragmented under pressure of programmatic planners and managers. Each national programme has developed its own report forms, without very much consultation or coordination with other programmes or with the line managers. As a result, health workers have to draft each week, each month, each quarter, and each year a multitude of reports with substantial duplication. In Pakistan, for example, before restructuring of the routine information system in 1992, more than 20 different report forms were supposed to be sent from each first-level care facility. One of the most pressing needs in restructuring existing information systems, therefore, is to streamline the routine reporting system. As much as possible, reporting for health facilities should be comprehensive and made through the regular line management channels. Comprehensive reports will avoid unnecessary repetition of data items and simplify transmission, and if properly designed, they can become tools for direct use of the information for health unit management (see Box 19).

Box 19   The monthly report in Pakistan

In 1993, as part of a comprehensive restructuring of the health information system in government management health facilities in Pakistan, the Ministry of Health introduced a simplified reporting system. Previously, health institutions prepared more than 10 different reports which were dispatched through a variety of transmission routes to their final destination. Under the new system, most services provided and resources used are reported through a single comprehensive monthly report. Epidemic diseases are reported through an immediate report, while the yearly report serves to update demographic and infrastructural information.

The new monthly report is intended to inform both system managers and care providers. In four pages, it presents a complete profile of the health unit in a logical order: the first page provides demographic information and information on stock levels of essential drugs and vaccines; the second and third pages summarize information on curative services focused on priority diseases; and the last page reports on preventive maternal and child health activities. Only those indicators needed for health system management have been included.

The report is designed in such a way that health unit managers can directly use the aggregated information for better planning and managing their facilities. For example, space and population denominators are provided to calculate coverage percentages. (As an example, the section on maternal care activities is presented in Annex 12). Empty space is provided to permit health unit managers to communicate specific problems in a less structured way to district health officers.

The report is prepared in three copies. One copy remains in the health unit for further use, and two are sent to the district health officer. The district health officer in turn keeps one copy, and sends the other copy to the nearest computer centre for data entry. This transmission mode allows for flexible and timely feedback, which can be given immediately by the district health officer based on the information contained in the report form, or later on after computerized data processing.

• Data collection instruments for system management
Much of the information needed for health system management, especially at the national level, will be generated outside the routine health information system, through various quantitative and qualitative methods (see Chapter 7). Yet routine data can also be collected directly by the health system level. For example, information on quality of care provided can be obtained from data collected by supervisors. Based on standard guidelines for curative and preventive services, supervisory checklists can guide the supervisors of the basic health services in assessing quality of care during routine supervisory visits (see example in Annex 11). Data are collected through inspection of patient/client records and services records, through actual observation of the health care provider, or eventually from patient/client exit interviews. The data from these checklists can be further aggregated and reported to regional and national levels for programme monitoring and evaluation.

Layout

The layout of reporting forms can be a major help in both accurate completion of the forms as well as direct use of the information by the care provider and the supervisor. Many of the rules to improve the design of patient/client and service delivery records also apply to report forms. As much as possible, the forms should be self-explanatory, minimizing the use of unusual acronyms. The logical order of the data is important. For example, the monthly report for first-level care facilities in Pakistan has four pages: the first page contains identification data, data on outreach activities, and data on resource management; the second and the third pages gather all the data on curative management of priority health problems; while the fourth page summarizes data on preventive care. If proportions or percentages have to be calculated, numerator as well as denominator data should be put together, so that calculations can be done immediately. For example, for calculation of coverage by essential services, both the number of visits as well as the data on target population should be reported together (see Box 19 and Annex 12).

An important aspect to be taken into account when designing report forms is that the same information often is needed at different levels of the health services: for national programme managers, for district supervisors, and most important, for the care providers themselves. As further explained, computerization at higher levels can avoid unnecessary and time-consuming copying of data. At the health unit level, the use of carbon copies is the best solution to eliminate the need for recopying data. Report forms provided with detachable carbon copies are more sophisticated but more expensive.

Computerization

Obviously, in the absence of computers at the health unit level in most developing countries, computerization of report forms is not relevant, except in larger tertiary care units where resource management systems and services delivery records have been computerized. Yet since data processing at the district or higher levels has been computerized, the layout of health unit report forms should accommodate computerized data entry at higher levels. For example, data to be entered in the computer could be boxed, underlined, or bolded, so data entry staff can easily identify them (see Annex 12).

Design and implementation of routine data collection systems

In the process of restructuring routine health information systems, design and implementation of a routine data collection system is the second step, following the identification of information needs and indicators (see Chapter 2). The health planner or system analyst in charge of this process will have to answer a certain number of practical questions. For example:

- How many and what type of data collection instruments will be needed to respond adequately to the defined information needs?
- Are existing instruments adequate, or do they need to be modified?
- If new instruments are needed, how will they be developed?
- How will the new data collection instruments be introduced to the care providers in charge of data collection?

The answers to these questions will obviously determine the scope and the time frame of the restructuring effort. As a general rule, adequate existing data collection instruments should not be replaced. If it is found that existing data collection instruments are totally inadequate to generate the required information, a long and tedious consensus-building process will probably be necessary to produce a new set of instruments, acceptable to both care providers and managers. If only part of the data collection instruments need revision, the task is much simpler and shorter. For example, maybe only disease surveillance data collection instruments need to be developed.

Independent of the length and complexity of the process, future data collectors and users of the health information system should be involved in determining the quality and use of the data generated when setting up the system. Careful consensus building for this step more than any other in the health information system design process is an absolute necessity. One of the main reasons why routine systems often generate data of poor quality is the lack of motivation of data collectors to fill out forms which they consider inefficient, redundant, and irrelevant to their own information needs. Also, for the same reason, where appropriate, design of data collection instruments should first of all favour effective patient/client and facility management, rather than data collection for the purpose of health system management. Our experiences in Cameroon, Chad, and Pakistan have shown that involving managers and care providers in the design phase and later on as trainers in data collection has a major positive effect on the regularity and quality of routine reporting.

We propose to structure the development (or restructuring) of the data collection system in three phases: (i) development of a set of data collection instruments, (ii) forms design and pretesting, and (iii) implementation of the new data collection instruments.

Development of a set of data collection instruments

The first phase in the redesign of the routine data collection system is to compare information needs and indicators at different levels in the health services system with the existing data collection instruments. A practical way to proceed is to set up a table which matches information needs and instruments (see Table 19).

Such analysis will also help identify redundancies in existing data collection. As the example shows, integrating the prenatal and postnatal registers into one maternal health register will eliminate the need for double registration and enhance continuity of care. Ho (1985) describes how in Maharashtra state (India), an initial review of existing data collection instruments led to a reduction of the number of registers from 46 to 7. But the first rule remains not to replace data collection instruments if they are responsive to the identified information needs.

An important aspect of improving the data collection system is to standardize case definitions, case management procedures, and data collection procedures. Without a definition of what is a new case of a disease and what is a repeat visit for the same episode, data on disease trends are difficult to analyse. For example, if in one health facility a case of tuberculosis is recorded as a new case at each visit, while in another facility it is recorded only once, comparing the number of cases detected in

Table 19 *Matching information needs and data collection instruments for prenatal care*

Indicator	From existing DCIs	Need for revision	New DCIs
1. Percentage of pregnant women registered in catchment area	Prenatal register	Include column to register catchment area women separately	Create maternal health register (see indicator 4)
2. Percentage of pregnant women registered in first trimester	Prenatal register	None	Create maternal health register
3. Percentage of pregnant women with at least two prenatal visits	Prenatal register	None	Create maternal health register
4. Percentage of pregnant women with at least one postnatal visit	Postnatal register	Combine prenatal and postnatal registers	Create maternal health register
5. Percentage of low birth weight babies in catchment area	Not available	Define catchment area, define low birth weight	Create child health register
6. Percentage of pregnant women with haemoglobin less than 10 g% upon first visit	Not available	Develop standard for Hb measurement and equipment	Create maternal health register
7. Percentage of pregnant women with adequate weight gain during pregnancy	Prenatal register	Define adequate weight gain	Create maternal health register
8. Percentage of pregnant women having received prenatal care according to standards	Not available	Develop quality standards for prenatal care	Create supervisory checklist

Source: Adapted from list of indicators of HMIS/FLCF in Pakistan.
DCI = data collection instruments.

each facility becomes totally irrelevant. Furthermore, judgements about quality of care are quite subjective as long as no standardized case management procedures have been defined.

Forms design and pretesting

Forms design can contribute greatly in ensuring better use of the information for decision making, especially for patient/client record cards and for reporting forms.

Once a consensus has been established on data collection instruments to be revised, abolished, or created, detailed design of the forms can be left to a technical team with specific skills and experience for this task. This team will have to address various issues related to the production form and the layout of each instrument. Typical questions to be answered are, What should be the logical order of items on the form? In what language should the form be printed? Will pictures be included on the form, and if so, which ones? For patient/client record cards, should the card be patient-retained or health unit-retained? For health unit data collection instruments, should registers be used or tally sheets? What data on the report forms will be entered in the computer? Should the forms be printed in colour? Should record cards be laminated? Most of these questions were addressed earlier in this chapter. Additional issues related to printing of forms and registers will be discussed in Chapter 10.

Part of data collection instrument design is the production of a set of instructions, explaining to care providers how to fill in the data items on the form. Designers need to decide if these instructions should be included on the form or provided separately. Instructions on the record card or in the register are more easily read by the data collector, but make the instrument more cumbersome and its production more expensive. If instructions are provided separately, they should be listed together in an "instruction manual" and be put in each health facility in a place easily accessible to all health care providers. It is also possible to combine both approaches.

Forms design is a multistep, iterative process. Pretesting is an absolute necessity before finalizing the design. A myriad of details on a data collection form need to be taken care of in order to ensure that data can be recorded unambiguously and that the form can be easily handled by the data collectors. How much space should be left open for each data item to be filled in? If multiple choices, are the choices offered exhaustive? How will wording on the form be interpreted by the care providers? How many pages should a register have? How sturdy should the material be in order to last through a specified time and what are the cost implications? Many of these questions can only be answered during extensive pretesting of the forms in health facilities.

No standard methodological rules on the number of facilities and the time period for pretesting exist. Ideally, the sample of health facilities for pretesting should be as representative as possible. Important variables to consider are the location of the facility (urban versus rural, different cultural settings, areas with different languages), staffing (competence and workload), equipment and supplies, and patterns of use. The time period during which pretesting takes place should be long enough to study all possible events related to the data collection process: patients' and clients' initial visits as well as return visits; stock management, including ordering, receiving, as well as issuing supplies; monthly or quarterly aggregations; and so on. A minimum of 3 to 6 months is suggested.

All aspects of the data collection instrument need to be scrutinized during the pretesting phase:

- Relevance: Are the data to be collected used at the point of data collection for patient/client or health unit management?
- Feasibility: Is it possible to collect required data on the form in a particular health unit? For example, to collect laboratory data, the health unit needs lab facilities.
- Burden: How much time and effort are needed by the staff to fill in the data collection instrument?
- Layout: Is the flow of data items logical? Is there place enough to fill in the data?
- Clarity: Are the instructions for filling in the form clear and helpful?

This information can be obtained through observation by an external review team and through direct comments provided by the data collectors. In order to better structure comments, a pretest review form was developed in Pakistan to be filled in for each data collection instrument by the staff of the selected health facilities (see Annex 13). Based on the pretesting results, instrument design can mostly be finalized and instructions prepared for implementation. In some cases when, based on the pretesting, the data collection instrument has been substantially revised, a second round of pretesting may be required.

Implementation of the new data collection system

The final step in restructuring the data collection system is to implement the new forms and procedures in the health units. This process involves at least three actions: (i) printing and distribution of new data collection instruments, (ii) training health personnel in data collection procedures, and (iii) discontinuing use of old instruments. These actions are narrowly linked to each other, but also to the next steps in the health information system restructuring: the new data transmission and data processing procedures. Often different managerial levels and staff of the health services are involved. Implementation therefore requires careful planning and overall coordination. Overall planning for implementation and coordination of health information system restructuring will be discussed in a more comprehensive way in Chapters 13 and 14. In the following section, we will discuss specific issues related to the implementation of new data collection procedures.

The complexity of the implementation process will first of all depend on the scope of the restructuring effort, both in terms of the magnitude of change compared with the previous system as well as with the number of health units involved. To change a few record cards in a local network of first level care facilities is simpler than to introduce a completely new set of data collection instruments nationwide. The specific change content is another factor: to introduce new patient/client data collection instruments is less disruptive than to change the reporting system.

Printing and distributing a new set of data collection instruments is a long and tedious process, and can become a serious bottleneck in the implementation process. Fortunately, with the tremendous increase in desktop publishing capacity of personal computers, composition of printed forms can mostly be done by the design team itself, which eliminates the involvement of specialized printing agencies in the design phase. Ideally, printed supplies should be ordered in large quantities to decrease production costs. This obviously requires careful pretesting of new forms, to avoid ending up with mountains of record cards rendered useless because a major data item was missing. The delivery date and distribution of the printed supplies need to be coordinated with the training plan, so that health staff can use the new instruments as soon as possible after training.

New data collection forms are rarely self-explanatory. Training of health personnel in data collection procedures before or at the introduction of new forms is therefore a mandatory step. How to organize such training is once again dependent on the scope of the restructuring effort. For major changes involving the reporting system, formal training sessions at the district level are probably the best training method. Training should include all concerned staff in the district and be concentrated over a relatively short period, so that the disruption in changing from the old to the new system is kept minimal. The training programme should not only explain how to fill in the form but also focus on how to use the information generated through the forms. Ideally, training in data collection should be combined with service delivery or resource management training. If the change concerns patient/client cards, training can be spread over a longer period and can be done eventually on the occasion of supervisory visits. Clearly written or printed instructions on how to fill in the forms should be available at the time of the training and be handed to the health personnel so that they can be consulted at any time after training.

A last issue is the switch from the old to the new system of data collection, particularly in case major changes are made to the reporting system on a nationwide basis. In our experience, problems arise if the implementation period takes too long. If old forms are discontinued before all health units have been trained, information gaps could be created, hampering smooth programme management. For example, vaccine stock management could become seriously disrupted. If old forms are kept operational together with the new forms, the change could be perceived as burdensome to the health care providers, undermining the credibility of the new system. Careful planning for printing of the new forms and training of the health personnel are therefore essential. For nationwide restructuring efforts, it is advised to implement the new data collection system districtwide. As soon as all district health personnel have been trained to use the new data collection instruments, all health units switch to the new system at the same time. In the other districts, the old forms can be maintained until the staff are trained.

Conclusion

To fulfil information needs at all management levels, national health information systems should probably generate information from a variety of data collection methods. What should be the composition of the blend? Nordberg (1988) points out that "we lack clear-cut answers to [a certain] numbers of questions." Are routine systems really much cheaper than surveys if health provider time for data collection is counted? Should more attention be given to the improvement of vital events registration? If surveys significantly increase our knowledge of health problems and health-related behaviour, how do we design and implement survey systems that can be managed by regional or district staff? Some of these answers will be provided in the next chapter on nonroutine data collection methods.

In the meantime, most national information systems in both developed and developing countries use a combination of data collection methods. In Canada, a survey was designed to fill the gaps left by the traditional reporting system (Carstairs & Heasman, 1987). In the Philippines, plans were developed to supplement the routine health unit-based system with population-based surveys (Magnani, 1990). Claquin, Reynolds & Marsh (1993) describe the advantages and disadvantages of different data collection methods for disease surveillance and recommend a combination of simple health unit-based reporting, sentinel site reporting, surveys, and outbreak investigations. Nordberg (1988) suggests reducing the volume of routine reporting systems and supplementing them with relatively inexpensive household surveys. Yet routine health unit-based data collection systems should remain the backbone of the national health information system. As we described earlier, well-structured health unit-based systems with an important outreach component in the community can be powerful management tools in assisting public health managers and care providers to make informed planning and management decisions.

References

Amonoo-Larston R et al. (1994). *District health care: challenges for planning, organisation and evaluation in developing countries*, 2nd ed. London, Macmillan: 256–279.

Anderson N et al. (1989). The use of community-based data in health planning in Mexico and Central America. *Health policy and planning*, 4:197–206.

Anker M (1991). Epidemiological and statistical methods for rapid health assessment: introduction. *World health statistics quarterly*, 44:94–98.

Brown RC (1990). A simple system of nutrition surveillance for African communities. *Journal of tropical pediatrics*, 36:162–164.

Carstairs VDL, Heasman MA (1987). Information strategy as a basis for measuring health promotion and protection. In: Abelin T, Brzezinski ZJ, Carstairs VDL, eds. *Measurement in health promotion and protection*. Copenhagen, World Health Organization: 365–383 (European Series, No. 22).

Claquin P, Reynolds J, Marsh D (1993). *Surveillance of morbidity and mortality. Module 4, Primary health care management advancement programme.* Geneva, Aga Khan Foundation.

de Kadt E (1989). Making health policy management intersectorial: issues of information analysis and use in less developed countries. *Social science and medicine*, 29:503–514.

Foltz AM (1993). Modeling technology transfer in health information systems: learning from the experience of Chad. *International journal of technology assessment in health care*, 9:345–361.

Frere JJ (1987). *Health and management information system for child survival project in Pakistan*. Technologies for Primary Health Care Project, United States Agency for International Development: 1–23.

Garenne M, Cantrelle P (1989). *Prospective studies of communities: their unique potential for studying the health transition: reflections from the ORSTOM experience in Senegal*. Workshop on Measurement of Health Transition Concepts, Regent's College, London, 1–12.

Garenne M, Parvez A (1991). *Report on levels and causes of infant and child deaths in Pakistan*. Islamabad, Pakistan Child Survival Project.

Goldman N, Pebley AR (1994). Health cards, maternal reports and the measurement of immunization coverage: the example of Guatemala. *Social science and medicine*, 38:1075–1089.

Graham W, Brass W, Snow RW (1989). Estimating maternal mortality: the sisterhood method. *Studies in family planning*, 20:125–135.

Green A (1992). *An introduction to health planning in developing countries*. Oxford, Oxford University Press.

Helfenbein S et al. (1987). *Selecting and collecting data. Technologies for management information systems in primary health care*. Geneva, World Federation of Public Health Associations (Issue Paper, Information for Action Series).

Ho TJ (1985). *Managing health and family planning delivery through a management information system*. World Bank Population, Health and Nutrition Department. Washington, DC, World Bank.

Husein K et al. (1993). *Planning and assessing health worker activities. Module 3, primary health care management advancement programme*. Geneva, Aga Khan Foundation.

Kark S, Berggren G (1981). *Community health project in rural Haiti*. Teaching notes. Boston, MA, Harvard School of Public Health: 1–64.

Kasongo Project Team (1982). *The Kasongo Project: lessons of an experiment in the organisation of a system of primary health care*. Antwerp, Public Health Research and Teaching Unit of Prince Leopold Institute of Tropical Medicine.

Kirsch TD (1988). Local area monitoring. *World health statistics quarterly*, 41:19–26.

Klaucke DN et al. (1988). Guidelines for evaluating surveillance systems. *Morbidity and mortality weekly report*, 37:1–18.

Kleczkowski BM, Elling RH, Smith DL (1981). *Health system support for primary health care: a study based on the technical discussions held during the Thirty-fourth World Health Assembly, 1981.* Geneva, World Health Organization (Public Health Papers, No. 80).

Lippeveld TJ, Foltz A, Mahouri YM (1992). *Transforming health facility-based reporting systems into management information systems: lessons from the Chad experience.* Cambridge, MA, Harvard Institute of International Development: 1–27 (Development Discussion Papers, No. 430).

Magnani RJ (1990). *Information systems development at the Republic of the Philippines Department of Health.* Manila, Department of Health: 1–20.

Murthy N, Patel KG (1988). *A computer based information system for health and family welfare: the Bavala experiment.* Ahmedabad, Indian Institute of Management.

Nabarro D (1987). Assessing health and monitoring progress: instruments for use at individual level. In: Abelin T, Brzezinski ZJ, Carstairs VDL, eds. *Measurement in health promotion and protection.* Copenhagen, World Health Organization: 533–543 (European Series, No. 22).

Nordberg E (1988). Household health surveys in developing countries: could more use be made of them in planning? *Health policy and planning,* 3:32–39.

O'Neill K (1993). *Community based surveillance: a critical examination of nine case studies.* London, London School of Hygiene and Tropical Medicine: 1–84.

Reynolds J, Bryant JH, Inam B (1988). Community based PHC management information systems guidelines for development of a model system. In: Wilson RG et al., eds. *Management information systems and microcomputers in primary health care.* Geneva, Aga Khan Foundation: 73–88.

Rodrigues RJ, Israel K (1995). *Conceptual framework and guidelines for the establishment of district-based information systems.* Barbados, Pan American Health Organization, Office of the Caribbean Program Coordination (document PAHO/CPC/3.1/95.1).

Scrimshaw NS, Gleason GR (1992). *Rapid assessment procedures—qualitative methodologies for planning and evaluation of health related programmes.* Boston, MA, International Nutrition Foundation for Developing Countries.

Shahidullah M (1995). The sisterhood method of estimating maternal mortality: the Matlab experience. *Studies in family planning,* 26:101–106.

Stinson W (1983). *Information systems in primary health care.* Washington, DC, American Public Health Association (Primary Health Care Issues Series 1, No. 6).

Taylor CE (1983). *Child and maternal health services in rural India: the Narangwal experiment.* Baltimore, MD, Johns Hopkins University Press.

Taylor CE (1992). Surveillance for equity in primary health care: policy implications from international experience. *International journal of epidemiology,* 21:1043–1049.

Thacker BS, Parrish RG, Trowbridge FL (1988). A method for evaluating systems of epidemiological surveillance. *World health statistics quarterly,* 41:11–19.

Tremlett G, Lovell HJ, Morley D (1987). Guidelines for the design and use of weight-for-age growth charts. In: Abelin T, Brzezinski ZJ, Carstairs VDL, eds. *Measurement in health promotion and protection.* Copenhagen, WHO Regional Office for Europe: 544–554 (European Series, No. 22).

United Nations (1991). *Handbook of vital statistics and methods.* New York, United Nations.

Van Lerberghe W, Mercenier P, Van Balen H (1987). Health care data collection and information system in Kasongo, Zaire. In: Abelin T, Brzezinski ZJ, Carstairs VDL, eds. *Measurement in health promotion and protection.* Copenhagen, WHO Regional Office for Europe: 635–642 (European Series, No. 22).

Woodall JP (1988). Introduction: epidemiological approaches to health planning, management and evaluation. *World health statistics quarterly,* 41:2–10.

World Health Organization (1990). *The role of research and information systems in decision making for the development of human resources for health. Report of a WHO Study Group.* Geneva, World Health Organization: 1–57 (WHO Technical Report Series, No. 802).

World Health Organization (1994a). *La fiche maternelle tenue a domicile: comment la mettre au point, l'adapter et l'évaluer. [Home-based maternal records: guidelines for development, adaptation, evaluation.]* Geneva, World Health Organization.

World Health Organization (1994b). *Information support for new public health action at the district level: Report of a WHO Expert Committee.* Geneva, World Health Organization: 1–31 (WHO Technical Report Series, No. 845).

Wyatt JC (1994a). Clinical data systems, part 1: data and medical records. *Lancet,* 344:1543–1548.

Wyatt JC (1994b). Clinical data systems, part 2: components and techniques. *Lancet,* 344:1609–1614.

Wyatt JC (1995). Clinical data systems, part 3: development and evaluation. *Lancet,* 344:1682–1688.

Wyon JB, Gordon JE (1971). *The Khanna study—population problems in rural Punjab.* Cambridge, MA, Harvard University Press.

7 Nonroutine data collection methods: an overview

Rainer Sauerborn

Definition and classification

As we have seen in the preceding chapter, routine methods use the ongoing documentation of health care provision or administration. In contrast, nonroutine data are collected ad hoc for a special purpose to complement and corroborate data gathered through the routine reporting system. Routine and nonroutine methods are complementary in several ways (see also Chapter 6, Table 17):

- The help managers answer different questions. Frequently, nonroutine methods are used to explore the underlying reasons for weaknesses uncovered by the routine system. For example, in Burkina Faso, routine reports showed that maternal and child health services were underused by children. A simple user survey showed that the rationale of taking well children to a clinic was not understood and that mothers had difficulty justifying their absence from home. A nonroutine method, the Expanded Programme on Immunization cluster survey, helps to assess the community effectiveness (impact) of the immunization efforts. Managers can then compare the impact of their programmes with process quality (cold chain maintenance) and output (number of doses delivered).
- The methods are complementary in the source of information: routine methods are generally facility-based and collected on the subpopulation of users of health services. In countries where health care use is low, facility-based routine information systems generate a very biased view of health problems of the population for which the health care team is in charge. In contrast, nonroutine methods are generally community-based. Fig. 12 provides a pictorial view of the relationship between the health service (shaded rectangle in the centre) and the population it is in charge of. Health services cannot be run in a meaningful way without some knowledge of health-related beliefs of the population, factors that increase or prevent the occurrence of disease, and factors that influence the demand for health services (left side of Fig. 12). On the other hand (right side of Fig. 12), health care managers are interested in knowing the outcome of health services as their ultimate yardstick of success: Did health improve as a result of health care? Are consumers satisfied with services? Rather than being descriptive and static, the model is meant to be dynamic, looking at the interaction between health services activities and population characteristics.
- Routine and nonroutine methods are complementary with regard to the instruments used to collect data. Routine methods consist mainly of a set of recording and reporting procedures for use by care providers and health services managers. Nonroutine methods fall into three

Fig. 12   *Health system model*

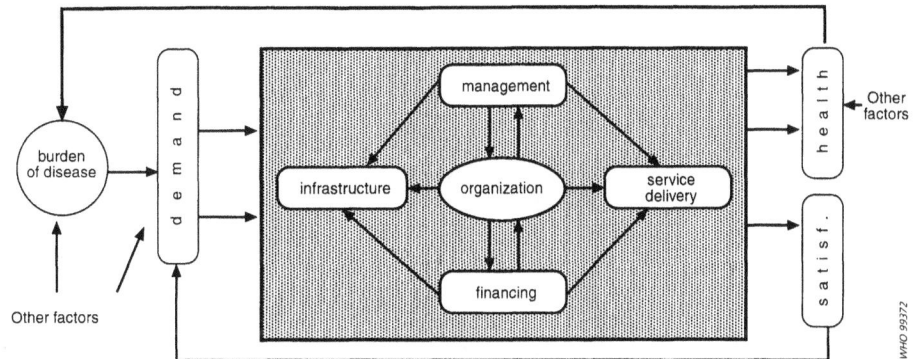

Table 20   *Nonroutine methods, disciplines, and types of data generated*

Nonroutine method	Predominant discipline	Examples of data generated
Demographic surveillance	Demography	Programme impact: age, sex, and cause-specific mortality; age-specific fertility
Survey	Epidemiology, sociology, economics	Perceived morbidity and disability, health care choice, household health care expenditures
Rapid assessment procedures	Anthropology, management	Perception of service quality and prices, health-related beliefs and practices

broad categories: rapid assessment procedures, surveys, and demographic surveillance. Table 20 provides a synopsis of the methods, the predominant discipline from which the data collection and analysis tools are borrowed, as well as examples of the type of data they generate.

In the remainder of this chapter, we briefly review these three main nonroutine methods, in turn. For in-depth treatment, we refer the reader to standard books and articles in the list of references.

Rapid assessment procedures

Need for rapid assessment procedures

Health care managers and providers must have an understanding of the sociocultural setting in which health services are embedded and of the health-related behaviour and practices of the target population to be able to design and implement effective health care interventions. As an example, the WHO Special Programme for Research and Training in Tropical Diseases incorporated a social and economic research component as early as 1979. The idea that more health can be gained by improving the delivery of existing interventions rather than by improving the efficacy of the interventions themselves was first formulated by Tugwell et al. (1985) and later by Vlassoff & Tanner (1992).

The dilemma health care managers faced was this: routine reporting does not provide the kind of insight into the behaviour and practices needed to increase "community effectiveness" of health interventions.

115

On the other hand, social science research—both classical sociological and anthropological research—is too expensive and takes too long to be of immediate use for decision makers. Scrimshaw and Hurtado (1987) therefore proposed to apply qualitative tools in a very focused way to examine local decision algorithms and perceptions with regard to a very limited range of problems. They called the approach rapid assessment procedures. Examples of such assessments include social risk factors for diseases (e.g. exposure to infection with schistosomiasis), community perception (acceptance or rejection) of preventive or therapeutic measures, use of and compliance with care (e.g. whether a drug prescription, is, in fact, filled, and if so, whether the drugs are taken in the dosage and for the duration prescribed), satisfaction with the quality of health care, a local vocabulary of health problems, and more.

The term "rapid assessment procedures" comprises a variety of methods, the bulk of which draws on qualitative research techniques, such as informal and formal individual interviews, focus group discussions, participant and document analysis (for an overview, see Scrimshaw & Hurtado, 1987, and Khan & Manderson, 1992). Other techniques frequently subsumed under rapid assessment procedures are more formal quantitative tools such as clinic exit interviews and checklists for infrastructure, equipment and supplies.

Definition and classification

While there is a lot of debate as to the most appropriate definition, most authors would agree that the key elements of rapid assessment procedures are (i) a short interval between data collection and presentation of results, (ii) a methodological pluralism combining qualitative methods with quantitative ones (well described in WHO, 1991), and (iii) orientation towards action which implies that decision-makers and clients (population) participate in defining the issues to be studied.

Table 21 lists the methods commonly subsumed under rapid assessment procedures. We have put the two survey techniques in brackets, since we do not think they fulfil the criterion of being "rapid". We will treat them below.

In the following sections we sketch the strengths and weaknesses of these methods. Again, for in-depth treatment we refer the reader to overview articles in the reference list at the end of the chapter.

Table 21   *Overview of methods subsumed under rapid assessment procedures*

Methods used for rapid assessment
Participant observation
Individual interviews
Focus groups
Review of reports and other documents
Checklists of facilities, equipment, and supplies
(Clinic exit surveys)
(Household surveys)

Participant observation

Brief description
Trained observers follow an interaction between two individuals, usually patient–provider encounter. They usually do not take active part in the interaction, nor do they intervene by asking questions or making comments. They take careful notes. Videotaping is usually considered too intrusive and costly to be useful.

Type of information than can be obtained
Observation is widely used to assess quality of care. Observed practice is compared to agreed-on standards of care, both in its technical/medical and human dimensions, for example the quality of communication and interaction between provider and client (Reerink & Sauerborn, 1996). In addition, observation has been used to establish patient flows and waiting times in clinical care settings.

Examples
Sauerborn et al. (1989) observed client–provider encounters in antenatal clinics in rural Burkina Faso to examine whether clients were properly screened for risk factors, such as previous pregnancy complication, anaemia and oedema. They found that those factors were only assessed in a minority of encounters. More troublesome still, even in cases where risk factors were identified, women were not given the appropriate special care.

Nicholas, Heiby & Hatzell (1991) used direct observation to validate supervisors' impressions of health workers and found that supervisors frequently and substantially overestimated the quality of performance, in the case of classification of dehydration by a factor of 10.

Individual interviews

Brief description
This technique is closest to standard anthropological methods. Individuals are selected intentionally to capture a large variety of experiences of interest. Interviews are usually held in settings familiar to the interviewees (their house, for example, or a nearby place in the village). No questionnaires are used, and the conversation flows freely. However, interviewers do have an interview guideline in mind and lead the conversation to certain relevant issues. Interviews are usually tape-recorded and transcribed. The transcribed text is then coded, using a set of codes that "mark" text that reveals key concepts. The analysis and tabulation of qualitative data are well described in Scrimshaw & Hurtado (1987) and Miles & Huberman (1984). As a rule of thumb, an hour of interview requires 7–8 hours of transcription, coding, and analysis.

Type of information that can be obtained

— reasons for health-seeking behaviour, for example for noncompliance with drug regimen, for not using preventive health services;
— satisfaction with health care;
— household strategies to cope with illness-related expenditures and production loss (Sauerborn, Berman & Nougtara, 1996);
— generating local vocabularies;
— generating hypotheses.

For instance, Hielscher & Sommerfeld (1985) carried out informal and formal individual interviews as well as focus group interviews to examine whether folk beliefs and etiological concepts of schistosomiasis impede the implementation of a control programme. They found that cosmopolitan and folk medicine are not mutually exclusive, but are viewed as complementary. Healer shopping was a frequent type of behaviour, based on perceived effectiveness of treatment, rather than on "affiliation" with an etiological model. The study concluded that health education without treatment would not be acceptable to villagers, a finding that was used by the schistosomiasis control programme managers to link any information, education, and communication measure with mass treatment.

Focus groups

Brief description

Focus groups involve a small group of participants (7–12) from the target population. A facilitator uses a pretested interview guideline to explore the participants' views on the subject of interest. The choice of participants is usually done purposefully rather than randomly, the objective being to have a wide range of opinions to stimulate discussion. Care should be taken in the selection of participants to avoid heterogeneity that might impede discussion rather than stimulate it (e.g. including men in the discussion of sexual behaviour of women, or including members of the upper social classes who might dominate the discussion or intimidate other participants). A second person takes notes during the meeting, observes nonverbal communication and is in charge of the complete transcription of the session using his or her notes and the tape recordings (where appropriate). A typical focus group session lasts about an hour and a half. In most cases, several groups are convened two to four times each for discussions. As a rule of thumb, 1 hour of discussion entails 5 hours of transcription and analysis. Add to this the time needed to prepare the interview guide and train facilitators and note takers, and it is obvious that this technique is not entirely "rapid". Khan & Manderson (1992) noted that "the advocacy of focus groups has been at least in part a consequence of their *apparent* economy" (our emphasis).

Although focus groups have been used in sociology and marketing for more than 70 years, they have recently—somewhat uncritically—been applied to social and behavioural research, especially in health and education. Anthropologists in particular observe with discomfort how their discipline is "hijacked" for short-term applications, with a "separation of anthropological theory and method, and a truncation of techniques and skills in applied contexts, specifically for rapid research" (Manderson & Aaby, 1992). Despite the large number of published studies, it is surprising that little attention has been paid to assessing the validity and reliability of seasonal effects, and generalizability. For an overview of these methodological issues the reader is referred to Kirk & Miller (1986). The most appropriate way to take this weakness into account is to combine the method with others, quantitative or qualitative, and to look for consistency or lack thereof—a technique called triangulation (Khan & Manderson, 1992).

The type of information that can be obtained

Similar to individual interviews. Focus groups are more efficient at extracting vocabularies, beliefs, and practices. They are not useful for sounding out very controversial or sensitive issues.

Example
Arhin (1994, 1995) conducted focus groups in Ghana to understand which form of payment for health care was favoured by the villagers and how much they would be willing to pay[1] for four specific packages of care. The results informed policymakers that community-based health insurance was indeed possible in rural Ghana and guided the premium setting and basic benefit package design.

WHO's rapid evaluation method

Brief description
The rapid evaluation method is a specific type of rapid assessment procedure that focuses on evaluating the performance and quality of health services (Anker et al., 1993). It is facility-based and uses a variety of the methods described above. It uses the same methods as described under rapid assessment procedures, with the addition of household surveys, which we do not consider to be a rapid technique and therefore discuss in the following section. The rapid evaluation method was first used to assess the performance of maternal and child health and family planning services, but was subsequently extended as a tool to evaluate any health service or programme (WHO, 1993). The rapid evaluation method starts by establishing an "issue-information matrix" with health planners, providers, and community representatives. It lists the problems perceived to be most urgent (left column) and the sources of information to describe and analyse the issues. The third dimension is the type of method applied to gather information from the data sources.

Example
Table 22 reproduces such a matrix from WHO (1993).

Surveys

It is beyond the scope of this book to provide a general review of household surveys as data collection tools. We refer the reader to the excellent overview articles of Ross and Vaughan (1984) and Kroeger (1985). In this section, we briefly review the different types of surveys health care managers can use. Since household surveys have been already well described, we will focus instead on the description of user surveys (or clinic exit interviews), and of standardized "international" multipurpose surveys and discuss their usefulness in complementing information from routine sources.

Household surveys

Single-purpose random sample household surveys can generate data on perceived illnesses, health care-seeking behaviour (e.g. the percentage of those who report an illness seeking various care options), and health care expenditures. A number of other health service, household, and individual characteristics can be used to look for associations with these variables. Although such surveys can produce data of high validity and accuracy, they are costly and time-consuming. There is also the problem of generalizability of the data beyond the source population to the national scale. It has therefore become increasingly popular to use

---

[1] For an overview of methods exploring the willingness to pay for health care, see Russel et al. (1995).

Table 22 An issue-information matrix developed in one country

Aspects of service / Health problem	Community action		Technical performance		Management				Resources
	Community KAPS*	Participation	Technical performance	Staff procedure	Planning, administration	Information	Supervision	Training	
Antenatal care	Attitude to referral; Knowledge of maternal deaths and high risk	Attitude towards ANC*	Risk identification; Risk management; Administration of tetanus toxoid; Frequency of ANC consultations RC OBS SQ EX	Antenatal target set	Coverage with ANC care; Risk; Follow-up	Number of supervisory visits	Adequacy of training; Understanding of job description; What to add to basic and post-basic training	Transport available; Budget for petrol; Availability of drugs and equipment	Availability of equipment and IV* sets, suction devices, ergometrine
Delivery care		What can be done?	Deaths? Causes? Constraints; Attitude to hospital	Referrals RC SQ	No. of village midwives registered RC SQ	Delivery records maintained; Deaths registered; Referrals recorded; Quality of records	Number of supervisory visits; VBA* supervision SQ RC	How much done for in-service VBA training?	
Postnatal care	Information received		Satisfaction with performing tasks	FP education and service; Number of PNC* RC SQ	Immunization start; FP given; Check-up RC SQ		Number of supervisory visits; VBA supervision SQ RC		
Family planning Fertility, Low coverage, Supplies	Knowledge of available FP services; Use of various methods of FP		Knowledge of FP targets; Satisfaction with FP coverage; Knowledge of eligible women	No. of clinics a week; Extent to which these clinics are advertized	FP targets set	FP records; Eligible couples recorded; FP coverage calculated	Number of supervisory visits; VBA supervision SQ RC		Availability of educational materials & contraceptive supplies
Immunization Tetanus toxoid polio	Awareness of tetanus and polio; Clinic schedule; Use/non-use; Knowledge of schedules	Possible support; Participation; Drop-out	Coverage: Dropout; Acceptance of policy of few contraindications	Tetanus toxoid as part of ANC; Education; Administration technique of immunization OBS EX*	Feedback received; Temperature of fridge recorded SQ RC OBS	Polio and TT* coverage; Use of data to determine non-coverage; Dropout rate	Number of supervisory visits; VBA supervision SQ RC		Availability of working fridge
Data collection method	FG*	FG	SQ*	various	SQ RC* OBS*	RC SQ	SQ RC*	SQ	OBS

*Abbreviations: ANC Antenatal care; EX Exit questionnaire; FG Focus group discussion; FP Family planning; IV Intravenous; KAPS Knowledge, attitudes, practices, satisfaction; KASS Knowledge, attitude, skills, satisfaction; OBS Observation of health facility; PNC Postnatal care; RC Record check; SQ Staff interview; TT Tetanus toxoid; VBA Village birth attendant.

standardized, multipurpose ("canned") surveys, such as the Demographic and Health Survey. These surveys offer the advantage of a national sample, thorough, well-tested methodology, and the flexibility to determine the time and geographical coverage as well as the content of the questionnaire.

Clinic exit surveys

Brief description

Clinic exit surveys (i.e. "exit polls" or "user surveys") are an efficient tool for learning about the perceptions of the subpopulation of those who use the health services.

Type of data information that can be obtained

Clinic exit surveys have been widely used to assess consumer satisfaction with health care and consumer perceptions of the quality of care (communication, advice given, appropriateness of price of drugs and fees, etc.).

Example

Sauerborn et al. (1989) interviewed all mothers who attended rural maternal and child health clinics[2] in Burkina Faso at the end of their visit in order to explore any difficulty the mothers might have with the organization of the clinics. They found that the timing of the clinics—in late morning—was very inconvenient for mothers. Mothers also reported difficulties complying with the fragmented schedule of child services scattered over the week (antenatal care, under-5 clinics, immunization sessions, curative care, cooking demonstrations).

Health care providers used this information to reschedule and reorganize comprehensive health services.

Demographic surveillance systems

The problem

Health impact can be defined either as a reduction of ill health or of fertility. As measures of ill health, we can use measures of morbidity, such as the incidence and duration of disease, the degree of disability it inflicts on the ill, or measures of mortality, such as age- and cause-specific death rates. The appeal of composite measures, such as the DALYs proposed in the 1993 *World development report*, lies in the fact that they yield a single indicator which incorporates disease, disability, and premature death. As measures of fertility, impact is expressed in terms of age-specific fertility rates and the total fertility rate as a single measure (so-to-say an integration of current age-specific fertility rates).

Estimates of health status play a pivotal role in health policy in several domains:

• Most health projects and policies state as their objective the improvement of health status, defined as a reduction in mortality, morbidity, or fertility indicators.

---

[2] Depending on how busy the clinics are and how many interviewers can work concurrently, it may be necessary to take a simple systematic sample, say, every second mother.

- Health care priority setting is based on cost-effectiveness studies, using the difference between current health status and estimated health status after the intervention as the effect variable. Far-reaching decisions to allocate resources are based on such estimations.
- Based on such estimates of cost-effectiveness, basic care packages are designed.
- In the context of improving health service quality, many consider the assessment of health outcomes as a crucial ingredient[1].
- Health status indicators are used for assessing a country's development progress in a broader sense (e.g. the infant mortality rate, the United Nations Development Programme development index).

Despite the importance of health indicators for policy design and evaluation, however, health status is rarely measured directly. Five arguments are frequently put forward both by national decision makers and by donor agencies:

- It is assumed that the health impact of interventions can be derived from expert panels reviewing research literature on the efficacy of interventions, defined as the effect on health status under controlled and optimal conditions (often in hospital environments with research staff supervising the correct application of interventions). "We know it works. Let's get just the implementation right, and we will have achieved improved health."
- The costs of assessing health impact are thought to be prohibitively high. Very sophisticated and costly research projects such as Matlab, Bangladesh, and Narangwal, India, where the cost of the measurement apparatus was US$ 48 per capita are frequently invoked to corroborate the argument that impact assessment is restricted to a few well-funded research projects.
- The time it takes for interventions to have an impact on health status (3–5 years) reduces the relevance of the data for decision makers who need immediate feedback on their programmes.
- It is not considered feasible to attribute changes in health status to changes in health care. Proponents of this argument rightly point to multisectoral influences on health status such as mother's education, land tenure, and income distribution and argue that it will be impossible to tease out these effects from health care effects.
- There are cheaper ways of obtaining valuable information on the effect of health policies, such as using Demographic and Health Surveys (see above).

We challenge below the assumptions underlying these five arguments based on innovative approaches to health impact assessment from several countries. Given that enormous resources are allocated on the basis of cost-effectiveness, it is worth taking a fresh look at feasibility to obtain the most realistic direct measures of health impact at a reasonable cost. We argue that prospective direct measurement of health status indicators provides more accurate and more relevant data on the effectiveness of interventions in a given country.

Efficacy versus community effectiveness of interventions

We define efficacy as the percentage reduction an intervention achieves on the target health outcome (i.e. measles immunization on measles incidence, oral rehydration therapy on death attributable to dehydration) under optimal conditions. The latter specification is of paramount importance since it points to the theoretical nature of efficacy. It tells the district health officer in Guatemala what oral rehydration therapy can achieve in a tertiary care hospital setting in a far away country (Egypt) using highly qualified research staff to monitor the dehydration status of patients.

Of course, the effect an intervention has at the community level is determined less by the efficacy of the interventions than by imperfect implementation due to resource constraints and cultural differences. Tugwell (1985) coined the term "community effectiveness" and delineated four factors that contribute to loss of effect: (i) low access to health services, (ii) poor provider compliance in diagnosing and (iii) in treating the health problem,[3] and (iv) low user compliance with procedures. These factors conspire so that the actual health impact of interventions (= community effectiveness) is likely to be much less than the estimated impact based on estimations of efficacy: in Burkina Faso between only 6% and 20% of the potential effectiveness of health care interventions is achieved at the community level.

The rationale for health impact assessment is threefold: first, it establishes a realistic outcome assessment of the community effectiveness of interventions for a given population or country; second, gains in health status can be related to improvements in health care inputs, access, and process (quality of care); finally, it allows us to look at health in a broader development context, as it is influenced by changes in other sectors: education, agriculture, and the economy. This may ultimately lead to a reordering of priorities for policies to improve health (e.g. educating girls may prove to be more effective than providing a denser net of health facilities).

Challenging the arguments against health impact assessment

The argument of attributability of change

The argument of attributability of change goes like this: health is influenced by a myriad of confounding factors unrelated to health care, such as education, agriculture, economics, equity, and so on. Any attribution of a change in health status to health care, therefore, is extremely difficult.

This problem of confounding variables can be tackled both at the level of the design of health impact assessment and at the level of data analysis.

The design should be a prospective population-based study. This would allow a before–after comparison. It would also capture seasonal variations in both health status and health care use. The problem with a single population is that while it may be plausible to relate change to a specific intervention, attribution of causality cannot be attributed with any confidence. First, a change in health status might have occurred anyway in the study population.

Second, changes in other sectors might have occurred, leading to improved health status. The addition of a comparison population enhances the plausibility of attributing changes in health status to intervention. Great care must be taken to choose a comparison population

---

[3] Provider and user compliance, in turn, can be subsumed under "quality of care".

which is comparable in social infrastructure, access to health and education, economic output, equity of wealth and income distribution, and so on.

Some authors raise ethical objections to the choice of a comparison zone, arguing that it is not possible to preclude interventions from a "control" population. The critical point here is to assess whether the intervention to be tested is "of proven benefit". If so, a "stepped wedge" design which takes advantage of staggered implementation of policies can be used (as in the Gambia hepatitis B trial and the Burkina Faso study). Another objection to the above design is often made on the grounds that no single zone chosen as a study zone will be representative of a country's population.

Box 20 presents the design of the Burkina Faso health care intervention study to show which tools were developed to generate reliable and accurate mortality and morbidity data.

Box 20   Burkina Faso health impact assessment

In 1988, the Ministry of Health decided to embark on a policy of user fees, community-controlled revolving drug funds at each of its peripheral health facilities, and quality enhancement measures. It asked the University of Heidelberg to provide assistance in setting up the measurement tools to pilot-test the effect that this policy had on the age-specific mortality rates (in addition to the effect on health care use and household health care expenditures) in the catchment population (26,000 inhabitants) of three "reformed" health centres in the district of Nouna. It was decided to choose a comparison or "control" zone of similar size where all the measurement tools were used but no change in policy was introduced. It was considered crucial for the replicability of the interventions on a national scale that the Ministry of Health maintain full control over the implementation of its policy and that the research team not inject any resources in the implementation process.

The following measurement tools have been implemented in both zones:

— a biannual exhaustive census of the study population which includes information on household production, sown area under cultivation by crop type, and assets;
— monthly vital events registration—information on the occurrence of deaths, births, and migration in each of the study villages is gathered by interviewers from "key informants", such as the village head, the traditional midwife, the imam, and so on. The interviewers then visit the households where such events occurred and collect further information required for the vital events register;
— verbal autopsies of each death;
— a monthly household survey which explores the occurrence of illness in the previous month, the number of days of work incapacitation, health care choice, and expenditures for each treatment episode;
— time allocation studies added to the household questionnaire once in the dry and the rainy season, respectively.

Data are entered by locally trained staff in a relational database and tabulated in the provincial health service headquarters of the study province.

The second way to tease out whether changes in health status are associated with changes in health care or in other sectors is at the analysis level. Variables assumed to influence health status (based on literature review) are used in a regression model either to control for them (ignoring their effect, if the focus is health care contributions to health status changes) or to analyse and quantify their effect (if the focus is a more holistic attribution of changes in any societal sector on health status).

The cost argument

While many would agree that such data are useful in designing and evaluating policy, skeptics will question whether such data collection can be done at an affordable cost to ministries and donors. In the Burkina Faso health care intervention study, the marginal costs for the health census and monthly vital events registration for a period of 3 years in both the intervention and control populations of approximately 26,000 inhabitants are US$ 60,000 per year. Are these costs affordable? To best answer that question, the costs of impact assessment need to be viewed in comparison with other health care expenditures and related to the population that is to benefit from the intervention as a result of the study. Such studies are undertaken to inform policymakers on national policy. It would not be appropriate, therefore, to relate study costs to the intervention and/or comparison populations alone. In the case of the Burkina health care intervention study, costs were related to overall health care expenditures. They amounted to US$ 0.00161 per capita or less than half a percent (0.44%) of total government plus donor health care expenditures in Burkina Faso (1992).

The fact that the Burkina Faso study has been fully integrated into the Ministry of Health structures carries several advantages:

— the study questions to be assessed have relevance for national policy-makers;
— policymakers are interested in a request to be informed on study results;
— local health staff and local facilities are used to a maximum, which lowers costs, fosters transfer of skills, and thus enhances the chances of sustainability.

The Burkina Faso study used one resident expatriate physician and two person-months of external consultants. It is planned that technical assistance will be phased out once data collection and analysis procedures are routinized.

The time argument

While it is true that any information on the health impact of a given intervention will not be available for at least 3 years, practical information on health care use and the process (quality) of health care delivery are collected during this "lag" period.

The argument that cheaper sources of information on effects are available

Demographic and Health Surveys and other cross-sectional studies can provide retrospective trends in mortality indicators and can assess current TFR. They cannot, however, provide data that evaluate the health impact of current programmes in a prospective way.

Conclusion for research and policy

The main strength of health impact assessment lies in its ability to generate mortality and morbidity data on effectiveness of interventions on the community. If a comparison or control zone is used, it is possible to produce current demographic indicators rather than rely on periodic retrospective estimations based on cross-sectional data (e.g. Demographic and Health Surveys). Costs can be kept at an affordable level and should be no major obstacle. The main challenge of impact assessment is to insure and monitor the proper implementation of interventions. Researchers should resist the temptation to finance or manage the intervention and thus create an artificial environment which is not replicable. An inherent problem with assessing the impact of interventions on mortality is the time it takes until statistically significant differences between intervention and control populations can be observed.

Given the crucial importance of country-specific data on mortality and morbidity for the assessment of the burden of disease, the cost-effectiveness of health care interventions, and the quality of care provided, governments in developing countries as well as donors working with them should consider using the longitudinal community-based measurement tools described in this chapter to obtain better data for better national policies.

In the absence of civil vital event registration, the only way to obtain data on the health impact of health policies and programmes is to set up demographic surveillance areas. Each country should explore whether the less expensive single surveillance zone or a representative multiple sentinel approach is more appropriate. The advantage of the latter is its representativeness for the entire population.

Link between nonroutine and routine methods: triangulation

Wherever possible, rapid assessment procedures data should be compared with findings from routine information systems and/or from other surveys. The link is not likely to be at the level of the database, but of design and analysis. As an example, in Nouna, Burkina Faso, the routine information system provided data on use of outpatient clinics by age. It was found that children used professional health services to a much lesser extent than adults. A qualitative interview study corroborated the underutilization and found that it was not due to a lack of knowledge on the part of villagers about the potential benefits of health care for sick children. Rather, villagers made hard choices in favour of maintaining household production. This was found to be the main reason they spent time and money on taking productive adults to health services, rather than "unproductive" children. It was concluded that even the most sophisticated information, education, and communication campaign would not be able to change villagers' priorities. Rather, policy was focused on lowering access costs for health care for children (Sauerborn, Berman & Nougtara, 1996).

Another widely used link between routine and nonroutine methods is in the area of vaccination/Expanded Programme on Immunization. Routine reporting provides data on the number of vaccine doses delivered, an Expanded Programme on Immunization cluster survey yields information on population-based coverage, whereas a sentinel surveillance system provides data on community effectiveness.

References

Anker M, Guidotti RJ, Orzeszyna S, Sapirie JA, Thuriaux MC (1993). Rapid evaluation methods (REM) of health services performance: methodological observations. *Bulletin of the World Health Organization*, 71:15–21.

Arhin DC (1994). *Community health insurance in Africa and its feasibility in Ghana*. London, London School of Hygiene and Tropical Medicine.

Arhin DC (1995). *Community health insurance in developing countries and its feasibility in Ghana. Final technical research report submitted to IDRC and UNICEF*. London, London School of Hygiene and Tropical Medicine.

Hielscher S, Sommerfeld J (1985). Concepts of illness and the utilization of health-care services in a rural Malian village. *Social science and medicine*, 21:469–481.

Khan ME, Manderson L (1992). Focus groups in tropical diseases research. *Health policy and planning*, 7:56–66.

Khan ME et al. (1991). The use of focus groups in social and behavioral research: some methodological issues. *World health statistics quarterly*, 44:145–149.

Kirk J, Miller ML (1986). *Reliability and validity in qualitative research*. Newbury Park, CA, Sage, 1–99.

Kroeger A (1985). Response errors and other problems of health interview surveys in developing countries. *World health statistics quarterly*, 38:15–37.

Manderson L, Aaby P (1992). Can rapid anthropological procedures be applied to tropical diseases? *Health policy and planning*, 7:46–55.

Miles MB, Huberman AM (1984). *Qualitative data analysis*. Beverly Hills, CA, Sage.

Nicholas DD, Heiby JR, Hatzell TA (1991). The Quality Assurance Project: Introducing quality improvement to primary health care in less developed countries. *Quality assurance in health care*, 3:147–165.

Reerink I, Sauerborn R (1996). Quality of primary health care in developing countries: recent experiences and future direction. *International journal of quality of health care*, 8(2):131–139.

Ross DA, Vaughan JP (1984). *Health interview surveys in developing countries*. London, London School of Hygiene and Tropical Medicine: 17–19.

Sauerborn R et al. (1989). Assessment of MCH services in the district of Solenzo, Burkina Faso—II. *Journal of tropical pediatrics*, 35(Suppl. 1):10–13.

Sauerborn R, Berman P, Nougtara A (1996). Age bias, but no gender bias, in the intra-household resource allocation for health care in rural Burkina Faso. *Health transition review*, 6:131–145.

Scrimshaw SCM, Hurtado E (1987). *Rapid assessment procedures for nutrition and primary health care—anthropological approaches to improving effectiveness of programs*. Tokyo, United Nations University.

Tugwell P et al. (1985). The measurement iterative loop: a framework for the critical appraisal of need, benefits and costs of health interventions. *Journal of chronic diseases*, 38:339–351.

Vlassof C, Tanner M (1992). The relevance of rapid assessment to health research and interventions. *Health policy and planning*, 7:1–9.

World Health Organization (1991). Epidemiological and statistical methods for rapid health assessment. *World health statistics quarterly*, 44:94–171.

World Health Organization (1993). *Rapid evaluation method guidelines for maternal and child health, family planning and other health services*. Geneva, World Health Organization (unpublished document WHO/MCH-FPP/MEP/93.1; available on request from Department of Reproductive Health and Research, World Health Organization, 1211 Geneva 27, Switzerland).

Data transmission, data processing, and data quality

Laura B. Shrestha and Claude Bodart

Introduction

In the most general sense, a routine health management information system is simply a process for collecting, processing, and disseminating information in a health system. This process uses staff, policies, and procedures, and may include varying degrees of automation (O'Brien, 1982). The primary role of an information system is to provide data that can be used to assist decision-making in the political as well as the management realms (Armenian, 1992), where decision-making is defined as the capacity to formulate alternatives, estimate effects, and make choices (Kraemer & Danziger, 1990). Because of the vast array of options they present, information systems are often perceived as overwhelmingly complex. However, an information system need not be complex to be effective. In fact, we argue in this chapter that, if designed appropriately, the system should facilitate decision-making.

As noted in Chapter 2, a health information system has an organized set of interrelating components that can be grouped under two entities: the information process, and the health information system management structure (see Fig. 2). Through the information process, raw data (inputs) are transformed into information in a "usable" form for management decision-making (outputs). The information process can be broken down into the following components: (i) data collection, (ii) data transmission, (iii) data processing, (iv) data analysis, and (v) presentation of data and information for use in health services planning and management.

For the remainder of this chapter, we contemplate two of the distinct, yet interrelated, components of the information process: data transmission, which considers how data are transferred among the interdependent actors in the health system, and data processing, or how the raw data are manipulated in order to transform them into useful information that is understandable to the maximum number of workers. In addition, we also consider data quality, that is whether the data collected accurately reflect the phenomenon they were intended to measure. Data quality is a condition which results from the effectiveness of the data collection, data transmission, and data processing components.

Data transmission

Functions of data transmission

In its simplest form, data transmission refers to the transfer of raw data from the lowest level to higher levels of a health system for the purpose of data processing. This function recognizes that raw data collected at the lower levels may not be in a form or of sufficient quality to be useful in determining appropriate actions. However, in recognizing that useful information is generated and used at every step in the delivery of health services, a more complete definition of "data transmission" would include consideration of how data are transferred among the interdependent parties in the health system to ensure that administrative, political, and management decisions are based on the best available information. First, however, raw data must often be processed into a form that decision-makers can actually employ.

As noted by Armenian (1992), data from a health information system are useful for both political decision-making (budget and resource allocation, jurisdiction of agencies, personnel selection, and legislation) and for management decisions (efficacy of patient care, effectiveness of public health interventions, compliance with standards, quality assurance, training, planning, and programming). The role of data transmission is to ensure that relevant data are available to the persons who make the actual decisions in each of these functional areas. As noted in Chapter 2, a health system consists of multiple participants who have different needs for health system information. Rational decision-making is required at three concentration levels (primary, secondary, and tertiary) for management functions related to patient/client management, health unit management, and health system management (see Fig. 3).

A well-designed information system will ensure that the data transmitted will be relevant not only for the decisions that must be made at higher levels but also for day-to-day management at the health centre level. This makes sense not only from the point of view of having an integrated health information system but also in terms of ensuring that the peripheral levels of the health system will have sufficient motivation to report the highest-quality data.

In developing countries, data transmission used to mean the transfer of paper documents from lower levels of a health system to a central unit. Now, however, the concept of data transmission is being completely revisited for at least two reasons. First, the trend is towards increased emphasis on local use of data; second, better information technology has reduced the technical and cost obstacles that block efficient data transmission. In the following sections, we consider two types of data transmission: vertical and horizontal. Fig. 13 highlights the distinctions between these two types of data transmission. Vertical transmission refers to the transfer of data between different levels of a health care system, whereas horizontal transmission moves between various health system actors and consumers at the same level. Both types of transmission allow feedback and information sharing between the participants.

There are numerous examples of horizontal data transmission, including transfer of data between, for instance, laboratory personnel and a care provider at a regional-level care facility, a private provider of contraceptives and a primary-level maternal and child health programme, the patient and her primary provider, and a surgeon and the internist.

Vertical data transmission

As already mentioned, vertical data transmission focuses on transfer of information between levels of a health care system. With respect to the

Fig. 13 *Horizontal and vertical data transmission*

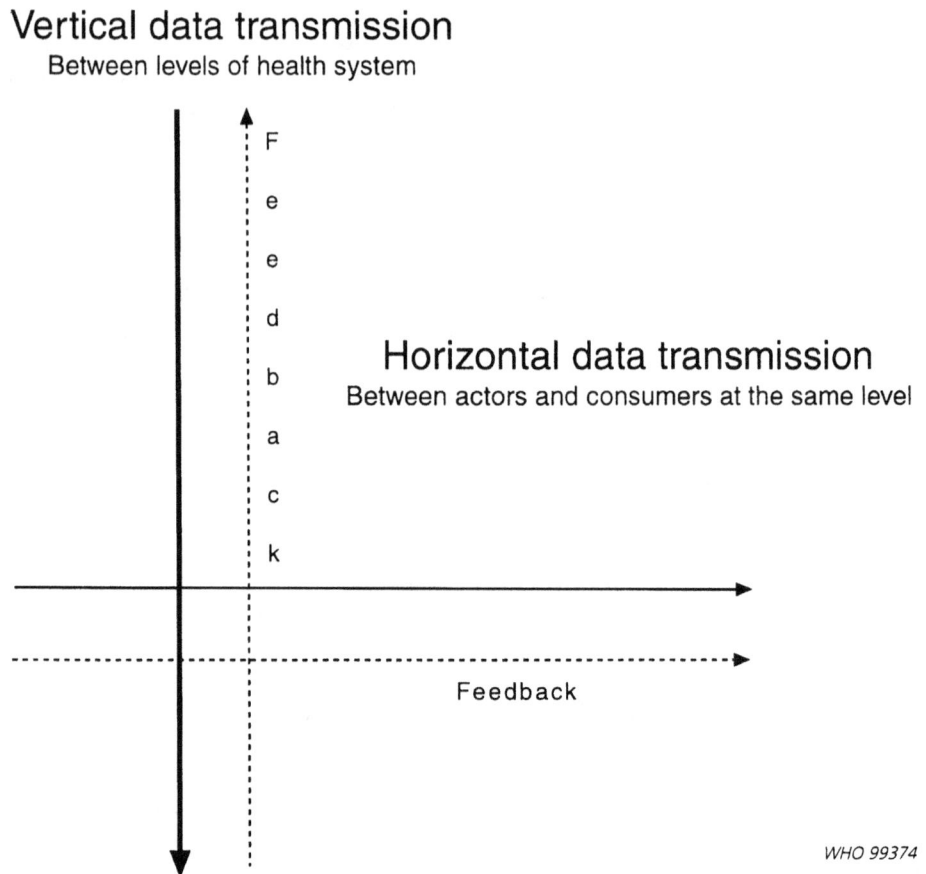

Vertical data transmission
Between levels of health system

F
e
e
d
b
a
c
k

Horizontal data transmission
Between actors and consumers at the same level

Feedback

WHO 99374

management functions described in Chapter 2, examples of vertical transmission include:

- *Patient/client management:* referral of patient records from a first-level generalist to higher-level specialists, or vice versa.
- *Health unit management:* transmission of detailed summary reports on the percentage of children immunized in a catchment area from health centre to district centre. Or, transmission of the health unit drug and medical supply usage reports to higher levels.
- *Health system management:* transmission of detailed summary sheets of disease incidence from health units and district hospitals to a central unit for disease surveillance. Or, transfer of data from a central unit to lower levels regarding changes in budgeting and financial resource allocation.

There are basically three levels of vertical transmission of data, as depicted in Fig. 14.

In most developed and developing countries, data transmission reflects the administrative structure of the health system. Panel 1 of Fig. 14, which is most prevalent in developing countries, represents the transmission of data through levels of the health system for processing purposes only, from the lowest unit to a centralized unit in the capital city. For example, panel 1 of Fig. 14 might represent data transmission in Viet Nam from the commune health centre level, to the district health

Fig. 14 *Types of vertical transmission*

Panel 1.

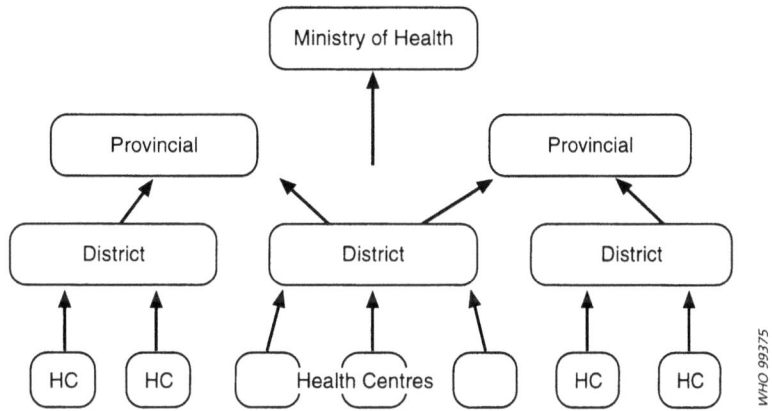

Panel 2.

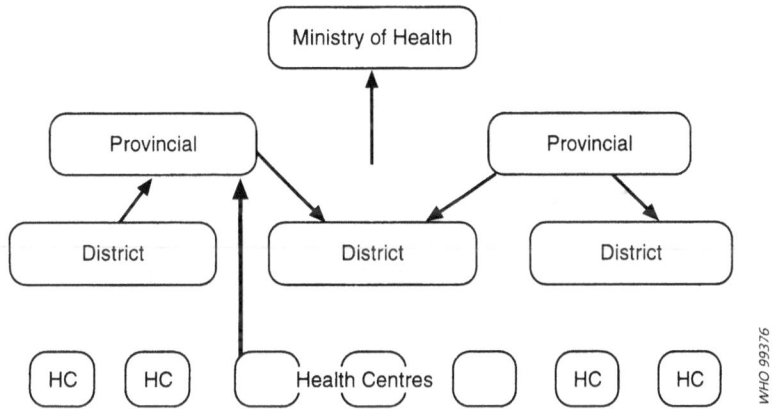

Panel 3.

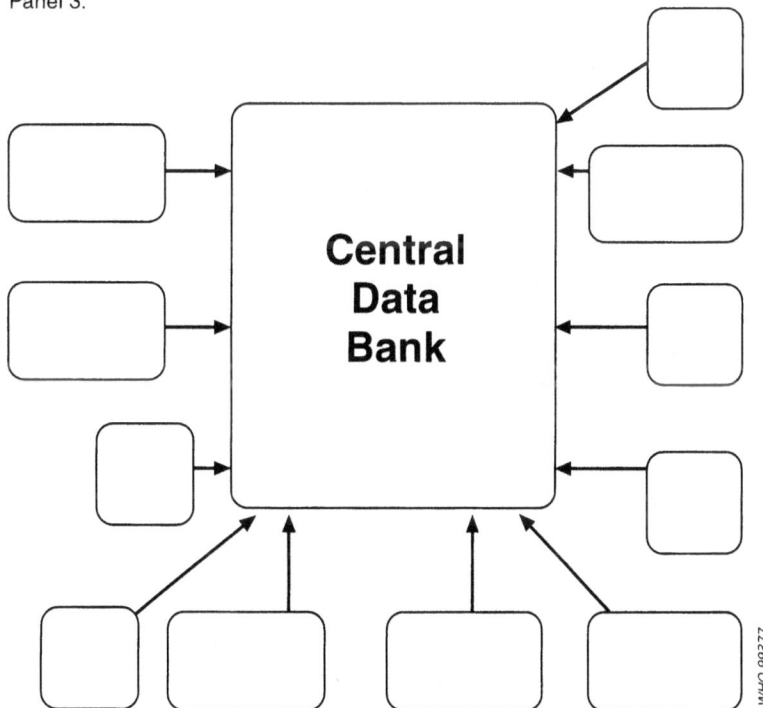

131

centre level, to the provincial health centre level, to the Ministry of Health level in Hanoi. When such a transmission occurs for processing purposes, there is an obligation to transmit the processed data back to the lower levels for feedback and to allow lower-level decision making.

The second panel of Fig. 14 represents an information system in which some administrative levels of the health system are bypassed in order to speed up the transmission of data between levels. The bypassed level gets information from the higher level. While not common in developing countries, such a system is being employed in Cameroon in an attempt to avoid delays in data transmission. Health centres report data to provincial levels, which, after processing, send information to the district level. In this case, the provincial level provides technological support to the district until the latter becomes computerized.

For both panels 1 and 2, the medium used for data transmission is usually paper, although some countries have begun to experiment with diskettes. In many developing countries in which the postal system is unreliable, staff use a variety of means to transfer data, for example arrangements with administrative authorities or with local transportation companies, casual trips to the district or regional capital, use of friends, and so on. In cases where supervision is regular, it is advisable to collect the reports and check the quality of the data provided during supervisory activities.

Panel 3 represents an information system in which units of the health care system are connected to a central data bank through modems and telephone lines. The use of such "wide area networks" is still in its infancy in the developing world, although some countries such as Côte d'Ivoire and Senegal are attempting to set up such systems. Wide area networks are attractive because of the speed of data transmission and the possibility of preprogramming processing procedures to make information instantaneously available for all decision-makers with access to the database. However, most developing countries will not be able to take advantage of this technology for many years, because of technical and cost constraints.

The main characteristics of the three types of data transmission are summarized in Table 23. In general, the selection of any of these types of information structures involves trade-offs. Data transmission along administrative structure lines may be the least complex, but it is often hampered by slow speed and lower-quality data. Data transmission via the bypassed administrative structure may be faster and may result in

Table 23 *Characteristics of vertical data transmission*

Type of vertical transmission	Along administrative structure	Bypassed administrative structure	Wide area network
Speed of data transmission	+	++	Instantaneous
Complexity	+	++	+++++
Data quality	+	++	+++
Accessibility of information	+	+	+++
Cost	?	?	?
Where in use?	Most developing countries	Some developing countries	Exceptional in developing countries; some experience at low scale

improved data quality, but the complexity of the system might increase. A wide area network may be best in terms of the speed of data transmission, data quality, and accessibility of information by users, but it also requires the greatest degree of technical competence on the part of the users. Finally, the costs of the three types of data transmission must be considered, but they are difficult to estimate and the literature on the subject is scarce. Although wide area networks are often perceived to be expensive, the cost entailed by filling out multiple, overlapping forms every month at the health centre level and retabulating the numbers at the next level is certainly high and should not be overlooked.

Horizontal data transmission

Horizontal data transmission, which refers to the transfer of data among actors and consumers at the same level of the health care system, has been increasing. This form of transmission has been necessitated by increasing intersectoral communication, greater recognition of consumer rights, and improvements in administrative support systems. The horizontal actors in a health system are numerous, and include community representatives, consumers, administrative and religious authorities, management boards, and nongovernmental health organizations, among others. There are three data-related functions that are served by horizontal actors in a health care system. First, they may provide data that are directly relevant to decision-making at the lowest levels of the health care system. For instance, community leaders might report that few pregnant women visit health centres for antenatal care services because of the perceived poor quality of the services. A direct decision to improve service protocols and information, education, and communication efforts in the community could result from this information. Second, they may provide data that are useful to inform decision-making but that require further processing in order to do so. For example, raw data sheets from local pharmacies might be useful when used in combination with facility records to estimate the percentage of women in a catchment area who are using family planning methods. Finally, horizontal data transmission ensures that community actors and consumers have access to compiled information from the health system. This function, which represents the use of information or "feedback" from the health care system, is discussed more thoroughly in Chapter 3.

Finally, there are a number of areas in the data transmission field that require further research. More specifically, there is only anecdotal information on the costs of developing and maintaining the data transmission mechanisms described in this chapter. A detailed analysis, which compares all costs associated with each of the systems, is necessary. Second, given that most developing countries continue to employ vertical data transmission systems, we need to understand precisely how the speed of data transfer can be improved and how better feedback mechanisms might help the lowest level of the health care system benefit from data compiled at higher levels. Given the increased importance of community actors in health care, a better understanding of methods that enhance horizontal transmission mechanisms is critical.

Data processing

The goal of data processing is to present information in a way that aids decision-making at all levels of the health care system. Data processing operations range from simple manual computations to sophisticated computerized processing, but generally involve at least two major steps: data cleaning and rearrangement of the information to form a summary set of variables conducive to analysis (Cleland, 1985).

Raw data, or data in the initial stage, often have inaccuracies or inconsistencies that must be evaluated and corrected. Common sources of error include missing or duplicate records, implausible values for a variable (for instance a pregnant woman aged 92 years), contradiction between two or more variables (age reported as 10 years in 1996 for a person born in 1926), and inconsistency with other known information (10,000 births reported in a given year even though census results indicate that only 2000 women of reproductive age live in the catchment area). As noted by Cleland (1985), "data cleaning" allows the transformation of raw data to a state in which analysis can be conducted smoothly with minimal distortion of results from errors. A number of procedures are available to resolve errors. Summary sheets may be compared with original registers of data. Procedures of "imputation", or assignment of values to missing or unstated codes, may be instituted through informed guesswork. Data in a computerized system can be cleaned by running data through several passes of an error-checking program. It must be noted that a data set is seldom error-free. Even if careful and thorough cleaning procedures are employed, it is likely that undetectable errors will exist. The goal is to try to ensure that the errors are small enough that they do not bias decision-making. One must also bear in mind the trade-off between improving data quality and costs (see Chapter 4).

The second major step in data processing is to rearrange the data to form a summary set of variables conducive to analysis. Often, this step will result in a set of tabulations and/or statistical analyses.

In sum, "processed" data have many advantages over raw data. Specifically, they ensure that extraneous values that could introduce bias into decision-making processes are evaluated and corrected. In addition, the process itself produces information that is useful for decision-making, and that is presented in a summary form that is most comprehensible to a wide range of players in the health care system.

The processing of data is not without its disadvantages, however. Both manual and computerized processing operations are subject to introduction of new errors by persons who are responsible for tabulation or data entry adjustments. Furthermore, the information could become meaningless for management decisions if the raw data are overly processed. For example, if we were to learn that the average income in an area of a developing country is US$ 1000 (in a country with a per capita income of US$ 500), we would normally conclude that families in this area are relatively well off in comparison with their compatriots. However, the "fallacy of the mean" shows that it is possible that one very rich resident may skew the average upward despite relative poverty among the rest of the sample.[1] Unit level aggregation of services can hide important information on specific areas or villages that are underserved (people living more than 5 km from the health centre, minority populations, adolescents for reproductive health services, etc.)

---

[1] For instance, in a village of 100 households, one household has an income of US$ 99,010, while the remaining 99 households have an income of US$ 10 each (approximately). The average household income in the village would still be US$ 1000.

Finally, as the saying goes, "garbage in, garbage out". Sophisticated data processing and application of fancy statistical techniques cannot increase the quality of the basic data. Processing of erroneous data can only result in biased information. Appropriate processing of good-quality raw data, however, enhances decision making, because it presents information in the form that is clearest and most useful for the health system personnel.

An example

Figure 15 shows how raw data can be processed into a graph that makes it easier for managers to make appropriate decisions. The graph with "processed" data provides the same basic data as the raw data, with three major improvements: (i) population data, which provide details on the number of children in the catchment area, have been integrated with the objectives of the measles immunization programme (number of doses of vaccines to be administered); (ii) the data show indicators of monthly and cumulative performance of the health centre; and (iii) the action level,

Fig. 15 *Processing of raw data for measles immunization coverage into usable information*

Panel A: Raw Data

	Annual	*Monthly*
Population in catchment area	11,000	917
Number of children <1 year: (4.5%)	495	41
Measles vaccination target (75%)	371	31
Action level: 50% of total children	248	21

	January	February	March	April	May	June
Doses administered	23	53	56	71	99	129
Action level	21	42	63	84	105	126
Vaccination target level	31	62	93	124	155	186
No. of children <1 year	41	82	123	164	205	246

Panel B: Processed Data
Measles Vaccination Coverage, January–June 1996

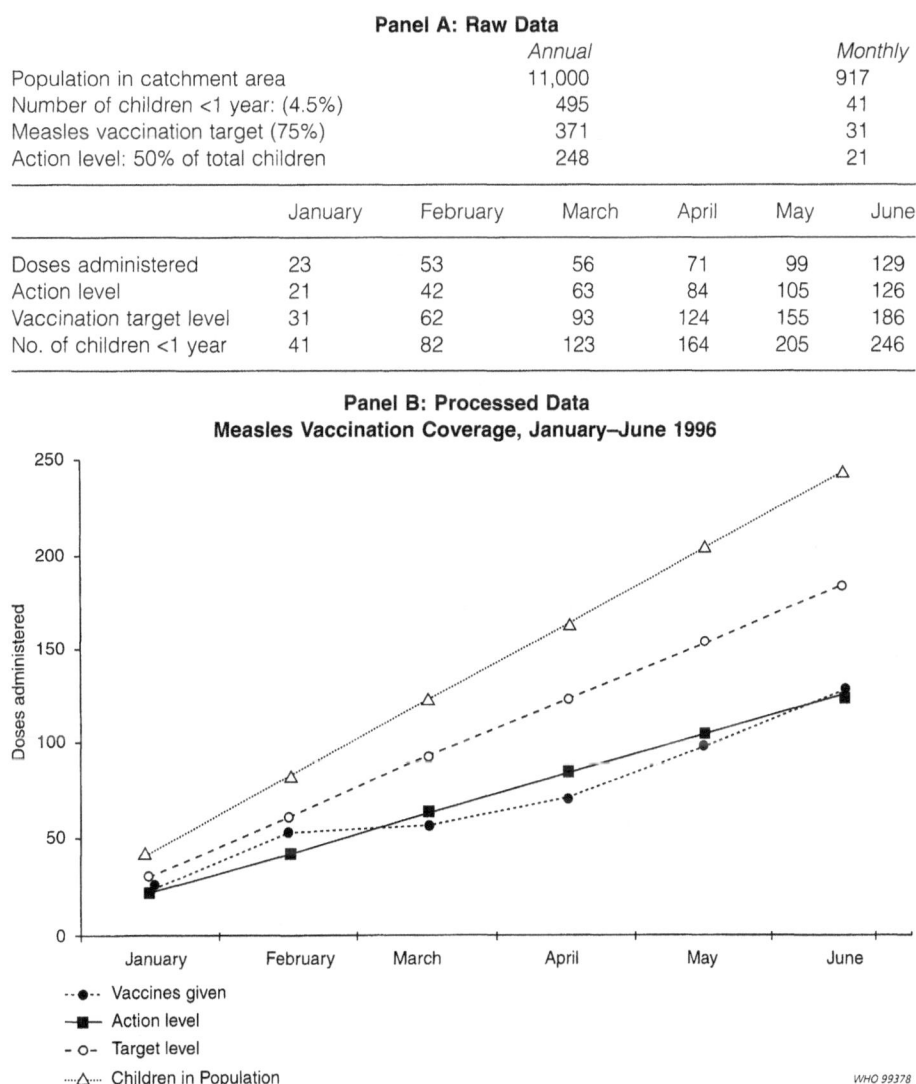

- ••• Vaccines given
- ■— Action level
- o- Target level
- △ Children in Population

WHO 99378

135

or the level at which an intervening action is to be implemented, is super-imposed onto the performance level in order to facilitate decision making.

Although difficult to assess from the raw data, we can draw a number of important conclusions from the graph: the number of vaccinations against measles that were provided by the health centre fell below the targeted number for each of the 6 months under study; the performance of the health centre fell below the action level in the months of March and April, which indicates that an interventionist strategy would be implemented following the fall-off in immunizations; and a stronger strategy would be necessary for the second half of the year to meet the objective of immunizing 75% of children against measles under the age of 1 in the year.

Computerized data processing

As mentioned earlier, data processing operations can range from simple manual computations to sophisticated computerized processing. Chapter 11 will provide a detailed description of computerization issues. In sum, it is critical in a developing country setting to achieve the right mix of computer and manual systems, and to ensure that they are fully integrated. Units that do not have computers must be able to produce compatible reports manually. Decision-making regarding whether or not to computerize, and at what level, should take into account:

— the availability of local resources to support computer equipment, software maintenance, and training;
— the volume of data to be processed;
— the complexity of analysis required;
— the costs of the technology vis-à-vis the cost and availability of skilled personnel to process the data manually.

With the rapid advancement of computer technology, however, the benefits of computerization in health information systems have become increasingly apparent. By the nature of the activity, data collection and analysis often involve the need to process large amounts of data quickly and accurately. Combined with time constraints, the large volume of raw, unprocessed data has often prevented managers from effectively using data to make informed decisions.

In addition to enabling the efficient and timely processing of large amounts of data for decision-making, computerization of data has other inherent benefits. The quality of data tends to improve with computerization since fewer staff are responsible for data input and tabulation, and staff are not required to make mathematical computations. Computerization also allows the production of a wide variety of outputs, including targeted feedback reports for specific topic areas (malaria surveillance, contraceptive distribution, etc.) and for specific areas (capital city, rural catchment area, and district hospital) from a single data set or through combining data sets. It may also eliminate the duplicate processing of work that is typically seen in many hierarchical data collection systems. Finally, computerization allows data sets collected for different purposes to be combined in a meaningful fashion. For instance, service statistics might be combined with data on health infrastructure, personnel needs, or financial management.

Data quality

Quality (or accuracy) of data refers to the degree to which the data or statistics measure what was intended to be measured when the data collection system was designed. It is important to keep in mind that the primary function of a health information system is to provide data that enhance decision-making in the provision of health services. By seeking to ensure that the system provides high-quality data, the health information system attempts to guarantee that decision-makers have access to both unbiased and complete information.

It must be recognized, however, that there is a trade-off between generating the highest-quality data and the costs associated with collecting it. As emphasized in Chapter 4, the higher the quality required, the higher the cost of producing the data. Since many planning and management decisions do not require a high level of precision, it is appropriate to consider what level of quality is required in order to support unbiased decision-making. Nevertheless, the level of quality of data from routine information systems in many developing countries is questionable and should be weighed against other methods of data collection.

A high-quality information system tends to be one that captures the underlying structural aspects of the health system. Rice and Anderson (1994) highlight three characteristics that should be present in a well-designed system of information flows: interdependence, interaction, and integration. Interdependence reflects the fact that health care employees belong to different worlds (medical and nonmedical), occupations (physicians, assistant midwives, administrators, and clerical workers), departments (antenatal care and medical records), and levels of the system (health centre and hospital), yet their work requires considerable interdependence across boundaries. Few medical care tasks can be performed without the cooperation of interdependent staff, yet the boundaries between groups may result in different understandings of the overall systems and organizational processes. The term "interaction" indicates that information flows within and across boundaries represent opportunities for gaining greater understanding of specialized but interdependent information and sharing of resources that can lead to cooperation and coordination. Integration ensures that, by providing geographically dispersed access to common and interrelated medical information, a health information system can create common databases that require the various players to cooperate. These interdependencies necessitate standardized forms, terminology, policies, and procedures.

Although designing a system that incorporates these characteristics does not guarantee that the system will produce high-quality data, it does recognize that data quality is multidimensional, with every step of the information system from design to actual decision-making having the ability to affect the level of quality of the information produced. It highlights that even the best-designed information system will not produce the required level of quality if the system has not been developed with and for the people who are supposed to run and use it. Furthermore, it recognizes that developing the right incentives structure to improve the quality of the data should be central in designing health information systems.

The following sections will analyse the impediments to quality data and will make suggestions on how to improve quality.

Impediments to good data quality

At least three sources threaten data quality: inappropriate data collection instruments and procedures (see Chapter 6), poor recording and reporting, and errors in processing data.

Poor data quality due to inappropriate data collection instruments and procedures

One important requirement of a well-planned and executed information system is the development of a set of concepts and classes to be covered, and adherence to these definitions throughout all stages of the collection and processing operations. These concepts provide the basis for development of question wording, instructions for data collectors, and specifications for editing, coding, and tabulating data. Only when concepts are carefully defined in operational terms and consistently applied can there be a firm basis for later analysis of the results. In addition to the imprecise definition of terms and lack of standardization, errors can also be introduced by overlapping category responses, by the inaccurate translation of material adopted from other contexts, or by leaving inadequate space for writing responses on data collection forms. Sometimes a well-designed instrument might be used in an inappropriate setting. For example, a sentinel surveillance system designed to clarify the mechanisms of HIV transmission in sub-Saharan Africa cannot be replicated in western Asia without significant modification of the data instruments.

The poor layout and quality of printed forms often contribute to low-quality data in developing countries. Where resources are scarce, forms are sometimes illegible due to the poor quality of the original form and repeated photocopying. In addition, instructions for filling out the forms are often lost in the process. (Chapter 6 discusses this topic in more detail).

Threats to data quality from poor recording and reporting

Failure to report data

Despite procedures for the timely transmission of data between different levels of a health care system, sometimes data transmission does not occur. Given the high recurrent costs of stationery (forms, operational cards, registers, etc.) and the inefficient supply system in many developing countries, the reporting health facility may lack access to necessary supplies. Or, data transmission may be hampered by the frequent absence of personnel in charge of the information system. Or, even if personnel are available, the high opportunity cost of time spent recording data on multiple forms coupled with the lack of incentives for reporting may hamper regular reporting. Another problem may be the lack of transportation and other means of communication (electronic data transfer).

An important related issue in a vertical data transmission system concerns what occurs at the higher levels when data are not received. In many countries, detailed procedures have not been established, and this results in ad hoc and inconsistent treatment of data. For instance, in addressing the question of how district level information technicians would handle the nonreceipt of a regular monthly form from the local level in Viet Nam, four different responses were received from four technicians in different parts of the country: (i) report it as missing data, and sum the total while excluding the missing locality; (ii) impute the previous month's value from the same locality; (iii) impute the value from 1 year ago (same month) from the same locality; and (iv) estimate a value based on the reported number in a neighbouring locality. Without having consistent protocols for the treatment of missing data and/or meticulous reporting of adjustments made to the data, it is very difficult to ascertain the quality of the final data.

Unintentional recording and reporting of inaccurate data
Unintentional errors are sometimes introduced into the data for innocent reasons. Staff may not have appropriate skills or supporting equipment to effectively carry out their data-reporting responsibilities. For example, it is not uncommon in developing countries for the same reporting forms to be used at different levels of the health care system. In Cameroon, nurses in health centres were required to classify diarrhoea among five health problems (shigellosis, amoebiasis, cholera, common diarrhoea, and other types of diarrhoea), despite having extremely limited access to diagnostic means. With computerized data entry, a clerk with limited experience may enter codes in a database by selecting from menu options that may not match the exact terminology used by the physician (Chamarro, 1992; McDonald et al., 1992).

Data reported by health facilities are generally based on data previously collected on operational cards, accounting forms, or registries during daily activities. Errors often occur during this internal processing of data, since forms may not be available or staff do not know how to fill them out correctly. For example, registers in maternity hospitals in Tunisia have columns for delivery complications (yes/no), obstructed labour (yes/no), and eclampsia (yes/no). Haemorrhage, which has recently been identified as the leading cause of maternal mortality in the country, should be identified as a delivery complication (yes), with "no" codes for obstructed labour and eclampsia. However, many midwives tend to check "yes" for delivery complication only if the complication was obstructed labour and/or eclampsia.

As another example, an informal small-scale study on the accuracy of data on immunization was carried out by health centre staff in the Democratic Republic of the Congo (formerly Zaire) in 1988. The unpublished study revealed that there was less than 60% correspondence between data on immunization coverage kept by health centres and the immunization cards kept in the households.

Figure 16 illustrates potential sources of error in recording clinical data that constitute multiple threats to data quality: misinformation from the patient, quality of clinical findings, error in recording patient data by providers, personnel error during diagnostic tests, and inaccurate interpretation of tests.

Intentional recording and reporting of false data
Information systems can significantly improve patient care, hospital management and administration, research, and health and medical education, but many systems do not achieve these goals. Often, such systems fail because of user resistance, even though the systems are technologically sound (see Kaplan & Maxwell, 1994).

One of the greatest fears of users is that information systems will monitor employee work, and that repercussions will occur if the employee does not attain a particular level on a performance indicator.

Fig. 16   *Sources of error in recording clinical data*

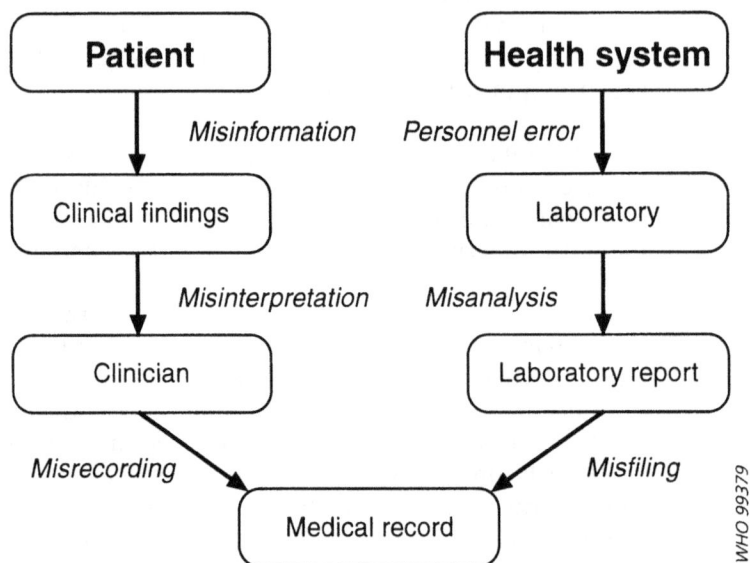

Source: Wyatt (1994).

Such concerns are not unwarranted. In Cameroon, posters were used to display a number of indicators that were discussed with community members. The performance of health centres was also compared during staff meetings, thus increasing peer pressure and leading to the reporting of false data. In fact, during an assessment in 1993, it was discovered that reporting of false data on coverage for preventive care was common.

Sometimes the health system is set up in such a way that reporting accurate data acts as a disincentive. Burnum (1989) suggests that US physicians deliberately misrecord patient data to avoid litigation. Nurses in Cameroon have underreported the number of patients treated because the fee paid by some patients was illegally kept by the health provider. Supervisors found that data on self-reported absenteeism were frequently falsified.

Data on the frequency of supervision are also frequently overreported. If supervisors monitor their own supervision, they have a tendency to exaggerate the number of supervisions performed. Asking those who are supervised to report the data does not solve the problem as they then face "moral" pressure from the supervisor to supply falsified reports.

Errors in processing data
Errors occur during the transfer and aggregation of data at all levels of the information system. Manual processing, which is common in most developing countries, involves tedious computations that often result in errors. As discussed earlier, accurate (if any) corrections rarely are made for missing reports. In Cameroon, for instance, most of the variations in measles immunization coverage over time were traced to the population denominator not being available when reports from health facilities were missing.

If computers are available, data processing operations typically involve a series of basic steps, each of which is subject to possible introduction of errors: editing, coding, data entry, and tabulating.

- *Editing.* Registers or forms are edited to correct inconsistencies and to eliminate omissions. During this stage, managers need to make decisions about the treatment of "unknown" responses in the raw data. Where information is lacking on one variable, can a reasonable entry be estimated based on other information supplied on the form? Although clerks can manually do the inputting if given detailed specifications for assigning characteristics, automated equipment is useful for greater speed and accuracy in the application of simple rules. Machine processing is designed to reject or correct a taped record with missing or inconsistent data and to assign a reasonable response on the basis of other information. However, there is considerable scope for error in such cases. In the United States, for example, an unusually large increase in the centenarian population was reported in the 1980 census. Upon further investigation, it was learned that over 25% of the "new" centenarians had been assigned to that category as a result of computerized imputation, and that many had other characteristics that suggested they were actually much younger.
- *Coding.* Coding is the conversion of entries on forms or registers into symbols. While many coding procedures are relatively simple, involving classification of individuals by sex (male, female), by location (village X, village Y), reason for visit (preventive, curative), and so on, some coding procedures are complicated and have the potential for significant error. For instance, when classifying cause of death according to the *International statistical classification of diseases and related health problems*, 10th rev. (ICD-10) (WHO, 1992) categories, it is relatively easy to confuse the coding of disease A37.0 (whooping cough due to *Bordetella pertussis*) with that of category A37.1 (whooping cough due to *Bordetella parapertussis*).
- *Date entry.* Data entry refers to the means of transfer of the data from the original document to the computer. The data might be typed directly into the computer, or microfilmed copies of the registers may be "read" by moving beams of light over coded responses. For manual data entry into the computer, many institutions perform double entry to reduce data errors. With double entry, a computer program accepts the record only if the clerk has entered it exactly the same way. This procedure minimizes the introduction of errors due to typing mistakes.
- *Tabulating.* A final step entails rearranging the data in order to provide the most useful charts and figures for decision makers. The potential for error is significant if the programmer provides incorrect instructions (to the computer) for the required tabulations. For instance, a programme manager might request information on the number of antenatal visits in District X (a rural, underserved area) in 1996. The programmer might incorrectly insert the code for District Y (an urban area of high access) for 1994. Without reviewing the coding from the programming, the programme manager might recognize that districts X and Y were confused, but is unlikely to know that the years 1994 and 1996 were also tabulated erroneously.

What can be done to improve and ensure data quality?

The following strategies can help ensure the availability of high-quality data at low cost:

Keep the design of the information system as simple as possible

Operational cards, registers, and forms should be designed simply with clear instructions. Valid, sensitive, and specific indicators must be selected to increase data quality. It is also important to minimize the number of levels in the information system in order to avoid errors during transfer and processing of data. In general, the collector and the user of data should be as close as possible. Indeed, in action-led information systems, the collectors and users of the data may be the same people. This will reduce errors in handling data and will improve the decision-making process, as data are more likely to be meaningful to the person who collects them. Data should be transferred first to the immediate supervisor of the staff reporting the data. If the use of computers is not appropriate, staff should use calculators to avoid many computation errors. The simplicity of the design of the information system can constitute a strong incentive for staff. For example, in Cameroon, the reduction of the number of monthly forms from 12 to 1 greatly reduced the complexity of and time required for data collection efforts.

Involve users in the design of the system

Involving users in the design of the system is an incentive in two ways: it helps develop an information system that is best suited to the user, and it increases ownership of the system. While involving users takes more time, it promotes general understanding of the system and improves the quality of the data produced. Furthermore, it ensures that the data collected are relevant.

Standardize procedures and definitions

Clear operational case definitions need to be developed. The case definition must match the diagnostic capabilities of different types of facilities. For instance, in Chad as in the lower levels of the health system in many developing countries, laboratory tests are rarely available, so suspected cases of malaria are reported as fever. For international purposes, national classification of diseases could be adapted to WHO's ICD-10 by using a similar coding system. Diagnostic and treatment algorithms are frequently used in developing countries, especially at the primary health care level, to standardize the decision-making of health personnel.

Procedures for filling out forms, aggregating and handling missing data, and so on need to be straightforward and clearly developed. If possible, instructions should be included in the forms since staff rarely refer to separate instructions.

Design of data collection instruments

Pretesting the content of data collection instruments and methods has proved to be very useful in providing a basis for decisions that must be made during advance planning for a health information system (see Chapter 6). Some examples are testing new data items, changing the wording of a question, or trying different types or layouts of registers or different data collection procedures.

Develop an appropriate incentive structure

The best incentive is to ensure that data collected are useful to the data collector. For example, it is not useful for the programme manager to know that he met only 50% of his measles immunization target if he did not have sufficient supplies with which to meet the target. Similarly, national level, aggregated data on prevalence of sexually transmitted diseases are not useful for a programme manager if he does not know the prevalence for his geographical area or for population subgroups within his district.

Regular supervision and feedback from supervisors also can be an important incentive for staff to report quality data, if the feedback is intended to improve performance rather than punish workers who do not meet prescribed goals for the month. However, it is important to exercise caution when developing and implementing incentive structures, to ensure that they accurately reflect the intended effects of the programme and do not introduce unintended consequences (see Box 21).

Monetary incentives based on reporting performances (percentage of reports arriving on time at the higher level) can improve both the regularity of reporting and the quality of the data if supervisors perform spot checks. In Pakistan, at least in the initial phase of implementation, the salaries of nonreporting health units were stopped. The motivational effects of decision tools, like posters displaying monitoring indicators or maps produced by a geographical information system, also merit additional study.

In the Democratic Republic of the Congo, regular cross-checking of data was performed by comparing immunization coverage from health centre data based on routine information and an annual districtwide survey. Although this had a motivational effect at the beginning, it dwindled rapidly; staff thought that it was not worthwhile to collect data on a routine basis because the cluster sampling technique would provide the data anyway.

Box 21   Examples of unintended consequences in incentive programmes

- Village health workers in Nepal were paid according to the number of children that they immunized. The result was that these workers reimmunized some children who had already been fully immunized because the children were in easily accessible locations. They also "invented" children by paying childless adults to sign a form indicating that their children had been immunized. The unused vaccines were discarded.
- Double counting of individuals is a common practice in localities where census enumerators are paid according to the number of persons that they enumerate.
- In the past, there were strong incentives in Bangladesh and India to encourage family planning workers to recruit as many new acceptors of permanent methods (and especially female sterilization) as possible. An unintended human rights consequence was that family planning workers began to pay a nominal fee to poverty-stricken women to meet their monthly quotas.
- During a rat infestation problem in China, the government instituted an incentive programme in which it paid a small fee for every rat killed. The consequence was that individuals began to breed rats in order to collect larger fees. In each of these cases, the reports arrived on time and apparently showed that the worker had met the reporting requirements for the given month.

Plan for effective checking procedures

Checking procedures should be part of the design of information systems; the challenge is to develop checking procedures at an acceptable cost. Supervisors should systematically devote part of their time to verification of procedures and providing feedback to staff. This is probably one of the most cost-effective ways to improve data quality. Targeted health information system supervision should only happen after the introduction of a new system or after changes are implemented.

From time to time the data should be cross-checked by collecting the same data through different means. Unfortunately, there are few examples that illustrate the use of such checks, and they are seldom built into the information system. One example comes from the United States, where the National Center for Health Statistics conducts a "follow-up" survey with the next of kin of a decedent in order to investigate the quality of information reported on the death certificate.

Training

Training is crucial for providing quality data, and basic training should cover the information system itself. Data collection instruments, data processing, analysis, and decision-making should be part of the national curriculum in schools of nursing and medicine. Refresher courses on the information system should be organized for all levels.

Experience from many developing countries demonstrates that training is crucial but not sufficient for improving the quality of data in the long run. Training needs to be organized in an environment that promotes quality assurance through a system of accountability, positive and negative incentives, and control.

Summary

This chapter has considered two distinct but interrelated components of information processes: data transmission and data processing. In addition, we have considered data quality, which hinges on the effectiveness of data collection, data transmission, and data processing components.

Data transmission considers how data are transferred among the interdependent actors in the health system to ensure that administrative, political, and management decisions are based on the best available information. We have highlighted how both vertical and horizontal data transmission mechanisms can help meet management needs for patient/client management, health unit management, and system management. It was noted, however, that a number of topic areas need further research. Specifically, to date, only anecdotal information exists regarding the cost of developing and maintaining the data transmission mechanisms described in this chapter. Second, given that most developing countries continue to employ vertical data transmission systems, they need to learn how to improve the speed of data transfers and how to use better feedback mechanisms so that the lowest level of the health care system can benefit from data compiled at higher levels. Finally, given the increased importance of community actors in health care, better understanding of methods that improve horizontal transmission mechanisms is important.

The third section of this chapter considered data processing, or how the raw data could be manipulated in order to transform them into useful information for the greatest number of actors in the health system. It described how data processing operations range from simple manual computations to sophisticated computerized processing, and generally involve at least two major steps: data cleaning and rearrangement of the information to form a summary set of useful variables. A brief introduction to the benefits of computerization for processing of data was presented, in preparation for more detailed analysis of this topic in Chapter 11.

The final section examined data quality, or whether the data accurately reflect the phenomenon they were intended to measure. Detailed descriptions of impediments to data quality and steps that managers can take to improve data quality were also provided.

References

Armenian HK (1992). Health information system: diversity of data and need for integration. In: Ties Boerma J, ed. *Measurement of maternal and child mortality, morbidity, and health care: interdisciplinary approaches*. Liege, Ordina Editions.

Burnum JF (1989). The misinformation era: the fall of the medical record. *Annals of internal medicine*, 110:482–484.

Chamarro T (1992). *Knowledge of transference in automating hospital operations*. Los Angeles, Nursing Information Systems, Cedars-Sinai Medical Center (unpublished report).

Cleland JG (1985). Data cleaning. Data processing. In: Pressat R, Wilson C, eds. *The dictionary of demography*. Oxford, Basil Blackwell, 49–51.

Kaplan B, Maxwell JA (1994). Qualitative research methods for evaluating computer information systems. In: Anderson JG, Aydin CE, Jay SJ, eds. *Evaluating health care information systems: methods and applications*. Thousand Oaks, CA, Sage.

Kraemer KL, Danziger JN (1990). The impacts of computer technology on the worklife of information workers. *Social sciences computer review*, 8:592–613.

McDonald CJ et al. (1992). The Regenstrief medical record system: twenty years of experience in hospitals, clinics, and neighborhood health centers. *M.D. computing*, 9:206–217.

O'Brien JA (1982). *Computers in business management*, 3rd ed. Homewood IL, Richard D. Irwin.

Rice RE, Anderson JG (1994). Social networks and health information systems: a structural approach to evaluation. In: Anderson JG, Aydin CE, Jay SJ, eds. *Evaluating health care information systems: methods and applications*. Thousand Oaks, CA, Sage.

World Health Organization (1992). *International statistical classification of diseases and related health problems*, 10th rev. Geneva, World Health Organization.

Wyatt JC (1994). Clinical data systems. Part 1. Data and medical records. *Lancet*, 344:1543–1548.

Population-based community
health information systems

David R. Marsh

Introduction

Population-based health and information systems serve defined populations which may be regularly censused, under demographic surveillance, or estimated. Community-based systems include local community participation in planning, managing, and responding to the system and its information. Population-based systems need not be community-based. For example, a district health system may be based on population estimates with little or no community involvement in its information. Similarly, community-based systems are not necessarily population-based. For example, a prepaid local health plan may seek beneficiary participation in policy dialogue, while remaining uniformed about the pressing health needs of local residents who are nonsubscribers. Population-based community health systems and the information systems that support them combine elements of both. They stress local participation in responding to the health needs of all in the defined population, often through household and neighbourhood level services, especially health promotion and disease prevention activities. Community members, often as volunteers, complement health personnel. Such systems strive for more than improving the population's health. They aim to develop local human resources and institutions.

The population-based community approach is common in research settings (e.g. Matlab [Bangladesh], Kasongo [Democratic Republic of the Congo], and Aga Khan University [Pakistan]), and in development programmes (e.g. private voluntary or nongovernmental organizations in numerous settings). On the other hand, large-scale examples linking communities to ministries of health do exist (e.g. guinea worm eradication programmes in many countries, the Health and Management Information System [Philippines], the "vital horoscope" [Islamic Republic of Iran], and the planned household health promotion service [South Africa]). This chapter describes examples of both. The more extensive examples from the nongovernmental sector highlight their important historical role and the potential for partnerships and information exchanges with government.

Information systems mirror activities. Two illustrations of population-based community health information systems (Table 24) include village volunteers mobilizing mothers for child immunization and household providers giving terminal care to dying relatives. Each is analysed according to the information framework presented in Chapter 2. The first example requires an interface with the ministry of health services for immunizations. The second activity may stand alone. The central information management strategy for improved Expanded Programme on

Table 24 *Community-based health information system: information framework*

Information step	Illustrative cases	
	Childhood immunizations	Home-based care
Activities	Volunteers perform household-level mobilizing of mothers for child immunization	Home caregiver provides care for dying household member
Information needs and indicators	Immunization status of each child <5 years. Completely immunized 12–23-month olds	QOC provided and index of care (4/5 parameters acceptable)
Data sources	"Road-to-health" cards and immunization outreach clinic	Volunteers perform monthly household observations and interview
Data flow and analysis	Data → volunteers' rosters: check immunization status by age → aggregated community coverage	QOC checklists: percentage of good QOC by trainee and by content area
Decision making	>12 months and incompletely immunized refer to outreach clinic	Refresh trainee; modify curriculum
Management	Supervisor performs monthly aggregegation/ support visit	Supervisor performs monthly aggregation/ support visit
Monitoring and evaluation	Lot quality assurance or end-line coverage survey	In-depth interview of care givers and patients

QOC = quality of care.

Immunization coverage might be a population-based roster for each volunteer listing all children and their updated immunization status, thereby allowing the volunteer to identify and mobilize those at risk. For supervising and supporting good-quality home-based care, the central strategy could be a brief checklist of measurable parameters of care by which the volunteers assess and support trained home-based care providers.

No population-based community health system stands alone. It needs to be linked to referral services for curative and rehabilitative care. In most developing countries, government health facilities provide these services, especially in rural areas. Thus, the district health model is an integral part of the population-based community health system. The focus has only shifted from the peripheral facility to their catchment areas, the communities they serve. The community adds another management level to the system, with its own information needs.

Essential public health functions

WHO is currently developing a concept and strategy which will define a set of the most essential public health functions which countries at all levels of development should ensure are carried out for the protection of the health of their total population. These concern health information management; environmental protection; health promotion and education; communicable disease control; health legislation; developing and implementing health policies, programmes, and services; developing human resources for health; assessing and standardizing health technology; occupational health; and delivering selected health services to selected populations. The essential functions may be carried out by government agencies and services, by nongovernmental organizations, by private sector enterprises, and/or by the community.

When the essential functions are selected, globally and within countries, they offer a clear basis for identifying the more important types of data to be maintained at each level of the health system. The community level functions will determine the critical types of health data to be captured and acted upon, or reported to higher levels. Examples include reporting births and deaths; notification of cases of infectious diseases and outbreaks; identification of high-risk children, pregnant women, and families; coverage and defaulters of critical services; coverage and quality of water and sanitation; monitoring air, water, land, and noise pollution; coverage of disadvantaged populations with health and social services; availability of functioning service facilities and staff; and availability of essential drugs (Sapirie, personal communication, 1997). Clearly, population-based community health and information systems are central to effective public health.

National programmes to eradicate guinea worm disease are a timely example of the community's role in essential public health. As recently as 1992 there were more than 22,000 known endemic villages; currently there are only 9865 (4404 of which are in a single conflict-ridden country). Regular use of data at all programme levels, as well as monthly feedback to communities, some of which are among the most remote in Africa, are keys to the eradication success to date. Regular data review and retraining sessions improved motivation among community volunteers. Intervention data included the availability of safe water, percentage of households with cloth water filter, and locations of unsafe water sources which may be suitable for chemical treatment (Seim, personal communication, 1997).

Clinical versus community approach

To understand population-based community health information systems, one must first grasp population-based approaches to public health. Their stories are intertwined. A scenario of a clinical encounter illustrating good and bad professional care can be a metaphor for good and bad public health practice. Wyon (1973) has eloquently compared and contrasted the tasks of the public health physician and the clinician. Each gathers data, interprets them, and makes recommendations—whether the concern is for a defined population or an individual.

Skilled clinicians do not just treat symptoms. Rather, they ask key questions, perform relevant physical examinations, and obtain essential laboratory investigations. For a patient with fever and shaking chills, a careful physician asks about cough, looks for rapid breathing, and examines a blood smear for possible malaria. He looks beyond what is immediately apparent to identify and treat the underlying problem rather than the symptoms.

How does this relate to a community's health? What if the public health practitioner assessed and responded only to readily visible "community" issues? Just as this would have been poor treatment in the above example (i.e. aspirin for fever), so it would lead to poor community medicine practice. Experience has shown that those at greatest risk and those with the worst health are often the least visible. These people are unseen because they are too poor to afford the health system, too uninformed to recognize their risk, too powerless to make decisions on their or their dependants' behalf, or too distant to access the health system. The public health practitioner who only considers evidence that is immediately apparent risks drawing erroneous conclusions.

Numerator and denominator analysis

Public health practitioners speak of "numerator analysis" and "denominator analysis". The former refers to collecting counts of health events, often from a health facility, say, numbers of cases of diarrhoea seen at a district hospital per month. These service-based statistics provide a partial, but incomplete (and possibly dramatically inaccurate) picture of the diarrhoea problem surrounding the hospital. For example, a cholera epidemic could ravage an inaccessible corner of the district while low numbers of diarrhoea cases survive to reach the facility.

"Denominator analysis", on the other hand, deals with rates of health events. Rates depend on both numerators, the counts, and denominators, the population at risk. District health information systems may rely on both facility-based counts (numerator) as well as estimates of relevant denominators. The population-based approach in the community allows for a more careful health assessment. For example, consider villages A, B, and C from which 30, 35, and 50 malnourished children, respectively, attend a nutritional rehabilitation centre. Numerator analysis identifies village C with the greatest child malnutrition problem and village A with the least.

A population-based community approach might describe a far greater (and different) malnutrition problem than facility-based data suggested. By encouraging each village to identify and characterize the nutritional status of its children, managers could find that villages A, B, and C really had 90, 75, and 60 malnourished children under age 5, with village A actually having the greatest problem. And its problem might manifest itself as more than childhood malnutrition because half of its cases had not accessed the system. The population-based community approach would therefore allow identification of all affected individuals, many of whom were invisible to the health system because of incomplete coverage.

Censuses are well suited for community mobilization, and data generated are invaluable for fostering self-reflection and problem solving. If the child populations of villages A, B, and C were 900, 500, and 1200, their malnutrition rates per thousand inhabitants would be 100 (90/900 × 1000), 150 (75/500 × 1000), and 50 (60/1200 × 1000), for villages A, B, and C, respectively. Thus, village B actually had the greatest malnutrition problem after correcting for the denominators. When the number of health events per population is known, one can compare and rank communities by their health status.

Why did village B have such a high rate of malnutrition? A basic community health approach might observe that the malnutrition rate was twice as high for girls as for boys. Communities contribute invaluably to deeper analysis through qualitative studies such as group interviews to identify normative practices and beliefs that might explain the gender differential. Discovering causation of malnutrition in these communities rests on the population-based community approach.

These questions of coverage, comparison, and causation are best answered by the population-based approach. Moreover, they are difficult, if not impossible, without community involvement. Incomplete coverage means an incomplete health system (recall the pitfall of an incomplete clinical encounter). Health officials who are unable to compare cannot validly measure the distribution of disease or monitor the effect of the health system's response. Furthermore, without clear notions of causation and risk, they cannot understand local health phenomena or target interventions. Interestingly, not all agree that epidemiology is key to peripheral health service management and planning. Unger and Dujardin (1992) argue that the minimum package of activities at peripheral facilities is unaffected by variations in disease frequency. This may be true enough perhaps at the facility level, but the variations among communities, households, and individuals uniquely signal health needs and guide services. Population-based community approaches are eminently suited to address these variations.

History: population-based community approaches

The roots of the census-based approach to health care date back 70 years to the Peking Union Medical College where John B. Grant and others extended the health care system to households (Wyon, 1994). Shortly thereafter, John E. Gordon pioneered household surveillance for scarlet fever in Romania in the 1930s, epidemiological surveillance during World War II, and the Khanna population study (Wyon & Gordon, 1971) in the 1950s and 1960s in rural Punjab, India, measuring the impact of household level services on fertility and mortality. Soon to follow was the Narangwal health services experiment of Kielmann et al. (1983), also in Punjab during the 1960s and 1970s.

Meanwhile, Sidney Kark and others developed the concept of community-oriented primary care, first in South Africa during the 1940s and 1950s, and later in Jerusalem during the 1960s (Tollman, 1991). Essential to this concept were combining epidemiological and clinical skills for a defined population, involving community for specific interventions, and measuring the impact of interventions (Abramson & Kark, 1983).

Frederiksen (1973) and other epidemiologists (Dunn, 1973; Taylor, 1973; Wray, 1973) debated the applicability of census-based approaches to public health in a seminal epidemiological surveillance symposium. Based on observations from Uttar Pradesh, India, Frederiksen reported an exponential decay in health facility attendance with increasing distance between residences and the facility. In addition, he cited the reemergence of malaria in Ceylon (now Sri Lanka) coinciding with replacing house-to-house surveillance with health centre-based surveillance. Thus, he boldly proposed a multipurpose household-level surveillance system akin to the then familiar unipurpose model in public health for malaria eradication. Possible aims included providing family planning services, conducting surveillance for public health threats such as plague and cholera, measuring demographic trends, and, of course, eradicating malaria. He observed that his proposal depended on a census-based approach. While fertility rates could be calculated on the basis of a population sample, the reduction of fertility required wide coverage.

Starting in 1958, the Kasongo project (Democratic Republic of the Congo) sought to facilitate community-based health care among a defined population of 195,000. Using a bottom-up approach to discover community needs, the programme restructured the existing system, including the traditional practitioners, and extended geographical coverage (Darras,

Van Lerberghe & Mercenier, 1982). Community involvement was encouraged through family registration at the initial census and maintained through domiciliary visits by bicycling *animateurs de santé* (health promoters) and monthly health committee meetings. Clinic-based *fiches opérationnelles* (operations forms) tracked essential clinical data which were summarized monthly. Managers calculated coverage from facility-based outputs and the baseline census, by geographic region (Abelin, Brezezinski & Carstairs, 1987). While this approach allowed neither targeting services to individuals nor precise estimates of coverage, it was affordable, and communities at risk could be identified.

In the 1970s and 1980s, lay reporting stressed community-level data generation and use. Lay reporting systems were used in Kenya, where chiefs and administrative officers registered births and deaths; China, where, since 1979, rural practitioners monitored birth and death registration, infectious diseases, immunizations, and family planning; and the Philippines, where household members recorded and basic health workers weekly transcribed information about illnesses, births, deaths, pregnancy outcomes, and immunizations (Interregional Meeting on Lay Reporting in Information Support, 1985). Health officials reported that such lay reporting systems raised the health consciousness of community members, especially where proper fora (community assemblies, primary health care committees, council meetings) allowed information feedback, discussion, and response.

The 23-year Jamkhed project (Arole & Arole, 1994) in Maharashtra, India, extends this technique and holds promise as a model which combines population-based community health and development approaches. Basic assumptions are that (i) most villagers have practical intelligence, with or without formal education; (ii) medical curricula are largely irrelevant to most health needs of rural India; (iii) most health problems can be met by local solutions; and (iv) villagers can learn to perform basic public health tasks. Central to the programme are annual surveys of every household to identify and respond to risk groups and to monitor progress. Targeting women for training as illiterate household-level health workers, the programme enhances their status, augments their household's income, improves the population's health, and strengthens community problem solving. The programme is now being replicated in over 200 Indian communities. Another recent Asian example, from Pakistan's Northern Areas (see Box 22), demonstrates how community involvement permeates the health and information system.

A strategy for community level social development was undertaken in Thailand in the early 1980s under the auspices of the Rural Poverty Eradication Programme by the National Economic and Social Development Board. This strategy enabled communities to assemble basic data on the health and social situation in their village. Nine desirable characteristics of Thai society and 32 indicators (Box 23) of basic needs enabled village committees to determine their priority needs and problems. With the advice of the subdistrict council, a development plan was drafted which contained the activities the villages were able to undertake. The villages thus were able to carry out problem identification, planning, specifying the types of activity and support needed, and evaluating the status of their "basic minimum needs". In this way they became more aware of the problems of their village and the level of their achievement (Nondasuta & Piyarata,1987; Royal Thai Government, 1988).

**Box 22   A population-based community health
information system in the northern
areas of Pakistan**

AW Khan, M Rahim, A Mir, S Wali, A Hussain, JC van Latum,
Aga Khan Health Services, Northern Areas, Pakistan

The Aga Khan Health Services began its primary health care programme in 1988 using community collaboration as a fundamental programme principle. Communities identify primary health care workers for training as voluntary community health workers or birth attendants. Lady health visitors, attached to preexisting health centres, are accountable to local health boards comprised of community members. Programme directors collaborate with the regional health board, also comprised of community members.

Community members and professional staff developed a comprehensive, concise, population-based community management information system to enable planning based on information. It is primarily picture-based as most volunteers are illiterate. Community health workers track births and deaths and morbidity due to diarrhoea and pneumonia. They assign cause(s) of death using structured verbal autopsy interviews. Birth attendants use illustrated antenatal care registers for collecting relevant pregnancy-related information, including outcome. Lady health visitors aggregate, analyse, and respond to the population-based community data monthly with the volunteers. This system has quickly identified outbreaks of pneumonia, cholera, and measles. Community volunteers also join lady health visitors for annual health surveys to supplement this system.

Health centre staff further aggregate and analyse data, sharing it with the health board, which then sets programme objectives, targets, and policies. Examples include an inquiry into risk factors for spontaneous abortion and improved publicity for immunization sessions. Similarly, data are further compiled and discussed with the regional health board, decisions of which include better collaboration with Ministry of Health partners and implementing birth attendant quality assessment studies. Community members undergird this system throughout. Indeed, they are regularly invited to continuing education sessions for Aga Khan Health Services staff, particularly those dealing with management information systems, to improve their communities' use of health data.

The 1978 Declaration of Alma Ata (WHO, 1978) codified much of the above experience as primary health care: universal coverage at the household level of essential services serves as a strategy towards equity in health. The notion has stimulated much health system dialogue and experimentation in the developing world, and millions of lives have been saved (Berggren, Ewbank & Berggren, 1981). But untold millions in the poorest countries of Africa, Asia, and Latin America remain outside their health systems. Indeed, wealthy countries are not spared such inequities. Increasingly, further health care reform relies on strategies invoking "defined communities" or "universal coverage" in both developing (Bryant et al., 1993) and developed (Institute of Medicine, 1984; White & Connelly, 1991; Showstack et al., 1992; World Federation for Medical Education, 1993) countries. Expecting small communities to reach all their residents at risk is unlikely without a population-based community approach.

Box 23   Indicators of basic minimum needs in Thailand

1. Weight and height for children under 1 to 5 years are commensurate with established standards.
2. Weight and height for children 5 to 14 years are commensurate with established standards.
3. Infant birth weight is not less than 3000 g.
4. People do not have severe cases of diarrhoea or malnutrition.
5. Houses are made of materials of not less than 5 years' durability.
6. House interior is clean, and the vicinity is kept orderly with a garbage container and no stagnant or dirty water.
7. Latrine meets sanitary standards.
8. Sufficient safe drinking water (2 litres/person/day) is available.
9. Children under 1 year receive vaccination against pertussis, tuberculosis, tetanus, diphtheria, polio, and measles.
10. Children and youth have the opportunity to receive compulsory education.
11. Primary school children receive vaccination against tetanus, typhoid, pertussis, and tuberculosis boosters.
12. People over 12 years of age are literate.
13. People have adequate information on occupation, prevention of disasters, and consumer protection.
14. Pregnant women are vaccinated for tetanus, checked four times before giving birth, and receive birthing services and a check-up from a government worker or a trained traditional midwife within 6 weeks after giving birth.
15. There is no theft, rape, crime, or bodily harm committed.
16. Travelling late at night is safe.
17. Adjustments in the soil are made for raising plants and animals, crop rotation, protection against soil erosion, and adjustment of acid soil.
18. Good species of plants and breeds of animals are used.
19. Chemical fertilizer which is appropriate for the soil and plants is used, and organic fertilizer is used for soil adjustment.
20. Protective measures are taken against harmful plants, insects, and animal and plant diseases.
21. People raise, treat, and reproduce animals.
22. Couples have no more than two children and are able to choose and practice more than one method of birth control.
23. People are members of groups which assist in improving economic and social conditions.
24. Each person participates in their own development and the development of their community.
25. People participate in supporting and maintaining public property, including that built by the government and community as well as natural facilities.
26. People participate in supporting and keeping cultural treasures in an appropriate condition.
27. People participate in taking care of natural resources.
28. People use their right to vote for subdistrict leader representative, subdistrict council, village leader, and village committee.
29. People are able to draw up a plan, implement the plan, and establish a system to maintain the work results by themselves.
30. Absence of addiction to alcohol, gambling, or severely addictive substances.
31. People participate in activities on important religious days.
32. There is moderation in these ceremonies according to religious principles and traditions.

One current hopeful example is South Africa's household health promotion service, now under discussion in the country's newest and poorest province, Mpumalanga. Each worker is slated to cover 200 households (about 1200 people), providing health education and gathering information for the health services system. Paid ZAR 100 (about US$ 23) for 30 hours of work per week, these individuals must be literate, nominated by the community they serve, and residents. These population-based community health promoters will be trained by the provincial Department of Health, Welfare, and Gender Affairs and supervised by retrained existing cadres, special auxiliary services officers, and assistants. The supporting information system is presently under review (Bam, personal communication, 1997).

Rationale

"Five E's" communicate five key facets of population-based community health information systems: epidemiology, equity, empowerment, effectiveness, and efficiency.

Epidemiology

Epidemiology is the foundation. Epidemiology is the study of the distribution and determinants of disease among human populations; literally, it is "the study of what is on the people" (from the Greek, *epi, demos,* and *logos*). Epidemiology provides the skeleton for population-based health programmes and their supporting information systems. Ethical and economical programme content is guided by epidemiology as are the related management, research, and policy implications. Equity and empowerment comprise the ethical dimension of our population-based programmes. Effectiveness and efficiency, or the ratio between effect and cost, comprise the economic dimension (Fig. 17). This model embraces the key requisites of primary health care. Affordable programmes must be cost-effective. Equitable programmes target risk groups and must be

Fig. 17 *Community-based health information system: basic principles supporting multiple aims*

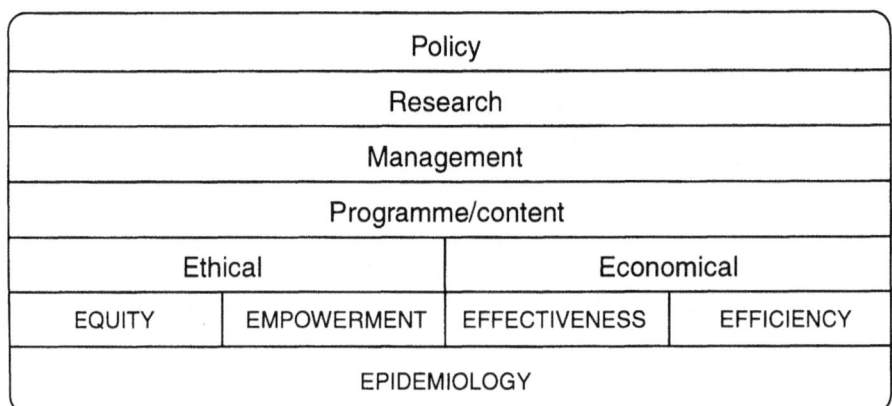

Policy			
Research			
Management			
Programme/content			
Ethical		Economical	
EQUITY	EMPOWERMENT	EFFECTIVENESS	EFFICIENCY
EPIDEMIOLOGY			

WHO 99380

154

accessible. Programmes that empower communities are likely to be acceptable since communities participate in guiding them.

Equity

In every community there are groups whose needs are relatively neglected: women and girls, the poorest members, and ethnic minorities. For example, in rural areas of Bangladesh, the risk of dying from severe malnutrition is twice as high for girls as for boys. In one of Jakarta's slums, 37% of children from the poorest families were moderately to severely malnourished versus 19% of children from the most affluent families. In Sudan, traditionally powerful ethnic groups were receiving 120% of standard food rations (Save the Children, 1992).

Without information from all segments of the community, these inequities cannot be demonstrated. Unless samples are extremely large and rigorously selected, they may be biased against minorities and the most mobile or isolated residents. Enumerating every member of a community (or at least all members of specific risk groups) enhances the likelihood of identifying and responding to those in greatest need.

A census-based monitoring system helps avoid what the *State of the world's children* (UNICEF, 1991) called the "fallacy of the average":

"Average levels of immunization coverage, educational achievement, or under-five mortality ... can and do mask serious disparities of many kinds—between boys and girls, between urban and rural, between different regions of a country, between different ethnic or cultural groups, and especially between different economic strata of society. ... A national under-five mortality rate of 50 can mean 30 for the majority in the mainstream of the nation's life and 150 among the ethnic minorities, the geographically isolated, or the politically disenfranchised. ... The monitoring process should therefore focus more on measuring how many fall how far below the average, and on identifying who they are, where they are, and why they are being marginalized by progress. ... This kind of monitoring is more likely to lead to a reaching-out to the unreached."

Taylor (1992) defended surveillance for equity in primary health care. Citing experience in China, India, Haiti, and elsewhere, he observed that health systems that reached every household in a community could demonstrate improved health among the unhealthiest members. Information from such surveillance galvanizes communities, nations, and donors to action.

Empowerment

Residents are empowered by a community-based information system if they are involved in its development and implementation, they receive and have the ability to interpret the information it generates, and the health interventions meet the needs identified by the information system.

A prerequisite for step 1 of empowerment, however, is enfranchisement. That is, a community will not support the development of a health and information system unless it is perceived to address important local problems. Community priorities are not necessarily those of a "standard maternal and child health package" offered by the health services.

Defining a package of health services is best determined by dialogue, rather than cost-effectiveness analysis. For example, community residents often want water, curative care, interventions against endemic diseases beyond the scope of most programmes—or even volleyball courts.[1] Thus, it is important for service providers either to incorporate into their programmes, or to advocate for, interventions which address these felt needs. They must also illustrate to community members, through population-based health information, how other interventions (perhaps not identified by the community) can also save community lives.

Private voluntary organization experience from Jakarta slums is relevant (Kay & Galvao, 1995). At the start of a health project, community residents stated that their major health problem was dengue. Although interventions against dengue were not initially envisioned, health programme managers opted for outreach workers distributing a mosquito larvicide during home visits to promote other interventions. After this affirmation of both community empowerment and programme responsiveness, managers used data derived from the community health information system in a series of fora to stress that immunizable diseases were responsible for much child mortality in their areas and that programme interventions were saving children's lives. By the end of the programme, community leaders chose to designate part of their small endowment fund to help institutionalize a health coordinator position within the municipal health department. This person would supervise community outreach workers (similar to those previously provided by agency staff) and afford community representatives a channel through which complaints could be aired if municipal health personnel failed to staff the local monthly community health posts. The community was empowered to mobilize for continued access to immunization services.

Community support for an information system also entails active participation in selecting outreach workers and detailing their workload (e.g. household visit schedules) and compensation. Community members should also have input into how outreach workers will be supervised in collecting data, communicating with families, and delivering services. For community empowerment to occur, supervision must also focus on ensuring that data are regularly fed back to the community (ideally to all groups) and that community members are trained to interpret data (e.g. through use of simple, graphic techniques). Unless community groups who traditionally have been disenfranchised are involved in collecting, reviewing, and interpretating data and in decision-making, it is unlikely that community empowerment will lead to greater equity.

Effectiveness

The census-based approach can increase outreach, coverage, and impact. That is, rosters which classify beneficiaries by risk status naturally enhance programme effectiveness since effort focuses on those in need. Moreover, such individuals contribute relatively more than their pro rata share of ill health. Census-based monitoring systems can meet their objectives more quickly than those which rely on data from surveys alone.

---

[1] Surprisingly, group discussions with Jamkhed residents discovered a need for a volleyball court! Yet this led to useful problem solving: how to have post-game tea across castes? Had this nonhealth perceived need been omitted, an important opportunity for community mobilization would have been missed.

Box 24   The role of population-based community health information systems in the urban primary health care programme of the Aga Khan University

M Lobo, The Aga Khan University

The Aga Khan University's department of community health sciences has improved the health of approximately 50,000 residents in seven Karachi squatter settlements since 1986 through providing effective, equitable primary health care, targeting women and children. An information system identified risk groups and measured indicators. A baseline census registered all families in a family folder. The programme trained community members (mainly women) as modestly paid community health workers to perform monthly visits to 100–125 households each for service provision and information update. Monthly reviews at each field site identified risk groups (malnourished or underimmunized children and pregnant women, for example) for interim follow-up or referral to supporting facilities. One community health worker at each slum, assisted by a team doctor or nurse, monitored information quality and guided its analysis and review with the community. Quarterly programme level reports generated overall indicators, the number of which gradually decreased with experience. Baseline under-5 mortality rates had decreased from 177 to 98 by 1992.

The programme provided services and opportunities for teaching and research, of which tracking cause-specific mortality was central. Health centre staff investigated all deaths by structured verbal autopsy interview. Between 1990 and 1992, 156 (36% of total) under-5 deaths had multiple causes of death. Diarrhoea, malnutrition, low birth weight, acute respiratory infections, and vaccine-preventable diseases played roles in 41%, 24%, 22%, 13%, and 2% of child deaths, respectively. Programme responses to such data included strengthening promotion of oral rehydration therapy; narrowing the target of growth monitoring and promotion to <3 years from <5 years; developing a low birth weight protocol; targeting children <2 for a pilot acute respiratory infection programme; and expanding the programme to address water and sanitation. Leading causes of adult (age 15–59) mortality (3.6/1000) between 1990 and 1992) were ischaemic heart disease, tuberculosis, burns, and maternal causes. Follow-up epidemiological studies continue to define each.

Data from census-based systems have been used to facilitate programme evaluation and research (see Box 24). The conclusions recently put forth by a working group from the National Research Council (Commission on Behavioral and Social Sciences, 1993) provide a strong rationale for using census-based data in evaluating the impact of basic health projects, especially on child mortality: declines in mortality rates should remain the ultimate indicator of the effectiveness of child health interventions in Africa; more emphasis should be given to age-specific mortality rates in stating programme goals; and there is a need for more long-term studies that include regular collection of vital statistics, routine surveys of service use, and quality of care.

Mortality rates can certainly be estimated through surveys. However, unless samples are very large and selected adequately to represent minority groups, it is difficult to reliably assess changes in infant, child, and maternal mortality or to determine whether rates differ between groups. Ultimately, a census-based system, which also affords the opportunity to target services, may be only a little more expensive than a series of large surveys.

Longitudinal data allows examining the temporal distribution of health events to guide programmatic response and generate explanatory hypotheses. The clustering of winter births in Nasirnagar, Bangladesh (Fig. 18), for example may relate to the cultural practice of marriages after the November–December harvest. Pregnancy-related care should reflect this seasonal pattern.

Efficiency

In any health programme, it is important to weigh the costs of monitoring and evaluation systems against other programme components, notably services. Generalizing the costs of census-based systems is difficult because of their variability from one setting to another. Key

Fig. 18   *Monthly distribution of births over 5 years, Nasirnagar, Bangladesh*

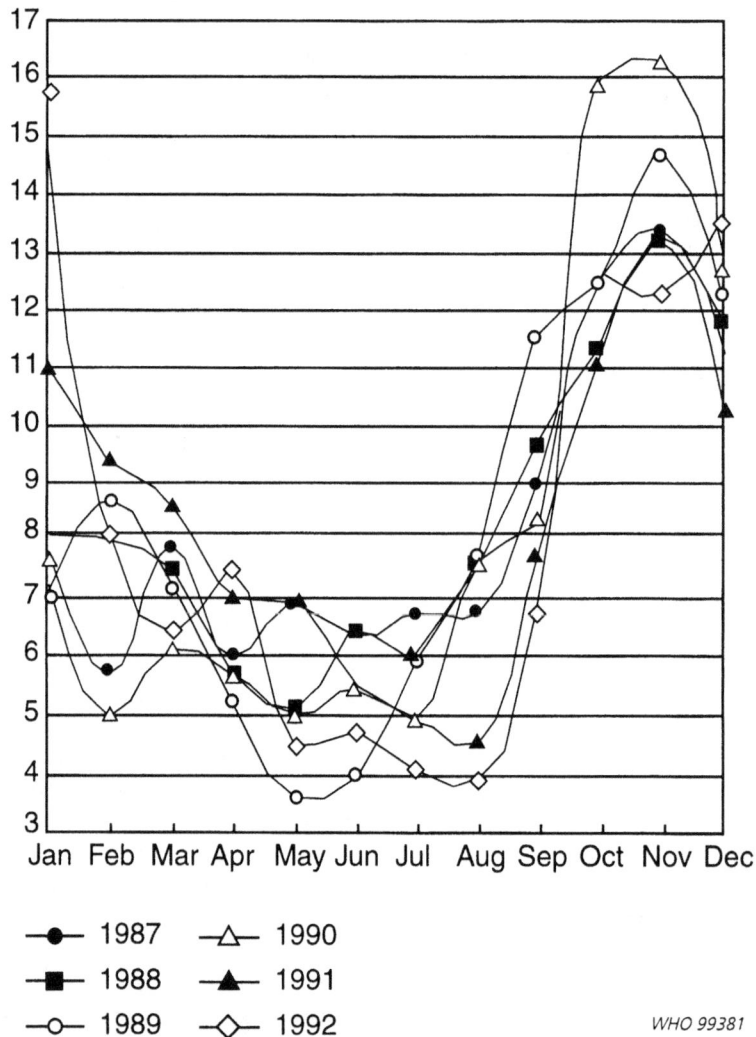

Legend:
—●— 1987   —△— 1990
—■— 1988   —▲— 1991
—○— 1989   —◇— 1992

WHO 99381

Source: Save the Children/USA.

determinants of cost are whether outreach workers are volunteers or salaried, the intensity of supervision, the frequency of home visits, and the role of computerization. Community-based private voluntary organizations often estimate that information systems represent 5–10% of total programme costs.

The costs of implementing and maintaining a census-based information system should certainly be recorded and analysed. Such analysis should be in relation to the cost of service delivery in areas with and without such systems. Zayan, Berggren & Doumbia (1992) examined the costs of immunization in rural Mali, comparing populations fully enrolled in a population-based community information system with those not enrolled. Immunization costs per thousand immunized were US$ 1470 in the enrolled versus US$ 2789 in the unenrolled population. Twenty-two per cent of immunizations in the enrolled population were attributable to the census-based health information systems. That is, they would have been missed through the standard government approach.

Variations of a community-wide census are possible. A "minimal" census-based information system might track indicators related to only one or a few phenomena impacting health using trained, preexisting community groups. A women's group might initially track its members' practices of exclusive breastfeeding, for example. With increased experience and confidence in problem definition; establishing information needs; data collection, manipulation, and analysis; and response, the group might enlarge its scope to include women outside the group, as well as deal with other issues.

Development of population-based community health information systems

Although the broad strategies to achieve equity in health are similar, each health system reflects local health priorities, culture, and resources. Amidst this diversity, however, certain health information system elements are constant because the questions are similar regardless of setting. Planners need information to identify and prioritize health problems. Supervisors need information about the number of births or service coverage in their community. Resident home visitors need information about whom to visit. Mothers need information about the next vaccination opportunity. On the other hand, criticism is in order if health information systems demand too much data or require extraordinary effort.

An understanding of the basic "generic" system is invaluable for health information users to interpret others' field experiences and consider applying such systems to other settings. The following sections follow the conceptual model from Chapter 2, although at the community level and especially at the household level, there may be blurring of the steps.

Determining community health activities

Health activities are determined through various methods and strategies. Some are implemented as part of a national programme. Some are driven by donors. Others arise from a local situation analysis. Combinations are common. Many private voluntary and nongovernmental organizations are skilled in mobilizing communities for a health situation analysis which often involves a census or survey. Indeed, such organizations often seek to include Ministry of Health counterparts in such training. The Aga Khan Foundation recently published a useful series of nine modules, the *Primary health care management advancement programme*, to help primary health care management teams collect, process, and analyse useful management information. Each volume is a balance of limited theory with vocabulary, clear practical steps to accomplish given management tasks, and copious examples of forms, indicators, and other primary health care information. Module 2 in this series details how to assess a community's health needs and coverage. The Save the Children/USA guide (Daniel, 1990) and accompanying training manual are similar private voluntary organization contributions which provide detailed instructions for conducting a census step by step.

Autodiagnostica (autodiagnosis) was a participatory process used by Bolivia's Warmi project (Howard-Grabman, Seoane & Davenport, 1994) to help women characterize the maternal and perinatal health care needs in 50 isolated altiplano villages. The steps included discovering attitudes regarding pregnancy and birth, and related problems; identifying vocabulary; and designing interview formats to broadly explore the issues, share findings, and prioritize them. The Bolivian flag (three horizontal stripes of red, yellow, and green) served as a cultural strategy to help the women prioritize (red = top priority, for example).

In Chile, the Ministry of Health has a long tradition of ensuring the coverage of essential health needs of the population through a pyramidal system of health services it owns and operates. In rural areas, health posts provide primary health care. Staffed by a trained, locally recruited auxiliary, each post delivers services to 1000 people, or to those within 12 km (2.5 hours walking). A key task is a detailed assessment of the catchment area's health needs. A detailed plan of the area is drawn showing houses, ways of communication, and natural obstacles. The assessment of local health, economic, and environmental conditions is made through household and community surveys which are repeated every 2 years. The main community problems are summarized, and high-risk families are identified. Thirteen local health programmes (child health monitoring, pregnancy monitoring, responsible fatherhood, immunization, etc.) respond to the identified needs (Sapirie, personal communication, 1997).

Indicators

Indicators allow managers to compare actual programme implementation and results to work plans and predictions. The PHC-MAP (primary health care monitoring and evaluation programme) series (Franco et al., 1993) provides a helpful discussion of their use. Obviously indicators relate intimately to activities. Outcome indicators track change in health status and are best selected from standard measurements of mortality, fertility, and the like. Output indicators measure goods and services produced by the health system. They measure coverage, use and quality of care of services produced. They also track changes in knowledge, practice, and skills. Community input is important here. For example, a current private voluntary organization programme in Malawi aims to reduce sexually transmitted disease and HIV infection. A variety of indicators could measure sexual behaviour, depending upon the cultural context: percentage of females over 18 years at marriage, percentage of females not initiating sexual activity before age 18 years, or percentage of unmarried females using negotiating skills around sexual activity, to name a few.

A good example of a tracking device for coverage and outcome indicators is the Islamic Republic of Iran's "vital horoscope" (UNICEF, 1994). This community device was developed for the most peripheral health unit, the "health house." The 50 × 70 cm display of seven key tables tracks community population, births, deaths, and family planning coverage. Specifically, it can generate percentage by age group, dependency ratio, percentage of married women, natural population growth, crude birth rate, general fertility rate, total fertility rate, percentage of deliveries performed at home or by untrained birth attendants, percentage of low birth weight, percentage practicing family planning by each contraception method, crude death rate, age-specific death rates, and cause-specific maternal and under-5 mortality rates.

Many developed and developing countries employ home-based maternal records. A review (Shah et al., 1993) of experience in eight countries (Egypt, India, Pakistan, Philippines, Senegal, Sri Lanka, Yemen, and Zambia) showed that the records increased people's participation in their own care, stimulated timely and appropriate intervention if a problem developed, encouraged continuity of care throughout the woman's reproductive cycle, linked various health care facilities, and taught beneficiaries. Although indicators of antenatal risk were only weakly predictive, the information system successfully increased mothers' knowledge of pregnancy-related danger signs. Such forms tracked health status and guided response at the individual and the community level. WHO has suggested register headings to capture key aggregated community information from individuals' records, including tetanus vaccination, prenatal care, postnatal care coverage, and birth outcome (WHO, 1994).

The search for simple, reliable, acceptable, affordable, and valid indicators continues in the field of child development. A WHO collaborative study (Lansdown et al., 1996) recently determined 13 to 19 key psychosocial milestone indicators for children in China, India, and Thailand. Not surprisingly, the items varied across cultures and between rural and urban settings. While the indicators (which were studied among 28,139 children) await further validation, they are being incorporated into the child home-based records. There are several pertinent points: the list of useful health indicators will remain a work in progress; indicators may not be identical among different communities; indicators guide both personal and community decisions; and experience will refine the value of indicators.

Data collection

Save the Children/USA serves as an illustrative case. Its population-based community information systems attempt to resolve the tension inherent in balancing efficiency and equity. In brief, the system serves six levels of information users (Table 25). Each user is also an information provider to all levels. The flow and use of information throughout the system are accomplished with the help of several data collection instruments (Table 26): cards, forms, rosters, registers, and reports. The information may be transmitted and stored orally, in writing, and electronically. The instruments support and are guided by a series of information "activities" (Table 27) which in toto describe the population-based

Table 25 *Levels of health information users*

1. Families
2. Resident home visitors (health workers/volunteers)
3. Supervisors and community leaders
4. Health coordinators and district health officers
5. Field office directors and ministries of health
6. Home office staff and donors

Source: Save the Children/USA.

Table 26 *Data collection instruments**

- Home-based records: *immunization card, growth-monitoring card, home visit card, women's health card*
- Visitor-based reports: *pregnancy/birth card, death report form, child roster, and women's roster,* training session attendance form, visitor's work form
- Supervisor- and community-based records: *supervisor's roster*
- Impact-area or district-based records: *family enrollment forms, birth registers, death registers, migration reports,* reports from home visitors' rosters and from *supervisors' rosters*
- Field office- and ministry of health-based records: summary reports of health outputs and population health status
- Home office- and donor-based reports of health project outputs and population health status

Source: Save the Children/USA.
*Instruments in italics are discussed in the text. These forms are representative only. All forms are not used in all settings, and some programmes have developed different forms.

Table 27 *Health information activities and level*

Community:
— Promote community demand for health information;
— map and house numbering;
— enroll each family;
— count the population from the enrollment forms; identify age–sex profile;
— create children's and women's rosters, copying their names from enrollment forms;
— create and distribute the home-based instruments.

Resident home visitors:
— Visit homes regularly to promote health behaviours, to update rosters from home-based instruments, and to report pregnancies, births, deaths, migrations.

Supervisors:
— Supervise resident home visitors and monitor project output through rosters; control information quality through supervised visits to samples of homes; report achievements and remaining work to families and resident home visitors;
— collect reports of pregnancies, births, deaths, and migrations from resident home visitors;
— report results of supervision at regular intervals to coordinators and district health officers;
— register reports of births and deaths: report vital events monthly to families, resident home visitors, and community leaders; analyse birth and death rates by population group: report results of analysis at least annually to all levels.

Coordinator and local management:
— Computerize data, if applicable, for more frequent, complete, and detailed reporting;
— summarize monitoring and supervision reports at quarterly intervals and report to all levels with appropriate commentary concerning the programmatic implications of the findings.

Source: Save the Children/USA.

community health information system. The activities involve characterizing the population; identifying risk groups; reaching each household with health information and services; assuring services of good quality; empowering each mother to act on her own and her children's behalf; maintaining an accurate characterization of a dynamic community; and measuring programme effects in terms of coverage, behaviour change, and vital rate change.

Just as the health system responds to information gleaned from the whole community, so the health information system must be capable of providing this. Family enrolment forms proved to be an effective data collection instrument completed during a baseline census. Data collectors allot each mother and her children one form on which they note each family member's name, birth date, sex, relationship to head of household, immunization status, and optional socioeconomic data such as education and occupation. The aggregated family enrolment data provide an instantaneous glimpse of the age–sex composition of the community.

Certain segments of the population are biologically at high risk and thus targeted by primary health care: women of child-bearing age and children under 5 years. The family enrolment forms guide assembly of women's rosters and children's rosters. Resident home visitors use these notebooks to identify individuals at high risk and to track interventions on their behalf. For example, the women's roster includes identification number, name, birth date, birth-spacing training, and details for three successive pregnancies. The child roster includes identification number, mother's name, child's name, birth date, immunization dates, completed vaccination status, and growth monitoring.

Vital events inevitably change the community structure, and the one-time family enrolment will need revision. Resident home visitors can keep the information up to date by completing vital event cards. The death report form includes identifying data, date of death, date of completion, cause of death, and immunization status. The pregnancy/birth card contains mother's identifying data, expected date of delivery, reminders for at least three prenatal visits, immunization reminders, and outcome. The migration reports note the details of moves within the impact area or permanent migrations into or out of the area. These vital events require ongoing updating of family enrolment forms and rosters.

The Save the Children/USA project takes advantage of the ultimate "health worker" residing in the household: the mother. She uses several health information systems instruments. She has a women's card to track her health history, especially the reproductive and family planning aspects. Each child has an immunization card (often provided by the government) documenting all immunizations. Likewise, each has a growth card or road to health card which records the weights periodically measured during the first years of life. Often these two cards are combined into a single instrument. The home visit card, one per family, records the date, training content, and ancillary observations of each household visit by the resident home visitor.

Just as resident home visitors need to remind mothers to receive prenatal care and to obtain immunizations for their children, so supervisors need to support the resident home visitors in performing their activities. The supervisor's roster focuses the supervisor's attention on areas and individuals most in need of support. For each resident home visitor, it

Table 28   *Community-based health information system: examples of levels, users, uses, and supervision**

Level	User	Instrument	Question	Periodicity	Quality control
Household	Mother	Immunization card	Which child needs which vaccine, when?	Continuous	RHV tracks vaccine schedule of each child
Household	Resident home visitor	Home visit card	What health promotion activities do I need to stress with this family today?	Quarterly	Supervisor notes proportion of children whose mothers have received ORT training on supervisor's roster
Neighbourhood service area	Resident home visitor	Death report form	Who died, when, and of what?	Quarterly and as needed	Supervisor compares expected to reported deaths on supervisor's roster
Neighbourhood service area	Resident home visitor	Child roster	Who are the children in my neighbourhood service area?	Continuous and quarterly	Supervisor compares reported visits to actual numbers of children under 5
Community	Supervisor	Child roster	What is the measles vaccine coverage in this zone?	Quarterly and annually	Health project coordinator compares with coverage data from baseline family enrollment
Impact area	Health project coordinator	Death registers and birth registers	What is the infant mortality rate in the impact area?	Annually	Donors, home office, and ministry officials compare to baseline and official national statistics

*Assumes a quarterly household visiting schedule.
ORT = oral rehydration therapy; RHV = resident home visitor.

lists the number of children followed; reported and expected births; reported and expected deaths; mothers trained and yet to be trained in oral rehydration therapy; children completely and not completely immunized; children weighed and not weighed; children gaining and not gaining; and children visited and not visited.

Table 28 provides additional examples of the interplay between users, instruments, and activities. More than one user can access the instrument at the same level; for example, both the mother and the resident home visitor use the immunization card to decide who needs immunizations. Also, the frequency of each activity varies with its urgency, and quality control checks are integrated for each example. What is lacking in this schema, however, are the explicit decisions based on the information. Table 29 details some of the decisions generated from village health promoters' (equivalent to resident home visitors) rosters in a Malawi child survival programme.

Data transmission

The extent of data transmission depends on the context. The Warmi project noted above sought community-based solutions for a geographically isolated setting; thus data transmission beyond the community was limited. However, no matter how constrained the setting, all information systems involve at least two layers: the point of contact and the aggregate. The contact point in population-based community health systems is often a household visit, but it may be a service-based contact as in a

Table 29 *Chilipa impact area health information system at the village health promoter level*

Information	Information source	Information frequency	Decision	Information flow	Flow frequency	Supervision and frequency
<5 growth static	village GM by VHP	monthly	home visit	monthly report	monthly	HSA, 2–3/months
<5 growth faltering	village GM by VHP	monthly	refer to HC	monthly report	monthly	HSA, 2–3/months
<5 behind on immunizations	transferred from RTA from <5 outreach clinics	monthly	refer to HC or outreach	monthly report	monthly	HSA, 2–3/months
<5 died	common village knowledge	as needed	home visit for verbal autopsy	death report and monthly report	monthly	HSA, 2–3/months
>5 years of age	from birth date recorded at enrollment	monthly	cross out name			HSA, 2–3/months
Birth	common village knowledge	as needed	home visit	enroll in roster, birth report, and monthly report	monthly	HSA, 2–3/months
Lacking education in ORT, WASH, AIDS, FP, etc.	roster	as needed	home visit to teach and urge to attend health education	number trained by content into monthly report	monthly	HSA, 2–3/months
WRA pregnant	common village knowledge	as needed	home visit to recommend ANC	monthly report	monthly	HSA, 2–3/months
WRA behind on TTV	TTV card	as needed	home visit to recommend ANC	monthly report	monthly	HSA, 2–3/months
Pregnancy outcome	home visit and common knowledge	as needed	home visit to recommend PPC	monthly report	monthly	HSA, 2–3/months
Lacking perinatal training	roster	as needed	home visit to train	monthly report	monthly	HSA, 2–3/months

Source: Save the Children/USA's child survival programme in Mangochi District, Malawi.
ANC = antenatal care; FP = family planning; GM = growth monitoring; HC = health centre; HSA = health surveillance assistant; ORT = oral rehydration therapy; PPC = postpartum care; RTA = road traffic accident; TTV = tetanus toxoid vaccine; VHP = village health promoter; WASH = water, sanitation, and hygiene; WRA = women of reproductive age.

contraceptive distribution or a facility-based distribution as in a revolving drug fund managed by a village health committee.

On the other hand, in Malawi, a private voluntary organization is collaborating with the Ministry of Health to transform its population-based community health information system into a districtwide sentinel surveillance system to monitor vital events, contraceptive prevalence, child nutrition, and other health events in rotation (Rubardt, 1996). Participating communities need the data from their village just as the district health officer needs the aggregated findings. Eventually, this may serve as a national model. Similarly, the Philippines piloted community health data boards in northern Mindanao as part of a larger national system, HAMIS (health and management information system) (Remotigue et al., 1994). These were intended to guide actions at the levels of household, *purok* (typically a 45-household community),

165

barangay (typically seven *puroks*), health station (the peripheral government facility serving typically three *barangays*), municipality, and Ministry of Health. Although they were widely implemented between 1991 and 1993, few community data boards remain. Nonetheless, the model remains a rare example of a seamless information system from household to district and beyond.

Data processing

Data processing at the individual level involves comparing individual variables with a desired state. Data processing at the community level involves computing sums, calculating proportions and percentages, and comparing these with target indicators. This is best done manually at the household and village levels. Indeed, the paper and pencil approach is well suited for aggregating tallies to calculate indicators using sub-tallies of multiple communities. The HAMIS community data board manual explains the four "C's": coding, counting, computing proportions, and combining values for aggregation, noting that the rural health midwife at the peripheral Ministry of Health facility performs 588 computations (28 indicators/*purok* × 21 *puroks*/facility) quarterly (Remotigue et al., 1994).

Computers offer certain advantages, including rapid, accurate manipulation of large quantities of data, easy subgroup analysis, compelling graphics, identification of variant values,[2] and even suggested programmatic response (Cibulskis et al., 1993). Of note, HAMIS (above) relied on computers for aggregation above the health centre level. Computerization should only be considered when the underlying manual system is functioning well. Moreover, not all problems benefit from computers, especially in settings of budgetary constraint, tenuous electrical supply, scant technical support, and extraordinary training demands. On the other hand, there are many health and demographic surveillance software programs available.[3] However, none of them is completely "bug"-free or meets all users' needs. Two are highlighted here: ProMIS, a demographic and health software (see Box 25), and the Deschapelles "facility- and community-based health and demographic software", which offers an exciting look to the future (see Box 26). A third case notes how a poor, rural community (plus some rather extraordinary circumstances) opted to computerize its immunization data.

Computers can play central roles in many aspects of population-based community health programmes: disease surveillance, management, information sciences, research, policy guidance, and demographic surveillance for equity. Managers must weigh their pros and cons. As the information age permeates the global village, the pros will loom ever larger.

---

[2] The PHC-MAP series (module 5, *Monitoring and evaluating programmes*) includes programmable spreadsheets which identify values exceeding user-determined thresholds.

[3] Examples include The Population Council's (NY, USA) *Household registration system* currently used in Navrongo (Ghana), Conlan Associates' (Farmington, CT, USA) *Health registration system*, Save the Children's (Westport, CT, USA) *ProMIS* as well as software developed in other settings, including Hôpital Albert Schweitzer in Deschapelles and Cité de Soleil in Port-au-Prince (Haiti), Matlab (Bangladesh), and the Health Systems Development Unit of the University of Witwatersrand for Agincourt.

Box 25   ProMIS

Save the Children/USA has designed a public domain health information software package, ProMIS (programme management information system). This population-based tool manages census data and monitors indicators, and is well-suited for most settings with a fully functioning manual family enrollment system.

Core data collected during family enrollment include location identification number, full name, date of birth, sex, and relationship in the family. Vital events (births, deaths, and migrations) to track population movements are entered on a routine basis. ProMIS can produce longitudinal descriptive statistics, such as crude and age-specific natality and mortality rates. In addition to the demographic core, ProMIS stores other information specific to individuals in the population in various modules, such as child immunization, growth promotion, pregnancy monitoring, and cause of death. As for the demographic data, ProMIS also prepares statistical reports based on these health indicators, such as rates of immunization, cause-specific mortality, and malnutrition. Moreover, through an accompanying feature, users can define their own modules to track additional variables of interest. Programmes have often added family planning-, vitamin A-, and/or acute respiratory infection-related indicators. Planning for educational and microenterprise indicators is ongoing.

An additional key feature of ProMIS is its ability to produce rosters of individuals meeting user-specified criteria. For example, ProMIS will generate a list of children under age 5 with their vaccination status or a list of women of child-bearing age and their pregnancy outcome histories. These lists are central to direct care to those at greatest risk.

Additional ProMIS features include (i) pull-down menus and on-screen windows; (ii) data storage in dBASE-type files; (iii) data-exporting utility common to statistical software packages for more detailed analysis; (iv) language independence with French-, Spanish-, and English-language files built in; and (v) error-checking utility. ProMIS will run on an IBM-compatible 286 (or faster) computer. A programmer is not required.

Feedback and use

Without feedback and use at the local level, the "community" system is merely extractive and short-lived. Feedback is usually spoken and/or graphically displayed. Each method has various forms. Community health committees or health boards are common receptors of health information. Often community leaders take part in such fora and then pass on the information through traditional channels, including village meetings, religious leaders, women's groups, and farmers' clubs.

Graphically displayed information takes many forms. The Aga Khan University piloted community growth charts on which weights of all children were plotted. This reinforced families' understanding of the different growth channels as well as boldly highlighted the extent of malnutrition so as to mobilize response. The Warmi MotherCare Project again used the Bolivian flag colours with which to make a coloured

---

**Box 26   Linking community-based and facility-based
health information systems in rural Haiti**

W Billingsley, Hôpital Albert Schweitzer, Deschapelles, Haiti

The Hôpital Albert Schweitzer (HAS) serves a defined population of approximately
200,000 within a 610-square-mile intervention zone in rural Haiti, 90 miles north-
east of Port-au-Prince. The hospital maintains a community health and development department to administer six outlying dispensaries, a veterinary medicine unit,
community health and nutrition surveillance, and a unit to implement wells, water,
irrigation projects, and other health-related agricultural activities.

In 1993 the hospital initiated a practical information system to provide data for decision making for the board of directors and its professional staff. Motivated by equity
and accountability, the goal of the system was to strengthen planning through tracking health (both population-based community preventive and hospital/dispensary-
based curative) and demographic events. The key to accomplishing this task was
to register every individual within the hospital's district, assigning a unique identifier
to each that allowed linking the population-based and facility-based data sets. This
family registration resulted in a manual roster for each defined locality within the
HAS district. Health agents used the rosters to record vital and health events in
their locality, such as births, deaths, immunizations, vitamin A distribution, family
planning, and nutritional status. These rosters have helped to increase the immunization coverage rates from approximately 45% to 85% within a 2-year period.

The computerization of these manual data allowed merging the facility-based and
population-based data. This, in turn, has strengthened individual and community
assessment and treatment in the HAS district. For example, for the patient at an
HAS facility diagnosed with or exposed to tuberculosis, a report can be printed of
all persons residing within that person's household, including the tuberculosis
status of each. The health agent responsible for that household uses the printout
to guide follow-up. Moreover, the integrated database also allows calculating
disease-specific incidence and prevalence rates by community, since ICD-9 codes
are used throughout the HAS district.

Needed steps include linking the laboratory data and a more detailed death report,
including direct, indirect, and underlying cause of death. The health information
system is a model for a comprehensive, integrated curative and preventive health
system.

"mountain", a band for each malnutrition category. Rural Haitians,
accustomed to round flat bread, intuitively understand "pie" charts and
the proportions they represent. World Relief (see Box 27) is currently
field testing an interesting version of culturally sensitive bar charts.
Method of presentation makes a difference. Rink, Swan & Stansfield
(1993) reported that rural Malawians grasped a proportion better
through measures of beans than through pie charts. They suggested that
everyday objects are preferable for demonstrations.

One innovative strategy, the Philippines' HAMIS community data board,
deserves special comment. Constructed on a 4 × 8ft sheet of plywood,
the permanent board includes a map of the community, a title, a key,

---

Box 27   Community-based, practical health information systems for Mozambique and Honduras

O Wollinka, World Relief

World Relief's 1995 child survival project in Mozambique's Mabalane and Guija Districts (total population approximately 125,000) seeks longitudinal, population-based, health information for community action. What are the chances of success in a setting of such extreme poverty relying on preliterate volunteers? Key operational tactics are likely to allow the information system to both be feasible and to save lives. These include (i) simple preliterate forms with pictures which require dots rather than numbers; (ii) limiting each volunteer's catchment area to 10 families; (iii) limiting data collection to every third monthly home visit; (iv) supplementing counts with routine qualitative community-based inquiries to explain findings and pretest programme responses; (v) presenting coverage findings to communities through simple "coverage graphics" (i.e. covering a sketch of children or households, as appropriate, with a darkened transparency representing the proportion protected by the relevant service); and (vi) monitoring key indicators with back-up, mid-term, population-based surveys.

Corresponding strategies in a child survival project in the Francisco Morazan and El Paraiso Departments of Honduras (total population approximately 50,000) include (i) integration with the Ministry of Health's system, including its forms; (ii) adopting a sentinel household-based system for quarterly tracking of project objectives; (iii) prompt feedback to the community through growth-monitoring sessions, supplemented by posted graphs of key indicators introduced sequentially; and (iv) selecting "attendance at growth-monitoring session" as the first graphed indicator to enhance the likelihood of greater participation at subsequent feedback sessions.

---

and a house-shaped data card for each of the (approximately) 45 households. These "roofed squares" are 2 to 3 inches on a side, with five rows (one for each quarter and total) and nine columns (one for each health concern). Each quarter, a household visit determines the status of each concern according to predetermined definitions (green = safe, yellow = improving, red = danger, blue = not applicable), and the data cards are coloured in. Relying on a strategy of "social pressure", these publicly placed data boards motivate individuals to "catch up with their neighbours". Moreover, the household level data are then counted and transformed into indicators which are posted as coloured pie charts in every community and health facility.

Literate groups and especially cultures familiar with targets from past or current command economies often readily understand more abstract data presentations, including bar charts, graphs, and even tables of counts and percentages. A poverty alleviation and nutrition programme in rural Viet Nam (Stornin, Sternin & Marsh, 1996) worked through the existing socialist community infrastructure, the head of which was the commune's Communist Party chairman. Graphical data displays and carefully crafted tables literally transformed party headquarters.

Decisions based on collected, transmitted, analysed, and "fed-back" data are as varied as the contexts from which they stem. Tables 25 and 26 list some examples. Decisions from Bolivia's Warmi project (Howard-Grabman, Seoane & Davenport, 1994) included requesting a town ambulance, implementing creative payment schemes for complicated deliveries, initiating family gardens to improve mothers' nutrition, and instituting adolescent sex education. A clustering of reported diarrhoea episodes in Deschapelles, Haiti, resulted in identification and control of a contaminated water source (Berggren, personal communication, 1996). A similar outbreak in Pakistan's Northern Areas (see Box 22) proved to be cholera. It was met with massive community education, strengthening of peripheral facilities' ability to handle severe dehydration, and disinfecting household water containers. Health volunteers in a malnutrition alleviation programme (Sternin, Sternin & Marsh, 1996) in Thanh Hoa Province (Viet Nam) discontinued home-based group nutritional rehabilitation when the prevalence of severe malnutrition dropped below 5% since household visits were more cost-effective than 2-week classes for small numbers of children. A Filipino man, Camiguin, constructed a toilet when he compared his household's "red" marker to those of his neighbours in the HAMIS project (Remotigue et al., 1994). The Aga Khan University implemented injury surveillance when an adult mortality review indicated road traffic accidents high among causes of male deaths and burns high among causes of female deaths (Marsh et al., unpublished, 1996). The health volunteers of Dur Mohammad Goth opted to identify and track all newborns to improve their immunization coverage (see Box 28).

Monitoring the information system

Kaye and Galvao (1995) provide helpful supervisory techniques such as enrollment validation surveys to measure coverage, tables comparing observed and expected vital events to highlight variance, and linking pregnancy and birth tallies to identify possible data gaps. Their case of interpreting infant mortality details the many threats to validity that the programme manager confronts during the analysis and interpretation of key vital indicators. Lot quality assessment (Galvao & Kaye, 1994) is a useful technique to quickly identify community health workers who need further support in maintaining complete and up-to-date health information records.

Beyond validating an information system's data are questions of its efficiency. Are the data used? Is the effort worth the cost? Useful questions for district health management teams' problem solving are: Which health data actually drive decisions? If we could obtain only 3 (or 5 or 10) indicators, which would they be? How could we improve the completeness, validity, timeliness, analysis, and response to each of these essential indicators?

Conclusion

Population-based community health information systems grew from a need to achieve equity in health in a participatory, accountable way. Advocates of social justice seek to provide services to those most underserved and to empower the powerless. The planning cycle of community diagnosis, risk group identification, response implementation, and monitoring rely on population-based community health information systems. Problem identification is guided by local ecology, community perceptions, and baseline census supplemented by other surveys. Risk group identification directly depends on the baseline census and longitudinally

---

Box 28   Community computers and immunization information in rural Karachi

A Javed Khan, The Aga Khan University

Dur Mohammad Goth is a periurban Balochi community of about 1500 persons an hour's drive outside metropolitan Karachi. The majority of its inhabitants continue to derive livelihood from agriculture. Local volunteer community health workers, with assistance from volunteer medical staff from the Government Civil Hospital in Karachi city, have run a maternal and child health clinic since 1982. The programme emphasized primary health care, especially immunization services.

After 10 years of operation, the community health workers suspected that many children from Dur Mohammad Goth and seven surrounding villages were missing immunizations. This suspicion was raised by survey findings from the Adventist Relief and Development Agency and heightened after the village was the site of a 1993 health system evaluation exercise by a supervised batch of final year medical students from the Aga Khan University. Meanwhile, one volunteer had received some training in computers during previous work in Karachi city. Thus, the volunteers decided to create a computer database of all children born since 1983 in these eight villages, monitor immunization status, and actively locate underimmunized children.

A census of the eight villages and vaccination records at the maternal and child health clinic in Dur Mohammad Goth provided the baseline information. Health workers eagerly learned to enter the data into Epi Info and to run simple frequencies and programmes to generate monthly reports. Indeed, initial immunization coverage was below 30% for the third dose of DPT (diphtheria-pertussis-tetanus) at 6 months and for measles at 9 months. This information prompted programme managers and community health workers to make the following decisions: (i) maintain the Epi Info immunization database as part of the primary health care programme, (ii) actively identify and immunize newborns according to schedule, (iii) actively identify and immunize children who missed their scheduled immunizations, (iv) encourage new health workers to learn Epi Info data entry and analysis, and (v) expand this service to 18 other villages in the area.

Immunization coverage (appropriate for age) between 1994 and 1996 was above 95% for BCG and the third dose of DPT and above 90% for measles.

tracking vital events and identifying pregnancies. Programme implementation rests on specifying individuals and individual groups for services as well as supporting individual workers and programme components as needed through analysing the appropriate aggregations and breakdowns of information. Programme monitoring and evaluation include many of the implementation activities as well as reviewing population level indicators to measure coverage as well as health outcomes. The central role of a population-based community information system at each step is apparent, all while demonstrating responsible stewardship before beneficiaries, intervention teams, peers, government colleagues, and donors. Population-based community health programmes and information systems may be the "worst systems—except for all the others", This aphorism, borrowed from Winston Churchill's defence of democracy, is fitting. Indeed, a population-based community health information system is admittedly a political venture based on those democratic principles which are increasingly valued and widely, and perhaps universally, applicable.

Open questions

Despite a global climate which is increasingly favourable to democratic principles, the health situation for huge regions and groups of people does not match expectations. Private voluntary organizations have taken the lead in health information systems which track individuals because of equity. But radically different systems or slightly modified ones may reach similar ends. We urge others to consider the following, and other, questions.

- How much equity can be achieved without a population-based community health information system?

This is a fundamental question. Are there communities or settings where facility-based or service-based or "other-based" health systems and information systems will achieve equity in health? In other terms, must we have household level services?

- How much can we streamline population-based community health information systems?

Invariably, start-up experience with household level information systems is overloaded with information. Even when managers know to expect this and try to avoid such overload, it often happens anyway. How can we reward managers who achieve the same results with fewer numbers and reprimand (gently) those who do not? The stakes are not trivial. Too much information deflects resources. It distracts and possibly demoralizes workers. One recent suggestion is to eliminate columns for the date of each child's individual immunization on household-level workers' rosters, substituting a single column for completed immunization. Should a health worker want the details, he could look in the local immunizer's roster. How many other columns can we eliminate?

- How can we focus, expand, and refine the target group?

Epidemiology, economics, and ethics compel us to define target groups that validly reflect the distribution of risk in a community. We commonly do not progress far beyond the census-based age–sex determinants: children under 5 years and women of reproductive age. Vitamin A distribution includes those in the 6th year. Promoting child nutrition may be best focused on those under 3 years. Beyond these are strategies to limit target groups to pregnant women and their young offspring. While this has the appeal of decreasing initial workload, the ultimate target group could potentially become as large as that identified by the traditional targeting strategy. Alternatively, the age risk factor could be narrowed while adding non-age factors, such as extreme poverty, previous child death, orphanhood, and the like. Village health committees could guide identifying households in need of additional services.

- What is the relationship between population-based community health information systems and research?

We have justified in part population-based information systems because they support research. At the same time we have shown that information is not always complete or correct, as shown by special studies. Moreover, some of the objectives of a population-based community health system are achieved by its information system somewhat irrespective of its accuracy. Where does research fit here? One dictum might be that until the information has reached the validity threshold for decision-making, research should not be contemplated. Another might be that information systems without paid household level workers are unlikely to achieve sufficient validity for research. Information collecting is resource-intensive.

- How do we invert the data collection/data response ratio?

Vast effort is spent in collecting, aggregating, analysing, and displaying data. Far less effort is devoted to interpreting the data and to making data-driven decisions. Analysis often is limited to such activities as transforming counts into rates, ratios, or proportions; it does not refer to explaining the result.

- Can more communities design, implement, and manage their own information systems?

Externally funded health and development programmes have many stakeholders to please. The information system, in part, serves the needs of funders who desire accountability from implementors on behalf of their donors. Many population-based community information systems are externally designed and managed or, at best, comanaged. Communities, on the other hand, probably need less rigorous systems. A woman's group that monitored a village's perinatal deaths might enhance safe motherhood more than volunteers' systematic mobilization of women for prenatal care as guided by rosters. Simpler, less precise systems may ultimately be more empowering. The crucial question then becomes, How can communities be convinced of the value and feasibility of data for decision making at the community level?

Acknowledgements

The author is indebted to Drs Jack Bryant, John Wyon, Warren Berggren, and Raj Arole for operationalizing "information for equity" and to Drs Theo Lippeveld and Steve Sapirie for their careful manuscript review and their suggesting numerous innovative government examples of community health information systems.

References

Abelin T, Brzezinski ZJ, Carstairs VDL (1987). *Measurement in health promotion and protection*. Copenhagen, WHO Regional Office for Europe: 635–642 (European Series, No. 22).

Abramson JH, Kark SL (1983). Community oriented primary care: meaning and scope. In: Connor E, Mullan F, eds. *Community oriented primary care: new directions for health services delivery*. Washington, DC, National Academy Press.

Arole M, Arole R (1994). *Jamkhed*. London, Macmillan.

Berggren WL, Ewbank DC, Berggren GG (1981). Reduction of mortality in rural Haiti through a primary-health-care program. *New England journal of medicine*, 304:1324–1330.

Bryant JH et al. (1993). A developing country's university oriented toward strengthening health systems: challenges and results. *American journal of public health*, 83:1537–1543.

Cibulskis RE et al. (1993). A knowledge-based system for monitoring immunization coverage in Papua, New Guinea. *International journal of health planning and management*, 8:59–69.

Commission on Behavioral and Social Sciences (1993). *Effects of health programs on child mortality in sub-saharan Africa.* Washington, DC, National Academy Press.

Daniel K (1990). *Measuring health—a practical guide to establishing a health information system.* Westport, CT, Save the Children: 45–78.

Darras C, Van Lerberghe W, Mercenier P (1982). *The Kasongo Project: lessons of an experiment in the organisation of a system of primary health care.* Antwerp, Public Health Research and Teaching Unit of the Prince Leopold Institute of Tropical Medicine, 9.

Dunn FL (1973). Limitations of epidemiographic surveillance. In: Frederiksen HS et al. *Epidemiographic surveillance: a symposium.* Chapel Hill, Carolina Population Center, University of North Carolina: 29–34 (Monograph 13).

Franco LM et al. (1993). *Monitoring and evaluating programmes.* Washington, DC, Aga Khan Foundation USA.

Frederiksen HS (1973). Epidemographic surveillance. In: Frederiksen HS et al. *Epidemiographic surveillance: a symposium.* Chapel Hill, Carolina Population Center, University of North Carolina: 1–28 (Monograph 13).

Galvao L, Kaye K (1994). Using lot quality assessment techniques to evaluate quality of data in a population-based community health information system. *Tropical doctor*, 24:149–151.

Royal Thai Government (1988). *Health and social development in Thailand.* Bangkok, Royal Thai Government.

Howard-Grabman L, Seoane G, Davenport CA (1994). *The Warmi project: a participatory approach to improve maternal and neonatal health—an implementor's manual.* Arlington, John Snow.

Institute of Medicine: Committee of Community Oriented Primary Care (1984). *Community oriented primary care: a practical assessment*, vols 1 and 2. Washington, DC, National Academy Press.

Interregional Meeting on Lay Reporting in Information Support to HFA Strategy Management, Manila, Philippines, 8–15 October 1985 (1985). Geneva, World Health Organization (unpublished document DES/LR/HFA/85. REPORT, Add. 1; available on request from Department of Health Systems, World Health Organization, 1211 Geneva 27, Switzerland).

Kaye K, Galvao L (1995). Management tools for improving the quality of health information in systems based on full enrollment and sentinel surveillance. In: Marsh DR et al., eds. *Everyone counts: population-based community health information systems—a reference compendium on the collection, analysis, and use of data for accountability in health.* Westport, CT, Save the Children.

Kielmann AA et al. (1983). *Child and maternal health services in rural India. The Narangwal experiment*, vols 1 and 2. Baltimore, Johns Hopkins University Press.

Lansdown RG et al. (1996). Culturally appropriate measures for monitoring child development at family and community level: a WHO collaborative study. *Bulletin of the World Health Organization*, 74:282–290.

Nondasuta A, Piyarata P (1987). Basic minimum needs. *World Health*, 14–15.

Remotigue T et al. (1994). *Health databoards for communities.* Manila, Department of Health, Republic of the Philippines and GTZ.

Rink B, Swan S, Stansfield SK (1993). Communicating coverage data with non-literate communities: beans, sticks, or pie charts? *Health policy and planning*, 8:57–60.

Rubardt M (1996). Sustainable population-based community health information systems in Mangochi, Malawi. Paper to be presented at American Public Health Association.

Save the Children (1992). *Program reports.* Westport, CT, Save the Children.

Shah PM et al. (1993). Evaluation of the home-based maternal record: a WHO collaborative study, *Bulletin of the World Health Organization,* 71:535–548.

Showstack J et al. (1992). Health of the public: the academic response. *Journal of the American Medical Association,* 267:2497–2502.

Sternin M, Sternin J, Marsh DR (1996). Rapid, sustained childhood malnutrition alleviation through a "positive deviance" approach in rural Viet Nam: preliminary findings. In: *Proceedings of Technical Advisory Group: The "foyer" method and child nutrition.* Carol Stream, IL.

Taylor CE (1973). Epidemographic surveillance and family planning. In: Frederiksen HS et al. *Epidemiographic surveillance: a symposium.* Chapel Hill, Carolina Population Center, University of North Carolina: 62–65 (Monograph 13).

Taylor CE (1992). Surveillance for equity in primary health care: policy implications from international experience. *International journal of epidemiology,* 21:1043–1048.

Tollman S (1991). Community oriented primary care: origins, evolution, applications, *Social science and medicine,* 32:633–642.

Unger JP, Dujardin B (1992). Epidemiology's contribution to health service management and planning in developing countries: a missing link. *Bulletin of the World Health Organization,* 70:487–497.

UNICEF (1991). *State of the world's children—1991.* New York, Oxford University Press.

UNICEF (1994). *Guide to filling the vital horoscope and extracting various indices.* Tehran, Ministry of Health and Medical Education.

White KL, JE Connelly (1991). The medical school's mission and the population's health. *Annals of Internal Medicine,* 115:968–972.

World Federation for Medical Education (1993). Edinburgh Declaration. *Medical Education* (suppl.).

World Health Organization (1978). *Report of the International Conference on Primary Health Care; 6–12 September; Alma Ata, USSR.* Geneva, World Health Organization.

World Health Organization (1994). *Home-based maternal records—guidelines for development, adaptation and evaluation.* Geneva, World Health Organization.

Wray JD (1973). A health information and service system. In: Frederiksen HS et al. *Epidemiographic surveillance: a symposium.* Chapel Hill, Carolina Population Center, University of North Carolina (Monograph 13).

Wyon JB (1973). Appropriate and effective health services in developing regions. In: Frederiksen HS et al. *Epidemiographic surveillance; a symposium.* Chapel Hill, Carolina Population Center, University of North Carolina: 62–65 (Monograph 13).

Wyon JB, Gordon JE (1971). *The Khanna study—population problems in the rural Punjab.* Cambridge, MA, Harvard University Press.

Wyon JB (1994). In Perry H. *The census-based, impact-oriented approach to child survival and its application by Andean Rural Health Care,* 86–93.

Zayan A, Berggren W, Doumbia F (1992). *The price of immunization and the value of information.* Westport, CT, Save the Children.

Management of health information systems

Eckhard Kleinau

Introduction

While information needs drive the design of health information systems—sometimes even beyond a sustainable level of sophistication—resource considerations are equally important in health information system design and implementation. As mentioned in Chapter 2, no two health information systems are alike, because needs and resources differ within every country. But conceptually, all health information systems need a management structure. This management structure includes a minimum of two components: health information system resources and organizational rules (see Fig. 19). The development of these components is country-specific and will vary in breadth and depth. Critical resources to consider include personnel, supplies, computer hardware and software, and financial resources. Organizational rules are necessary to ensure optimum use of health information system resources.

This chapter discusses health information system resources and organizational rules, including structures and procedures, essential for an effective and sustainable health information system.

Resource requirements

The design and implementation of a health information system should be driven not only by the perceived need for routine information, but also by available resources. A health information system succeeds or fails due to resource constraints at both the primary care level (the most important point of data collection in most countries) and the immediate support level (the district). Using the need for resources at the national level as a yardstick can easily result in an overly complex and ineffective system. Furthermore, donor funding, while often available for the design and implementation of a health information system, is not a reliable financial source for routine operations, and should thus not determine the complexity of a health information system.

For the same reason, prior to discussing detailed resource requirements, two resource scenarios are presented which take account of different economic means available to individual countries. The first, low-budget scenario assumes that very limited public resources are available for health information system personnel and operating costs. The second, high-budget scenario assumes that the public sector has sufficient resources to support a health information system with larger and more educated staffing at the peripheral and district levels, and extensive computer use at all support levels. In this high-budget scenario, managers and health

Fig. 19   *Elements of health information system (HIS) management*

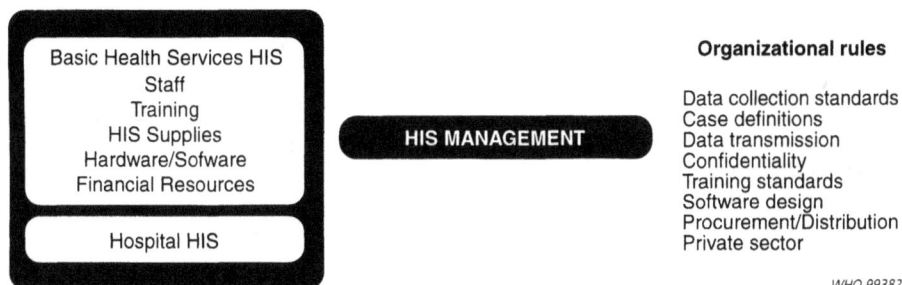

```
┌─────────────────────────────────┐
│  Basic Health Services HIS      │
│          Staff                  │
│        Training                 │            HIS MANAGEMENT
│      HIS Supplies               │
│     Hardware/Sofware            │
│     Financial Resources         │
│                                 │
│        Hospital HIS             │
└─────────────────────────────────┘
```

Organizational rules

Data collection standards
Case definitions
Data transmission
Confidentiality
Training standards
Software design
Procurement/Distribution
Private sector

WHO 99382

care planners would be prudent to emphasize more intensive use of the information provided by a health information system with a simple design, rather than trying to implement a health information system with a complex design that could ultimately use up resources and be difficult to operate effectively.

These resource scenarios determine the design and implementation of the various components of the information-generating process, such as data collection, data processing, and information feedback. Components can be scaled according to the resources (i.e. more or less staff time and training) or need not be fully implemented (i.e. routine data collection and a few rapid assessments, but no large surveys). Most countries will fit somewhere between the two extremes described by the budget scenarios. A summary of health information system resource requirements by resource level is shown in Table 30. Detailed cost calculations are provided later in this chapter in Tables 31, 32, 33, and 34.

Staff positions, roles, and responsibilities

In many countries, cumbersome data collection processes are typical for a health information system. Nurses can take several days to complete required reports—valuable time that could be spent caring for clients and patients. Therefore, in determining staff resources for health information system-related activities, it helps to remember that improving the health status of individuals and populations through the delivery of curative and preventive services and health promotion is the primary task of medical and paramedical personnel.

Primary care facility

In managing the effective delivery of curative and preventive services, clinical staff should spend only as much time as necessary on administrative tasks, including those for a health information system (Box 29). Collecting data that can and should be used by a facility to maintain and improve service delivery is an essential health information system function; collecting additional data can easily result in a waste of scarce human resources.

Facilities and offices at all support levels require staff that are responsible for health information system-related activities, but whether these activities are performed by the care providers themselves or by full-time dedicated staff depends upon the budget scenario and service characteristics (Kleinau et al., 1995). Primary care providers generally do not need dedicated staff, with the exception of large facilities. For patient/client

177

Table 30 *Health information system resource requirements under low- and high-budget scenarios (in 1997 US$)*

Health information system structure	Low-budget scenario		High-budget scenario	
Annual operating budget level (normalized per facility covered by health information system, without referral level)*	total including salary costs	US$ 232	total including salary costs	US$ 3790
	without facility salary costs	112	without facility salary costs	790
	district/reg./national salary	40	district/reg./national salary	340
	training	19	training	132
	computers	6	computers	108
	basic operating costs†	47	basic operating costs†	210
Per capita GNP	US$ 300		US$ 1000 or higher	
Staff at primary care level	• Facilities have few staff (1–2) of mostly auxiliary level training • 1 person spends 10% on record keeping • Reporting and monitoring of a few (5) key indicators • Salaries are low ($ 100/month)		• Facilities have a wide range of staff with senior level training (nurse, clinical officer) • 2 persons spend 20% on record keeping • Reporting and monitoring of 5 or more key indicators • Salaries are high ($500 per month)	
Staff at first referral level	• Mostly small hospitals with 50–100 beds, low occupancy • Each unit keeps their own registers • 1 person spends 25% on basic reporting		• Medium-size hospitals with 100 or more beds, central admissions • Units keep additional registers • 1–2 full-time MIS staff, since reports can be extensive (including *International Classification of Diseases* reporting)	
District staff	• HIS functions carried out by 2 district staff with other duties at 20%(salary $300) • Compile monthly/quarterly reports from about 30 facilities, monitor key indicators, provide simple feedback, maintain simple coverage maps, participate in general supervision		• Districts have 2 staff who spend 50% on HIS and 50% on other monitoring and evaluation activities (salary $500), a total of 3 trained in HIS • Thoroughly analyse 30 monthly/quarterly facility reports, maintain district profiles, complete coverage plans, data quality checks, participate in other data collection/surveys	
Regional/national staff	• HIS information flows directly to the national level; regions might exist but play no separate HIS role • 6 national staff spend 50% on HIS activities (salary $500) • Programmes rely mainly on the HIS for information		• HIS information might flow through regional offices (assumed 5) or directly to national level • 2 staff per region spend 50% and 10 national staff work full-time on HIS (salary $1000), perform detailed geographic analyses, conduct operations research • Programmes might have dedicated staff for monitoring and evaluation to conduct additional data collection	
Staff training	• District and national staff have an initial 3-day training every 5 years and a 1-day refresher per year • Computer training: 2 weeks initial training, 2 days annual refresher		• Facility staff have a 3-day initial training every 3 years plus a 1-day refresher every year • District, regional, and national staff have a 5-day initial training every 3 years and a 3-day annual refresher • Computer training: 2 weeks initial training, 5 days annual refresher, LAN administration, user support	

Table 30 (continued)

Health information system structure	Low-budget scenario	High-budget scenario
Data collection instruments and supplies	• Minimum of 6 generic register books are used and adapted by hand for clinic activities • Monthly or quarterly reports cover essential data only and are preprinted with 2 duplicates (facility, district, national) • Tally sheets are either reusable or hand-drawn • Key indicators are monitored on plain or engineering paper	• Minimum of 6 preprinted registers or individual patient records are used for clinic activities • Monthly/quarterly reports are short and preprinted with two duplicates (facility, district, regional/ national) • Tally sheets are printed and distributed • Key indicators are monitored on preprinted charts and tables
Computer equipment	• National health information system office has 4 personal computers used partly for general office tasks	• District offices have 2 personal computers that also do general office tasks; manual backup system exists • Regional offices have 2 computers • National level has 10 computers dedicated to HIS tasks
Software	• Software is off-the-shelf and a simple flat-file database (i.e. Epi Info) or formatted spreadsheets • Or a simple database, self-explanatory, error correcting, includes population denominator and incidence estimates, has a simple administrative/inventory module • Produces basic maps, charts, and tables by district, region, country	• Advanced database management software with complex programming language • Requires substantial time for software design and programming • Relational database with separate modules for service activities, demographic and incidence estimates, finance, personnel, inventory, other administrative functions • Provides basic maps, charts, and tables for district level; more complex outputs for regional/national level • Assumes skills to use additional analytic software.

*Since HIS needs vary widely between countries, it is difficult to estimate absolute budget requirements. Instead, costs are normalized by estimating an annual US$ amount per facility covered by the HIS based on direct costs at the primary level and all support levels for staff training, supervision, district, regional and national level operations. Referral facilities have more expensive systems; therefore, costs for hospitals are calculated separately. Hospitals usually receive proportionally more resources than the primary level, some of which should be used for a simple patient management system. Detailed cost calculations are provided later in this chapter.

†Basic operating costs include all HIS supplies for manual and computer operations, telephone, fax, electronic mail, and photocopies.

MIS = management information systems;

LAN = local area network;

HIS = health information system.

management, clinic staff responsible for specific services can perform data recording, including daily tallies of all service activities, as a routine part of their service delivery function.

Specific clinic staff should be assigned to compile service data for monthly and quarterly reports. This responsibility includes aggregating daily tallies from different services into running totals, transferring these sums into monthly reports, and updating charts and tables to monitor key indicators. For example, depending on the size of a facility and the budget scenario, one auxiliary nurse in a small dispensary might spend 2 days per month on this task, which amounts to about 10% of 22 total work days per month. Such a small facility might have a total of three

---

Box 29   Primary care facility

Staff time for HIS
- Clinic staff register patient/client level data as part of service delivery.
- Clinic staff tally service data daily.
- 1–2 designated clinic staff spend 10–20% on monthly/quarterly HIS report.

HIS responsibilities
- Aggregate daily service tallies.
- Prepare monthly/quarterly reports.
- Calculate area coverage for essential services and prepare maps.
- Monitor key indicators with charts, tables, "health flags".
- Present information to, and discuss with, facility management and community.
- Provide support to communities for surveillance.

---

paramedical staff, attend to 200–300 outpatients per month, immunize 20–35 children under 5 years of age for each month, have a small family planning clinic, and care for a few chronically ill patients through home visits. As a second example, a busy health centre in an urban setting could have 5 times the volume and staff, and require a total of 9 days every month to aggregate daily service tallies and to complete the monthly or quarterly report. This could be accomplished if two nurses or health technicians spend 20% of their time on the health information system task, which includes monitoring key indicators, and presenting and reviewing the information with other facility staff and management.

Referral-level facilities have very different information needs and data collection procedures, requiring more costly solutions.

District level

The district health office must provide health information system support for facility staff. The low-budget scenario might only provide for up to two part-time (20%) health technicians, nurses, or administrative staff who also have other responsibilities, while high-budget districts might afford 50% time for two staff members. Their main responsibilities would be to aggregate monthly or quarterly reports from facilities, monitor key indicators for the district and update annual district health profiles, maintain district coverage maps, and present a quarterly executive summary to the district medical offices and the district governing board (Box 30). Even though these functions could be carried out by a single staff member (40% time), this is not recommended. With two staff who can perform the same task, there is the assurance that work is completed even when one staff member is absent. District staff responsible for health information system management functions participate in facility and community support or supervisory visits, in which they verify data quality through spot checks of records and registers.

In most middle-income and in some low-income countries, data processing at the district level has been computerized. Computerized data processing tasks do not require specialized staff. With little additional training, these tasks can be performed by paramedic and administrative staff.

Box 30 District level

Staff time for HIS
- At least 2 health technicians, nurses, or administrative staff for 20–50% of their time.
- In large districts with more resources, a health information officer.

HIS responsibilities
- Aggregate and process facility reports (with or without computer).
- Monitor key indicators and prepare district health profile.
- Prepare and update district coverage maps.
- Present information to, and discuss with, district health management team.
- Supervise HIS activities at facilities.

Box 31 Regional level

Staff time for HIS
- For low-budget scenario, combine regional and national level HIS functions.
- At least 2 health technicians, nurses, or administrative staff each at 50%.
- For large regions with more resources, a health information officer.

HIS responsibilities
- Computerize aggregation and processing of district data sets.
- Monitor key indicators and prepare regional health profile.
- Analyse variations of indicators between districts.
- Prepare and update regional coverage maps.
- Present information to, and discuss with, regional health management team.
- Perform performance audits of district HIS activities.

Regional level

As more countries follow the model proposed by WHO to decentralize health administrative functions, responsibilities and resources will shift from regions to districts. In some countries (e.g. Zambia), regions have become part of the national level organization; in others (e.g. Ethiopia, Madagascar, Pakistan), they still represent a distinct level between the district and national offices. Combining regional and national health information system functions without a separate administrative entity may be the most efficient option in the low-cost scenario, since it avoids additional staff and operating expenditures, and shortens the flow of information between the district and central offices.

In larger regions that have distinct planning and implementation functions and the necessary resources, at least two staff responsible for the health information system are justifiable for about 50% of their time. Their responsibilities would be similar to those of national health information system offices and include preparing regional coverage maps, assessing interdistrict variations for key indicators, and presenting status reports to regional governing boards to guide decision making concerning public health (Box 31).

National level

Depending on the budget scenario, national health information system management functions are assured by a team of 6–10 professionals working 50–100% of their time (Box 32). The teams are composed of health planners, epidemiologists, statisticians, mid-level technical staff, and administrative support personnel.

Since routine health information systems in most countries have been computerized at national, regional, and even district levels, a specialized computer staff (e.g. systems analyst, local area network administrator, user support specialist, computer programmer) is required, at least at the national level. Many countries will not have the means to hire all this personnel, but some essential functions like local area network administration and user support can be carried out by administrative or technical staff who receive special short-term training. Other more specialized functions like systems analysis and computer programming are mostly needed at specific times, such as during the development phase, and could be covered by short-term consultants.

Training personnel

The effectiveness of a health information system in providing information support to decision-makers, managers, and care providers depends upon well-trained staff. Not only must the mechanics of data collection be mastered, but high familiarity with case definitions and service standards are equally important. (A more detailed description of training contents and strategies is provided below under organizational rules.) Thus, for a health information system to produce valid, reliable, and useful information, staff skills must be built and maintained through initial training, regular refresher courses, and regular follow-up with supervision.

There are several reasons why training health unit staff in health information systems should be combined with other technical and manage-

---

Box 32 National level

Staff time for HIS
- For low-budget scenario, a total of 6 staff for 50% on HIS (2 epidemiologists/statisticians, 2 mid-level technical staff, 2 administrative support).
- For high-budget scenario, a total of 10 staff for 100% on HIS (3 epidemiologists/statisticians, 4 mid-level technical staff, 3 administrative support).
- Team headed by health information officer.

HIS responsibilities
- Develop long- and short-term objectives and work plans for an HIS.
- Computerized aggregation and processing of district and regional data sets.
- Monitor key indicators and prepare national health profile.
- Analyse variations of indicators among districts/regions.
- Prepare and update national coverage maps.
- Assess on an ongoing basis information needs of data users and ensure adequate restructuring.
- Perform performance audits of district HIS activities.

ment topics. Not only are health information system operations very dependent on general service delivery skills, but an integrated training approach also reduces costs for transportation and course organization.

District, regional, and national level health information system personnel often might need short-term or long-term training in epidemiology, statistics, and use of computers. Computer training will vary in intensity by level. District staff in high-budget countries require at least an introduction to basic skills to use the computer for data entry and reporting, but could benefit from some exposure to word processing and spreadsheet use. These basic skills could be taught through hands-on exercises during general health information system training. Regional and especially national level staff need more intensive computer training, because they use more applications and should be able to support users in the districts and other departments of the Ministry of Health. Depending on the size of the national health information systems office and the computer technology, one or two persons should receive in-depth training in local area network administration and user support.

Health information system supplies, procurement, and distribution

Although a health information system might be well designed to generate relevant information and allow timely feedback at the facility, district, and national levels, it falls short of its goal if it fails to collect data at the point of service delivery, or to process data at the district, regional, or national level. To protect considerable investments in health information system restructuring, the government must budget for basic supplies at all levels to assure a functioning system. In addition, effective procurement, storage, and distribution systems are required to ensure that these supplies are available in a timely manner to the data collecting and processing staff (Box 33).

Box 33   An illustrative list of essential HIS supplies

- Patient/client records (under-5 cards, reproductive health cards, tuberculosis follow-up cards, etc.).
- Outpatient register and/or tally sheet.
- Inpatient register and/or tally sheet.
- Maternal care register.
- Special registers (family planning, HIV/AIDS, tuberculosis, other chronic illnesses and disabilities).
- Community outreach register.
- Coverage plan and map with communities, community-based workers, demographic data.
- Large-size paper to chart key indicators.
- Financial record forms.
- Drug stock cards.
- Health committee meeting register and facility/community action plan.
- Monthly/quarterly report forms.
- HIS user guide with templates.
- Writing utensils.
- Solar-powered calculator.

Facilities require sufficient supplies of patient/client cards, registers, and report forms. Patient/client cards, in their simplest and least expensive form, can be generated from blank notebooks. While this works well for first-level acute curative care, chronic diseases and preventive care need well-designed and preprinted record cards. In low-budget countries, blank registers can be provided to save costs. Facility staff can draw appropriate columns and titles according to templates in the health information system user guide. Countries with a high budget might opt to preprint most facility registers. This would ensure better consistency of data collection, but would increase costs substantially. Some economies can be achieved by combining information into one register rather than using separate ones. Another means of saving costs is to record data on tally sheets instead of registers, particularly for data to be aggregated. If printed on thick paper, tally sheets can even be reused if data are recorded with an erasable pencil. In order to reduce errors, report forms should always be preprinted. Sufficient quantities should be available to prepare two to three copies. More details on the format of various data collection instruments can be found in Chapter 6.

Other essential health information system supplies are writing utensils (pens, markers) and large sheets of paper to monitor key indicators such as Expanded Programme on Immunization coverage, health flags, and coverage maps. If resources are available, poster-size laminated (erasable) preprinted charts could be provided for monitoring key indicators and updating coverage maps. Each health facility should also have a user guide, both for data collection procedures, as well as for use of information. Finally, in order to reduce error rates, simple, solar-powered calculators are no longer a luxury in a first-level care facility, even in low-income countries. Their unit price has been substantially reduced in the last decade.

District supplies include tally sheets and preprinted report forms (if data processing is done manually). Districts also need to keep in stock all printed supplies required by health units.

In countries with high health information system budgets, it is worthwhile, even at the district level, to invest in communications technology, such as telephone, fax, and electronic mail. Also, a photocopier can greatly contribute to more effective and efficient data transmission. Annual operating costs for telephone calls, which includes fax and electronic mail (because they use the same phone lines), can be as high as US$ 240–1200. Except for regular telephone conversations, fax and electronic mail require stable and low-noise communications to work effectively. High-budget countries might be able to afford this technology, but since many countries will at best have only a telephone, these costs are not included in the calculations of a minimum budget in Table 31.

Even in low-income countries, national or regional health information systems offices should be equipped with modern communications technology, such as telephone, fax, and electronic mail (these costs are included in Table 31). Their responsibility to provide feedback to lower levels requires the availability of one or more heavy-duty photocopiers, or at least a stencil duplicator as a low-cost alternative. These offices are also responsible for developing, producing, and distributing guidelines and user manuals for the health information system. In addition to their availability in facilities and districts as reference materials, these

Table 31 *Detailed calculation of operating costs*

Low budget	Costs	High budget	Costs
Facility staff time: 1 auxiliary at 10% (= 18 hours if 22 days/month, ½ hour per day to tally = 11 hours/ month, 7 hours to do monthly report)	US$ 120	Facility staff time: 2 nurses at 20% (= 71 hours if 22 days/month, 1 hour per day to tally = 22 hours/ month, 16 hours to do monthly report, 16 hours on data use, mapping, charts, 15 hours for community surveillance)	US$ 3000
Registers*: 6 generic every 2 years, tally sheets, report (small volume) incl. carbon paper	40	Registers*: 6 printed every year, tally sheets, report (large volume) incl. carbon paper	180
Facility staff HIS training part of medical training (1 every 3 years)	10	Special HIS training of 2 staff per facility (3 days, 1 every 3 years)	100
Staff: district (2@20%), regional (0), national (6@50%)	40	Staff: district (2@50%), regional (2@50%), national (10@100%)	340
Staff training district (2), regional (0), national (6): 3 days initial HIS (1 every 5 years), 1 day/year refresher HIS; national/regional: 2 weeks initial computer training (1 every 5 years), 2 days annual computer refresher	9	Staff training district (3), regional (2), national (10): 5 days initial HIS (1 every 3 years), 3 days/year refresher HIS; national/regional: 2 weeks initial computer training (1 every 3 years), 5 days annual computer refresher, 4 week LAN administration (2 persons every 3 years), 2 weeks user support (2 persons every 3 years)	32
Supplies: district, regional, national incl. computer, photocopies, phone, electronic mail	7	Supplies: district, regional, national incl. computer, photocopies, phone, electronic mail	30
Manual system at district level, national level computerized, simple database for national office (5 computers with electronic mail, laser and dot matrix printer, accessories, 1 photocopier, 1 stencil duplicator, 1 fax, 5-year depreciation)	6	District, regional, and national levels computerized, relational database for district/regional/ national levels (3 computers, 2 dot matrix printers per district and region, 10 for national office, and 3 laser and 3 dot matrix printers, accessories, peer-to-peer network, 6 photocopiers, 5 fax, 5 electronic mail accounts, 5-year depreciation)	108
Annual total per facility	US$ 232	Annual total per facility	US$ 3790

*Outpatient, inpatient, Expanded Programme on Immunization/growth monitoring, maternity, family planning, infectious/chronic diseases.
LAN = local area network.

documents are also used in introductory and refresher training courses on health information systems. Countries with low health information systems budgets will probably have to obtain donor funding to produce manuals and guidelines.

Computer hardware, software, and maintenance

The use of personal computers slowly increased in developing countries during the 1980s, when they were mainly employed at the national level to process data and to perform other office tasks. High prices and difficulties in using the technology contributed to this slow growth, and the health sector, with its proportionally small share of the national operating budget, was less likely to be able to afford office automation. In the 1990s, increased performance and user friendliness, combined with a drop in prices and increased vendor competition, resulted in personal computers becoming widely available in developing countries. They are now found at the regional level as well as in district offices, when resources make this possible.

An overview discussion on purchasing computer hardware and software, as well as on maintenance issues is provided in Chapter 11.

Detailed health information systems budget calculations for operational expenditures

Because health information system needs vary widely between countries, it is difficult to estimate absolute budget requirements. Instead, costs are normalized by estimating an annual US$ amount per facility covered by the health information system, based on direct costs at the primary level and all support levels for staff training, supervision, district, regional, and national level operations. Referral facilities need more expensive systems to handle the greater variety of services and the larger volume, thus costs for hospitals are calculated separately below. In low-budget countries it might be appropriate to use two to three times the costs for primary-level facilities as a rough estimate of health information system costs for very small first-level hospitals instead of the higher estimates given here. Health information system development costs, but not initial design costs, are shown separately in Table 32, but are included in Table 31 as depreciation costs over a 5-year period.

Table 31 uses the same structural health information system elements as used in Table 30 in determining annual budget requirements per health unit covered by the health information system under the two scenarios. Total operating costs depend extensively on personnel costs at the facility level, which amount to about 50% under the low-budget scenario and about 80% for high-budget countries.

Low-budget countries are assumed to have 50 districts with 30 facilities each, equalling 1500 facilities. High-budget countries are assumed to have 100 districts with 30 facilities each, equalling 3000 facilities. It is further assumed that all health programmes are integrated at facility and district levels. However, at the national level some programmes will maintain separate technical offices with special information needs that

Table 32 *Development costs for a national health information system*

Low budget	Costs (US$)	High budget	Costs (US$)
Hardware regional, national	20,000	Hardware regional, national	100,000
Hardware districts	—	Hardware districts	1,200,000
Software development	20,000	Software development	100,000
Initial HIS design*	200,000	Initial HIS design*	400,000

*Not depreciated and not included in Table 28; consists of health information system planning, consensus-building process, technical assistance, development of materials and production (registers, reports, user manuals), general staff training (in low-budget countries health information system design is usually financed by donors).

might have to be satisfied by sources other than the health information system (i.e. the Expanded Programme on Immunization and immunization coverage surveys).

Resource requirements for a hospital health information system

Hospitals require an information system that serves primarily administrative and clinical functions and that can directly improve the quality of services (Box 34). Administrative functions include patient flow between registration and different departments, accounting and billing, and inventory control for the pharmacy. Clinical functions cover medical records, including results of diagnostic procedures, access to standard diagnostic and procedure codes (i.e. ICD-10), prompters for essential patient information (i.e. obstetric risk assessment), or automated alerts in cases of drug incompatibility and contraindications. Most of the latter functions require a computerized system. Hospital information systems monitor indicators such as financial status, quality of care, type and volume of services provided to referred and nonreferred patients, length of stay, case fatality rates, comorbidities, and severity of illness. How systems are implemented in specific hospitals varies greatly among the type of facility, the economic status of its client base, and the technology available to automate the system.

Box 34   First level referral facility

Staff time for HIS
- Patient reception, admission, discharge (no additional HIS staff)
- Clinical staff register patient/client data (out- and inpatients, no additional HIS staff)
- Medical records (no additional HIS staff)
- Pharmacy services (no additional HIS staff)
- Laboratory, X-ray and other diagnostic services (no additional HIS staff)
- Accounting and billing (no additional HIS staff)
- Human resources (no additional HIS staff)
- Clinical departments and ancillary services tally service data daily (no additional HIS staff)
- HIS or statistics personnel aggregate service data and compile monthly reports; in small hospitals, HIS tasks can be shared with other functions such as accounting or billing: 2 clerks, 1 HIS office manager
- Well-endowed hospitals have a computerized information system and dedicated personnel: 1 HIS office manager, 1 HIS assistant, 1 computer programmer, 1 local area network administrator, 1 user support specialist

HIS responsibilities
- Monitor essential hospital operations (admissions, length of stay, mortality, waiting and service times).
- Monitor the financial viability of clinical care and other services (cost recovery).
- Assess the functioning of the referral system.
- Present information to, and discuss with, hospital management.
- Use information for continuous quality improvement.

In many countries, referral hospitals have more extensive reporting requirements than do primary care facilities. For example, instead of reporting volume by broad disease categories, hospitals in Eritrea, Ethiopia, Madagascar, and Zambia submit case counts by ICD category (Kleinau, 1995a; 1995b). This seems feasible because hospitals usually have more human and financial resources to support extensive reporting, even though some of this information reported through a health information system might be of little direct use to the hospital (i.e. just providing an exhaustive list of rare diseases without any reference population).

To estimate resource requirements for a hospital information system, the following elements are considered: staff dedicated to health information system functions, training, system supplies, computer equipment and software, and financial resources. Resources and costs are estimated for a secondary hospital with about a 100–150 bed capacity and a volume of 4000–5000 discharges per year and 2000–3000 outpatients per month. A health information system in a tertiary facility would require about three to five times the resources and costs of a secondary facility.

Staff

All recording functions are routinely maintained by clinical and administrative staff, though data aggregation and reporting to hospital management and districts is done by dedicated health information system staff. All essential administrative and clinical services are listed because they provide the data for the system, but they do not require any special information system personnel. Health information system functions should be carried out by a separate hospital health information system office which reports directly to the hospital director.

Training

The validity and reliability of data collected by the hospital health information system depend on how well staff are trained in case definitions and proper registration of cases (for a more in-depth discussion, see the section on organizational rules). Trainees include staff from clinical services, ancillary services, and finance and administration. Training accounts for the large part of the health information system budget because of the large number of staff involved. Costs can be reduced if senior hospital staff themselves provide the training. Training should be in short sessions of less than a day, in order not to disrupt patient care.

Supplies

Registers, medical records, and index card systems are necessary for a patient/client management system, whether kept manually or computer-based, and they are essential to any useful hospital health information system that ties into a national system. Therefore, costs are estimated for all patient management and health information system supplies. Direct health information system costs include general supplies of stationery, data tally sheets, and monthly reports.

Computers and software

It would be unlikely for most smaller rural hospitals with low operating budgets and not much revenue from patient payments to use computers.

Some facilities might be able to afford a few computers to improve patient registration, medical record retrieval and administrative tasks. Patient registration still requires developing a simple database program because of the large volume. Development time should not be more than 2 months.

Hospitals with much greater resources and substantial cost recovery, which could include private and public facilities, might be able to afford a complete computer-based patient management system. This system is built around local area network technology that allows all clinical, ancillary, and administrative services to access the same patient/client information. In addition it helps to improve quality of care by standardizing diagnoses through instant access to diagnostic categories, physician reminders to complete essential assessments, or alerts in cases of drug contraindications. Extensive computer use offers many benefits, but it comes at a high cost and requires appropriate infrastructure and support personnel. Patient management software is expensive, too, and takes time to develop (3 months to a year) if an off-the-shelf computer program is not acceptable.

Detailed hospital health information system cost calculations

Tables 33 and 34 provide some rough estimates of annual costs for a hospital health information system. The first table only considers costs related to manual operations without computer technology and development costs. As for a basic health services health information system, personnel amounts to the largest cost item, followed by supplies. If all hospital staff need some refresher training in the case definitions and administrative tasks that are prerequisites for good data collection, then these training costs are much higher than training specifically targeted to a few health information system staff.

The design and development costs of a hospital health information system are estimated at US$ 20,000 in a low-budget country and US$ 50,000 in a high-budget one for both manual and computerized

Table 33 *Detailed calculation of operating costs for a hospital health information system*

Low budget	Costs (US$)	High budget	Costs (US$)
Staff time: 1 HIS manager at 50% ($200/m), 2 clerks at 100% ($100/m)	3600	Staff time: all full-time, 1 HIS manager ($1000/m), 1 assistant ($500/m)	18,000
Registers, tally sheets, report (small volume) incl. carbon paper, medical records	1200	Registers, tally sheets, report (large volume) incl. carbon paper, medical records	6,000
Facility staff training in case definitions, administrative tasks, data collection	1000	Facility staff training in case definitions, administrative tasks, data collection	5,000
HIS staff trained in reporting, analysis, interpretation, feedback	300	HIS staff trained in reporting, analysis, interpretation, feedback	2,000
Annual total per hospital	6100	Annual total per hospital	31,000

Table 34 *Development and implementation costs for a hospital health information system (HIS)*

Small computerized HIS	Costs (US$)	Large computerized HIS	Costs (US$)
Minimum hardware*	8,000	LAN-based hospital HIS*	30,000
	—	Complete hospital LAN*	80,000
	—	Computer staff: 1 programmer ($750/m), 1 LAN administrator ($750/m), 1 user support ($500/m)*	120,000
Staff training in computer use*	2,000	Staff training in computer use*	25,000
Software development†	20,000	Software development†	80,000
Initial hospital HIS design†	20,000	Initial hospital HIS design†	50,000
Annual average per hospital‡	2,160	Annual average complete LAN‡	45,260

*Costs are estimated over a period of 5 years. Hardware, staff, and training are per hospital.
†Software and initial HIS design are one-time costs. None of these costs are depreciated. Initial HIS design consists of hospital HIS planning, short-term technical assistance, development of materials and production (registers, reports, user manuals), and general staff training. The same design and software can be used in hospitals on the same level.
‡Annual average costs per hospital exclude initial HIS design. Countries with a small computerized hospital HIS are assumed to have 50 hospitals. Countries with a larger computerized and local area network based hospital HIS are assumed to have 100 hospitals.

systems. They include health information system planning, short-term technical assistance, development and production of data collection instruments, and general staff training. These costs are in addition to the development costs for the national system (see Table 32).

In some countries, a new hospital, especially if privately owned, might want to adopt computer technology on a small or large scale over the coming years. For these facilities, hardware, computer staff, and computer training are shown in Table 34, including systems design and development costs. Table 34 contains costs for a 5-year implementation period to account for the fact that computer equipment lasts at least 5-years, and that design and development efforts are only justifiable over a longer time frame. Any computer-related costs need to be added to the operating costs shown in Table 33.

Organizational rules

The mere availability of health information system resources as described in previous sections is not sufficient. A set of organizational rules is required in order to ensure optimum use of resources in support of the information-generating process. The following paragraphs present an overview of organizational rules for various health information system components.

Overall health information system management

One of the first decisions that countries face when reorganizing or strengthening their health information system is where to place the responsibility for managing it. The locus of health information system responsibility in the health care system determines the importance attributed to the information function of public health services and its leadership role. Most countries have a dedicated health information system service, division, or department within the ministry of health. In countries where the health information system unit reports directly to the secretary-general (or the equivalent highest decisional level) of the ministry, its cross-cutting role and leadership responsibility are clear. Where the health information system unit is attached to a technical service, for example disease control and prevention, the epidemiological surveillance function might be emphasized, but its leadership role in information management could be weakened vis-à-vis other services and programmes.

Experience from several countries has shown that placing health information system management on the highest level within the health sector hierarchy does express the importance of information in strategic planning and policy making. In Zambia the health management information systems unit is part of the Central Board of Health and thus plays a key role in health sector reform (Health Management Information Development Team, 1997). This and a participatory approach led to a clear vision for the role of the health information system and to a systematic and well-documented implementation process.

Overall health information system design and direction should be provided by a multidisciplinary committee to meet the needs of various users of information. A health information system steering committee has to set the long-term goals for a health information system and needs to decide which key indicators should be measured and which data are necessary. To be effective, data collectors as well as users at various levels should be represented on this committee. The role of the committee is to provide overall recommendations, to set general health information system policies, and to support the health information system manager, but its role is not to micromanage health information system functions. Examples of countries that opted for directing health information system development and implementation through a steering committee are Eritrea, Madagascar, Pakistan, and Zambia.

While the location of overall health information system management is primarily an issue on the national level, the management role at the district level is of crucial importance, as discussed in other paragraphs of this section. District health teams not only produce information but are also users. Chief medical officers need data for planning and managing district health services and for allocating resources where decentralization foresees such responsibilities. Assuring the quality of data should be a key responsibility of district health management teams because they directly control data collection by the health facilities.

Data collection standards including case definitions

Routine and nonroutine data collection instruments are described in detail in Chapters 6 and 7. Data are only comparable if they have been collected using the same approach, or if it has been validated that two approaches yield the same information. For example, indicators estimated from facility survey data will usually yield different results when evaluated with a supervision instrument. Or, procedures to calculate couple-years of protection need to be standardized in order to compare coverage for family planning services between districts.

Data collection standards include exact case definitions for clinical and other services. Dissimilar skill levels require that guidelines be adapted for all types of users. For instance, whereas in reference hospitals with experienced physicians and many diagnostic facilities case definitions can be adapted from ICD-9 or ICD-10, primary care facilities need symptom- or syndrome-based disease categories. Staff at ambulatory care facilities must know the difference between a new case and a return visit for the same illness. Further, though it might seem obvious, it is important that data be reported in the same way by all facilities. For example, if case load is reported by certain age groups, then all facilities need to comply; otherwise data cannot be analysed by age.

Data transmission, processing, and reporting rules

Data transmission and processing are described in detail in Chapter 8. Data will only be used if they are available in a timely manner. A clearly defined but realistic schedule must be developed by which all levels of the health system complete and forward reports in either paper or electronic format. Regardless of whether all points of service have provided reports on time (which in itself is one health information system performance indicator), subsequent levels must process data in conformity with the established schedule. Otherwise data arrival at other levels of the health system will be delayed as well. This becomes increasingly important as more and more levels become involved in a health information system. Experience shows that report arrival at the national level can be delayed for months, or even years, by delays at the first level.

A defined schedule is also important for regular feedback and supervisory activities, as both rely on the availability of information. While supervisory visits can take place without health information system data in hand, there is a missed opportunity for quality supervision, or for identifying where attention should be placed in quality assurance activities. Supervision and health information system feedback should be jointly planned following established schedules.

Service activities, including financial and stock reports, are generally reported on a monthly or quarterly basis. Staff inventories, equipment inventories, and reports about the physical condition of a facility can be reported annually. Whichever time period is chosen, a firm schedule should be developed and communicated to all units. If reporting intervals are long, necessary reminders must be included in the schedule.

The primary care level normally reports clinical data in less specific and far fewer disease categories than the referral level. It has to be decided whether reported case incidence statistics combine all level of care, or whether they are provided separately for primary care facilities and hospitals. If the national health information system office summarizes case reports from different types of facilities, disease categories have to be combined into broader groupings. The combination of primary care and hospital data is only appropriate if both provide similar types of care, for example ambulatory services, even though hospitals do so with more highly-qualified staff. Combining data from referred patients with data from primary care would be inappropriate.

Confidentiality and right to privacy

Clients expect that their privacy will be protected when they supply information to the service provider. Patient/client information does not leave the institution and is only divulged with patients' or clients' explicit knowledge and consent.

As a matter of principle, all client and patient data must be treated with confidentiality. This principle should not be broken even in the case of family members. For example, it is up to the woman to let her husband know that she uses birth control. However, there are a few exceptions where the right to privacy is superseded by the obligation to protect the public from serious health hazards. Certain illnesses with mandatory reporting fall into this category. Confidentiality requires a set of rules that can differ from country to country.

Often data gathered at the facility level are associated with research efforts. In general, it is inappropriate to use clients' data without their expressed consent. If such consent is not obtainable, all information identifying specific individuals must be omitted or completely disguised. All research activities must follow national standards of biomedical ethics.

Training design and standards, production, and dissemination of materials

Whether redesigning an existing health information system or introducing a new system, staff require introductory training as well as regular refresher sessions. Since training is often expensive, health information system design should be simple enough to require only a minimum amount of training for personnel to collect, process, and use data.

Ideally, health information system training for health unit staff should be combined with courses that improve clinical or other service delivery skills. This may be the only feasible option under the low-budget scenario. Initial training includes at the minimum 1 day of practical exercises in filling out registers, tally sheets, monthly or quarterly reports, and monitoring key indicators. If a higher budget permits more extensive initial training, the course can be expanded to 3 days. Such intensive training will focus particularly on the use of information for decision making at the local level. Topics would include preparing population coverage maps, estimating target populations, estimating the expected incidence for key diseases, preparing indicator charts, or discussing options to improve coverage and quality of services. Whether health information system budgets are low or high, staff should regularly and at least annually attend short refresher courses. Generally 1 day of health information system topics during general management or clinical refresher training is sufficient.

Training facility staff is mainly carried out by district health information system personnel with some assistance from the regional or national levels.

Initial training of district health information system staff requires between 3 and 5 days. District managers require an in-depth understanding of data collection procedures and use of the information at the facility level for a triple purpose: to use the information for district level management, to become trainers of facility staff, and to provide supportive supervision to the staff. The duration of the initial training and its frequency depend on the available budget, but every 3–5 years is appropriate.

Finally, national and regional health information system staff require extensive training. First of all, in order to become expert trainers for district staff, they need to have a profound understanding of the peripheral data collection system. In addition, they need training to assume their specific responsibilities at the national or regional levels in reviewing policies and establishing norms for data collection, flow, and processing. They need to carry out detailed geographic and trend analyses, and to provide information for high-level management decisions that impact on service access, quality, and equity. The role of regional offices varies between countries. In a low-budget health information system, information should flow directly between districts and the national office, thus eliminating the need to train regional staff. Very large countries and those with high-budget health information systems could require training regional level personnel, following the same content as national level staff.

Training materials should be simple and brief, and based upon practical exercises. The health information system instruction manual, describing all data collection instruments and data collection standards, should be the main reference document. The trainer's manual needs to be more complete and should include exercise workbooks and charts to explain key health information system concepts and information flows. All these materials are developed during the health information system design phase. Sufficient training materials should be available for refresher training and reprinted when necessary.

Computer use

Computer technology can greatly enhance and expedite data processing and the presentation of information in a health information system. It greatly reduces the time required for processing data at the district, regional, and national levels, as well as the number of errors inherent in a manual process. This does not mean that technology is a panacea for more fundamental health information system problems (e.g. lack of basic supplies at the point of data collection and an overly burdensome design).

Countries with a low-cost health information system use computers mainly at the national and regional levels, whereas most districts process data manually. Even countries that have the resources to computerize district offices should be prepared to process data for key indicators manually, as working conditions can be treacherous and repair services may not be readily available. If the health information system is totally reliant on computer technology, the system is likely to fail in the medium term. Therefore manual data processing should be taught at all health information system training courses.

Procurement and distribution system for health information system equipment and supplies (including computers)

In most countries, the general finance and/or administration offices of the ministry of health are responsible for procuring and distributing health information system equipment and supplies (computers, software, printed data collection instruments, and other supplies). Rules and regulations for health information system equipment and supplies are therefore the same as for other equipment and supplies. International tenders can save costs, provided large quantities are ordered and the purchase is tax exempt. If donors such as the World Bank are involved in initial procurement, additional regulations may apply.

Equipment should be standardized to facilitate maintenance and upgrades (i.e. same brand, similar configuration). This provides some assurance that parts can be used interchangeably. Standardization of software packages is required in order to allow for effective staff training. The same applies to printed materials such as registers, data collection forms, and report forms.

Printed health information system supplies are best distributed through the same supply system as drugs and medical supplies. Computer supplies should be provided through different channels. In countries with district level computerization, each district office should have an annual budget to procure computer accessories. This is feasible if budget responsibilities have been decentralized. In the other cases, national and regional health information system offices should function as suppliers. Supply management procedures must be communicated clearly to all concerned staff, recipients, and suppliers.

A maintenance and replacement policy and budget should be developed, as well as a process to correct equipment failure outside major cities. This is probably the greatest challenge to maintaining a computerized health information system, since maintenance and replacement costs are generally not affordable except in countries with considerable health information system resources. Initially donors might be of some help, but the government must eventually adopt a more sustainable solution. Providing districts and regions with budget autonomy is probably the best approach. In the case of a centrally managed budget, district computers can be out of order for extended periods.

Using private sector computer vendors for maintenance seems to be the most cost-effective solution. Private vendors obtain their revenues from sales, and can provide maintenance more efficiently on an as-needed basis.

Establishing a government-owned repair shop is less cost-effective, as such facilities cannot afford highly qualified technicians due to low public sector salaries. Also the operating costs to run a repair shop are very high, and require maintaining a large inventory of parts. Maintenance contracts should be avoided, as they are very expensive for the client and very profitable for the vendor (at least 10% of the purchase price on an annual basis).

Computers should be delivered with software preinstalled, especially to district offices whose staff cannot be expected to install software themselves. Staff training should be provided immediately after delivery of computer equipment, eventually with support from commercial computer vendors and donor technical assistance. Country experience has shown that staff have great difficulties using information technology if the equipment is delivered without appropriate staff training.

Continuous quality assurance of health information system operations and data

Training personnel at facilities and on all support levels by itself will not assure data quality and compliance with regular reporting. Training must be complemented by regular support and supervisory visits to facilities by district staff, and by performance audits of districts by national or regional offices. Visits should be structured, and should assess health information system operations systematically using a checklist. Part of the audit should be a random check of registers and medical records to verify numbers in monthly and quarterly reports.

Examples of questions that could be included in a facility supervision checklist follow. Most require simple yes/no answers. Not all areas need to be addressed during each visit; rather, the team should focus on areas that need improvement.

- Are registers kept according to national norms? Compare each register with its template and check.
- Are daily tallies kept for six key services? (Define six key services).
- Does a random check of two to three clinical activities show matching numbers between registers/medical records and the monthly report?
- Is the coverage map for the health facility up to date and is appropriate demographic data used?
- Are charts that monitor key indicators up to date?
- Is there evidence that the information generated is used (e.g. appropriate action taken if the threshold is reached)?
- Are sufficient health information system supplies available for the coming 3 (or more) months?
- Did health unit staff receive health information system training?

Examples of questions that could be included in a district performance audit checklist follow. Most require only a calculation of percentages.

- What proportion of facilities submit reports as defined by national norms?
- What proportion of facilities submit reports within the time frame specified?
- What proportion of facilities received a health information system supervisory visit during the previous 3 months?
- Did district staff correctly aggregate facility data into a district report based on a small random check?
- What proportion of districts have an updated coverage map and use appropriate demographic data?
- What proportion of districts have a chart with updated key indicators?
- What proportion of districts show evidence that information generated is used (e.g. appropriate action taken if threshold is reached)?
- What proportion of districts have sufficient health information system supplies available for the coming 3 (or more) months?
- What proportion of districts have staff trained in health information systems?

Role of and interaction with the private sector (nongovernmental organizations, private practitioners)

In most developing countries, nongovernmental organizations participate in a national health information system—especially when the government subsidizes this sector. These facilities face the same challenges as public sector facilities, and should be given the same support and supplies. The not-for-profit sector can contribute important experience to the design and implementation of a health information system, especially when community partnerships and surveillance are involved.

Health information system involvement by the private for-profit sector varies. In most countries it does not participate in the public sector system unless private practitioners claim reimbursement through public funds, such as social security. If such payments are involved, the public sector can impose and enforce reporting requirements. Otherwise the public sector has no leverage and cannot coopt private providers into reporting. This might be possible on a voluntary basis, but results are typically poor, as experience has shown.

Conclusion

Health information system management should and does, as examples for many countries show, assume leadership in providing an information-rich environment and in promoting the strategic role that routine information plays in planning and managing health services. The basis for health information system management is a solid management structure, including affordable health information system resources and a well-established set of organizational rules.

This chapter provided guidelines on how to plan, acquire, and manage health information system resources efficiently within a given budget situation. It also outlines how to establish various organizational rules that ensure production of quality and timely information. Health information system managers at national, regional, and district levels play a key role in developing and implementing these rules and adapting them to each country's setting.

References

Kleinau EF et al. (1995). *Measuring and improving service efficiency in public hospitals.* Boston, Harvard University, School of Public Health.

Kleinau EF (1995a). *Etude de l'informatisation du système statistique sanitaire du Ministère de la Santé de Madagascar. [Computerizing the health statistics system of the Ministry of Health of Madagascar.]* Antananarivo, Ministry of Health.

Kleinau EF (1995b). *Health management information system (HMIS) in the Southern Ethiopia People's Region: review and recommendations for a redesign.* Washington, DC, BASICS.

Health Management Information Development Team (1997). *Health management information systems: design and implementation plan for a DART-HMIS.* Lusaka, Central Board of Health.

11 Using computers in health information systems

Randy Wilson

Historical overview

The social sector in developing countries has been slower than other sectors, such as business, in taking advantage of computer technology, as is the case in industrialized countries. The health services borrowed applications from business during the early implementation of computers, for example from financial accounting, insurance, and inventory management. These were essentially vertical or task-oriented systems used primarily in the background of health service delivery (Greenes & Shortcliffe, 1990). Computerized systems primarily focused on the administration of hospital-based clinical services. In the early 1980s, new uses specific to primary health care began to emerge. One such development was decision support systems with computerized algorithms for disease diagnosis using minicomputers.

Research efforts in epidemiology and demography were among the first areas where computers became indispensable for population-based public health work. A variety of computerized applications have been used, principally for analysis of survey and research data. The public domain statistical analysis program called Epi Info, which is widely used in many developing countries, is an example of computer software developed by the Centers for Disease Control and Prevention in the USA to make this technology accessible to many health care workers.

Some of the first efforts using microcomputers to computerize routinely collected health information in developing countries focused on the entry and analysis of data on service statistics. Vertical programmes like the Expanded Programme on Immunization used computer software to process immunization reports. Essential drugs projects developed software for inventory control and international procurement management. Family planning projects produced software to track the recruitment and retention of contraceptive users and to manage contraceptive logistics.

A more recent trend is towards better integration of data on the full range of health services. This is partly a reflection of the changing philosophy about the delivery of health care services since WHO's declaration of health for all at Alma Ata. Thanks to increasingly powerful and easy-to-use relational database technology, health services are beginning to link together service statistics data on curative care, family planning, preventive, and promotional activities. These data can in turn be linked to data on resource utilization: personnel, infrastructure, equipment, and finance.

Another area with great potential began to open up with the rapid expansion of the Internet's World Wide Web in the mid-1990s—facilitating information exchange and online reference by health professionals around the globe. Web pages cover topics ranging from the specific, such as AIDS or family planning, to the general, such as the page maintained by the Centers for Disease Control and Prevention, which provides a wealth of information on a wide range of public health concerns.

The focus of this chapter is primarily on the use of computers in routine reporting systems for population-based health services. It does not cover the use of computers for medical research using online reference databases, as a differential diagnostic tool in individual case management, or for applications for medical practice and hospital management.

Rationale for using computers in health information systems

Wilson and Smith (1991) suggest: "The creative use of microcomputer technology is one of the most promising means of improving the quality, timeliness, clarity, presentation, and use of relevant information for PHC [primary health care] management." Recent experience, highlighted in some of the case studies included in this text, attests to the potential for this technology in the developing country setting.

At the same time it is important to ensure that computerization does not dominate the health information system improvement process. The majority of information users in developing countries have no access to computer technology, and the development and improvement of manual systems for the collection and analysis of data should be the primary focus. Computerization should only be undertaken when it supports the overall objectives of improving health surveillance and service performance.

Reasons for using microcomputers in a health information system include the following:

- Improving programme efficiency by processing and analysing large amounts of data quickly. Because manual health information systems are by nature paper-heavy, managers are often buried under mountains of data—much of which they are unable to navigate or effectively analyse and use for improved decision making. This often results in the phenomenon referred to as "information anxiety".
- Producing a wide variety of outputs and feedback reports targeted for many levels of the health system from a single data set or by combining data sets.
- Reducing the duplication of work which is typically seen in many hierarchical data collection systems. In such systems, each level of the hierarchy prepares similar analyses of the same data received from below. With the effective decentralization of computers and communications technology, data can be entered once, close to the periphery, and transmitted to higher levels on diskette or via modem. For example, each level can receive disaggregated data about the performance of individual health facilities. In traditional manual health information systems, this level of detail is often lost as each level in the hierarchy works with the aggregated data from the level below.

- Improving the quality of data collection through automatic validation during data entry and automatic preparation of immediate feedback reports on errors for individual health facilities.
- Improving analysis and information presentation to facilitate data interpretation and use for decision-making.
- Managing the data for monitoring the attainment of health programme targets and objectives.
- Developing decision support tools for planning increased service coverage and logistics (e.g. target cost from the futures group).
- Modeling and simulation to facilitate planning by analysing projected outcomes for given inputs and conditions (SUSPLAN, Afghanistan).
- Integrating service statistics data with already computerized data on demography, health infrastructure, and/or financial management.
- Decentralizing data analysis and use to reduce the data entry bottleneck at the central level and provide management information to district managers in a more timely manner. For this to work effectively, it is crucial to maintain compatibility of data at all levels, so that it can be aggregated for national planning and management.
- Training health personnel through computer-based interactive tutorials for self-instruction and continuing education.
- Accessing the Internet to search for information about new products and approaches to service delivery, and exchanging information with other health care workers around the globe.
- Improving data dissemination by providing online public access to data though Internet World Wide Web pages.

In addition to some of the direct reasons for using computer technology in primary health care work, a number of indirect benefits have been identified. From their experience in Haiti, Auxila and Rohde (1988) note that the process of computerizing in and of itself can in fact serve as an opportunity to review and improve dysfunctional manual systems and procedures. This runs counter to the conventional wisdom in the information systems field that suggests that there is little point in computerizing poorly functioning systems. Similarly, Sandiford, Annett & Cibulskis (1992) note: "The introduction of microcomputers provides the opportunity for a complete rethinking of information needs and a change of staff attitudes towards the utility of data". Another benefit is that the attraction of learning to use the technology can act as an important incentive to boost staff morale. However, this benefit comes with a caveat, as Sandiford, Annett & Cibulskis (1992) warn: "Unfortunately it would seem that the presence of a microcomputer in an office often correlates more closely with the status of the employee within that organization than with their ability to make fruitful use of the machine." In other instances, public sector employees, once trained and armed with very marketable computer skills, then abandon their jobs for much better paying private sector opportunities. Fig. 20 summarizes key steps in the computerization process.

Key issues to resolve with respect to computerization

What to computerize?

It is important to note that many common and useful applications of computer technology in the health sector have little to do with the development of a comprehensive health management information system. They include human resource management, bibliographic and document management, accounting, publications, surveillance data management,

Fig. 20   *The computerization process*

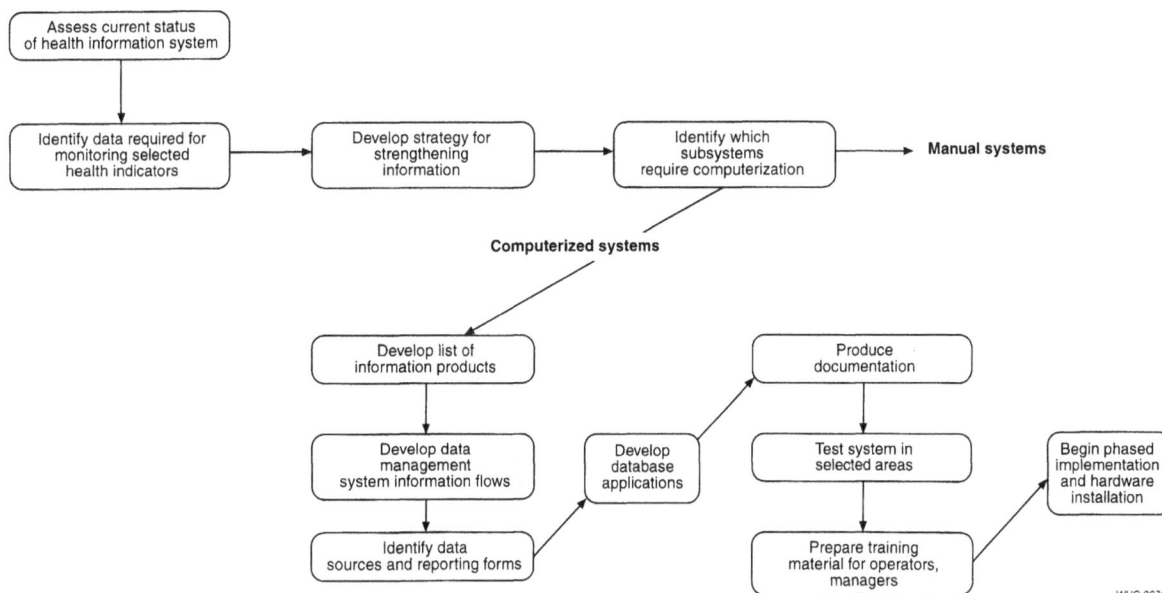

demographic (vital statistics) analysis and projections, survey data analysis, and inventory management, to name a few. The introduction of such applications can help prepare staff for developing more ambitious computer applications later on.

The focus of this chapter, however, is on the computerization of critical health information system functions. Key functions in typical sequence are:

— registering health facilities and infrastructure;
— registering health personnel and monitoring their training;
— monitoring service statistics on health problems, key interventions, and critical resources;
— managing logistics and stock;
— disseminating and archiving data.

What is the correct level at which to computerize?

It is critical in the developing country setting to achieve the right mix of computer and manual systems, and to ensure that they are fully integrated. This enables units which do not have computers to produce their analyses manually. Decisions about whether or not to computerize, and at what level, should take into account:

— the availability of local resources to support computer equipment, software maintenance, and training;
— the volume of data to be processed: with an extensive system, you may want to avoid the data entry bottlenecks often associated with highly centralized computer systems by decentralizing data entry.

Table 35 provides some guidelines about computerizing at different levels of the health system.

Table 35 *Computerization at different levels of the health system*

Level	Type of system	Issues
Health unit	Clinic resource management: inventory control, patient records, and financial management	Computerization at this level is probably not practical in most developing countries, except in the largest facilities with specialized staff to manage the system and considerable budget resources.
District	Disease surveillance, clinic activity reporting, districtwide logistics systems, population coverage	With the increasing decentralization of the management of health services in developing countries, there is substantial interest in computerizing at the district level. Computerization at the district level, if possible, is important, since it puts timely analyses in the hands of the managers who are directly responsible for supervising health care service providers.
Intermediate and national	Service statistics, logistics management, inventory control, geographic information systems, infrastructure management	Computerization is most practical and most common at these levels. Because of the physical distance from health service delivery structures, systems which are centralized at these levels need to focus on resolving 2 key problems: information dissemination (so that it gets into the hands of key decision makers) and feedback (so that the supervisors and service providers can use the results of central analyses without too much delay).

To computerize or to improve a manual system?

There is often a tendency to assume that a computer must be used in an information system. The decision to computerize should also take into account some of the following factors:

- *The complexity of analysis required.* This does not refer only to the complexity of statistical procedures being used, since many service statistics systems rely principally on sums, counts, and averages. More frequently this complexity refers to the number of ways in which the data must be presented after entry. An integrated service statistics system may need separate reports produced for each of the major health programmes, in addition to specialized reports for each level of the management hierarchy. Especially useful is the computer's ability to produce graphical output, which is very complex to prepare manually yet can greatly facilitate the interpretation and use of data (see, for example, Fig. 15 panels A and B in Chapter 8).
- *How well the existing system functions.* This often depends on how clearly defined the indicators are for the system, and how well standardized the mechanisms are for data collection. If health facilities send in reports on an ad hoc basis without standard indicators, it may be impossible to compare the data and useless to computerize. Keep in mind the adage, "If you can do it by hand, the computer might make it more efficient, but if you can't do it by hand, the computer is likely to make it worse."
- *The volume of data to be processed.* It is important not to get carried away with computerizing systems where the volume of data to be processed is very low. For rapid surveys, for example, you might want to use the researcher's rule of thumb, which suggests that it may be

quicker to analyse a simple survey with fewer than 200 questionnaires by hand than to put together a computerized system to do it.
- *The costs of the technology vis-à-vis the cost and availability of skilled personnel to process the data manually.* In a climate of shrinking public sectors, it is often not an easy matter to hire additional staff, even though this might be a cheaper option.

What type of infrastructure is required to manage computer system development and maintenance?

Often computerized systems development in the health sector is undertaken nearly exclusively with financial and technical assistance from donor agencies. The sustainability of such systems has been a serious problem in many countries. Although there are no simple solutions to this problem, at least two strategies should be considered to improve the system's sustainability.

- *Rely on locally recruited technicians to do all software customization and programming.* Most developing countries have a pool of reasonably skilled computer programmers whose skills can be upgraded to handle most health information system software development projects. Unfortunately, few of these people stay within the ministry structure because salary differentials between the private and public sectors are so great. When public sector employees cannot be retained, it is critical to develop mechanisms to provide ongoing private sector support to such development efforts. External technical assistance should focus on systems design and training.
- *Involve end-users in the systems design process from the earliest stages.* Developing software using a modular and incremental approach and installing it in small, manageable pieces helps to obtain end-user input on early modules, builds ownership, and provides useful insight into features which can be added to later modules.

Develop a heavily customized computer system or use off-the-shelf software for data entry and analysis

The data entry and computerized analysis needs of a given country's health information system are unlikely to be met by a single existing software package. There are a variety of approaches which can be used which are in between these two extremes, but the decision about which approach is most appropriate must be made very carefully.

- *Existing computerized systems developed for other countries can be modified to meet local needs.* If such systems were developed using simple tools for customizing data entry screens and creating new reports, much of the other logic and design elements may already be there. Much of the success of this approach will depend upon the flexibility of the tools used to develop the software in the first place and on availability of the source code for later in-country modification. This can be an appealing option because the overall structure of such systems is often quite similar, with databases maintained on the target population, health resources (personnel and facilities), and activity reporting. For the most part, however, such software will provide useful examples and lessons learned, but adaptation seldom works without the continuous support of the original developer.
  For example, a modular approach was used in developing the software for entry and analysis of routine reporting data from the Nigeria

family planning programme. A series of software packages were developed using files in a commercial database format and a commercial compiler. The packages are all built around a common menu system and use the same generic tools for report writing, data queries, and file management. Subsequently, modules were added for other primary health care activities. The software has since been translated and adapted for use in Turkey.

- *Use a variety of off-the-shelf software for data entry and analysis.* Several health programmes have had considerable success using simple software like Epi Info to create standard data entry and analysis utilities for routine reporting. End-users can then translate their data into spreadsheet formats to produce graphic analyses using their preferred software package. For example, the USAID-funded BASICS project has used Epi Info for standardized data entry and analysis of rapid assessments which are regularly conducted to evaluate health status and health service development. This approach is fine for simple data file structures, but has serious limitations for routine feedback reporting as data structures become more complex or there are requirements for files to be shared among many departments.

- *Develop a fully customized software package.* When the data entry and reporting requirements of a health information system become more complex, it is often necessary to resort to developing a customized software package. This usually requires the involvement of a software development team with a reasonable level of technical expertise, but can result in a product which simplifies work for end-users and can include a wide range of complex outputs. The computerized system (HMIS/FLCF) developed for the Ministry of Health in Pakistan is a good example of this approach (see Box 35). Several factors appear to affect the success of such an approach:

Box 35 Pakistan HMIS/FLCF: the anatomy of a computerized HMIS

The HMIS/FLCF produced as part of the Pakistan child survival project was developed using three software packages. The menus, data entry screens, validation procedures, and most tabular reports were developed and compiled using DOS commercial database and graphing software. Map output is produced using Epi Map.

Access to each of these modules is through a commercial database application. When a graph or map is desired, a database query selects the data to be displayed, and then either the graphing software or Epi Map is loaded with parameters to display the corresponding image. Once the graphic is viewed or printed, the user is returned to the main menu of the database application.

Variations of this approach have also been used in developing Windows-compatible software for the Nigeria essential drugs programme management information system (World Bank) and the Madagascar family planning management information system (USAID APPROPOP/PF). In these cases, the graphical output was greatly simplified because of the tighter integration of the graphing software within the Windows database application.

---

1. Use of high-level (fourth-generation) application development tools for software development. A range of commercial packages include powerful screen generators, report generators, query tools, and menu generators, that make it easier to maintain the software as information systems evolve. To enhance sustainability, it is important to resist the temptation to write the program code by hand, and to use the software's built-in tools as much as possible.

2. The availability of competent computer programmers locally to carry out program maintenance and upgrades over time. This reduces costly reliance on foreign consultants and increases the sustainability of the system. It is important for this local technical input to begin early in a system's development, so that common standards can be agreed upon for future development.

3. The degree to which the system's data can be exported for use with other software and shared with other departments. Giving user departments ownership of subsets of the data which they need to conduct their work using the software tools that they are familiar with can go a long way towards building long-term support for a system.

4. Developing and introducing the system in modules, simple ones first, so that end-users can gain experience with the software as it develops. In addition to reducing the initial data entry bottleneck, this approach produces some very useful input from users which can then be incorporated into the development of later modules. In the Pakistan HMIS/FLCF, a health institutions database module was introduced first to allow computer centres around the country to input key information about health facilities before they had to respond to the pressure of entering routine reporting data coming from the facilities.

5. The extent to which data entry and analysis can be decentralized. This reduces the data entry bottleneck and puts the information first in the hands of the managers with direct line responsibility. Early experience in Pakistan suggests that district health offices which were computerized were the first to have complete data sets and were able to keep them up to date. It is, however, important to ensure adequate infrastructure to support computerization down to the district level and to develop well-tested routines to transmit data to higher levels without significant delays.

6. The degree to which training is provided to data entry staff and management. This should include general computer literacy as well as specific training on the use of the software and the information generated by it. Computer operators need to know how to use their software efficiently, and managers need to rely on the information it produces in order to keep pressure on staff to keep it up to date.

Software and hardware options

With computer technology advancing extraordinarily rapidly, it is difficult to develop more than general themes to guide decisions in these areas.

Software

One of the first decisions that must be made in planning computerization of a health information system is to what extent you will develop your systems in DOS or in the graphical environment. The requirements

---

Box 36   A common computerization scenario

The Ministry of Health has a limited number of computers, most of which have been donated by different agencies for specific purposes pertaining to the various special programmes they are supporting. They were not intended to support the overall health information system. The machines and accessories are of many different types and ages, and there is a wide variety of software in use.

The health statistics division has some modern equipment, but they have yet to establish standard data formats for storage and processing, and there is a huge backlog in analysing and producing reports from the routine data which is collected. The provincial and district health services have no access to computers, although some of the larger hospitals have independently acquired computers which are used for locally developed applications, primarily of an administrative nature.

In general, staff have not been trained systematically to use the software available. Most learn on the job. Very little expertise exists within the Ministry of Health, although there are a number of staff who could be trained to become quite accomplished systems developers. Computer-related functions are not reflected in job descriptions or unit procedures manuals. Several staff who succeed in achieving some competence in computer use have been lost to the private sector.

External assistance has not really helped the situation. Often donor agencies have included computer equipment and software in projects without clear justification, and their procurement regulations have precluded the possibility of establishing uniform standards for hardware and software.

Many computers are not functioning properly for the lack of relatively minor maintenance, since no budgets have been established to cover operating costs. Program and data corruption due to viruses is common. At the same time there is sincere interest within the Ministry of Health to improve the use of informatics and to connect with the global Internet and World Wide Web.

---

of the software that you intend to use should be the guiding principle in the selection of hardware. Sometimes this process is not nearly as straightforward as one would think (see Box 36). Establishing and documenting software standards early will greatly enhance system integration and maintenance later on. Following are some guidelines.

Office automation software

Select a standard suite of software for this purpose, even if your computers are initially used mainly for data entry. This should include at a minimum a word processor and an electronic spreadsheet package. The former is essential for report preparation, systems documentation, and curriculum development, whereas the latter is an invaluable tool for modelling, managing budgets, and complex graphics work. These suites often include some presentation software and a database manager, which are discussed below. If you are planning a network, good integration of these packages with network services such as electronic mail and the ability to query specialized database servers are also important considerations. In addition to providing a similar interface, these suites have the advantage of costing a good deal less than the sum of the costs of the individual packages.

Network or stand-alone?

This is a key decision to make before developing the software for a health information system. Will several people or departments need to access the same data simultaneously? Will it be easier for many data entry clerks to enter records onto the same shared database on a local area network or can the data be pulled together from different computers later using floppy disks? How timely does your information need to be? Do you wish to establish remote links from other regions and pick up the data automatically on a daily or weekly basis forming a wide area network such as that developed in China for collecting epidemiological data? With network operating systems coming down in cost and becoming simpler to install and administer, it is probably worth the investment to consider this option at the central level where large amounts of data tend to accumulate and many organizational units may want access. These systems do require special skills to set up, and they tend to make software development a bit more involved because programmers may need to build in utilities for file and record locking which they would not have to worry about with a single user application. Fortunately, basic networking capability is now built into operating systems, so that organizations can make the jump to simple networking with the addition of network cards and cabling at a later date.

Application development tools

Most health information system software has been developed using third- and fourth-generation commercial database management software for microcomputers. These applications have proved to be a reasonable compromise between cost and user friendliness. Lower level languages such as C or Pascal have also been used, but these often require a much higher degree of computer programming skill and tend to be more difficult to modify and maintain. High-end commercial client-server database systems have tended not to be used because of the high costs of the software and the hardware platform needed to run them on (see Box 35 on the Pakistan HMIS/FLCF for an example of how a commercial database program was used for application development in Pakistan). Most health information system applications have been developed with software that can also compile executable files which can be installed with no royalties or licensing fees on any number of computers. This also provides better data security, since end-users cannot change the program logic or database structures.

Database query tools and report writers

Whatever software is selected for database application development, it is important to incorporate easy-to-use tools for end-users to query the data and produce their own custom reports. Software is available commercially that produces powerful and reasonably priced report writers that can be integrated into compiled software written in other languages—this supports a variety of data file formats. The advantage of this approach is that many of these dedicated report-writing packages read data from the databases, but users cannot modify the data files as they could if they had interactive access to the complete database software.

207

Statistical analysis

A well-designed health information system often relies upon data gathered from surveys and medical record reviews in addition to routine data collection. To enter and analyse survey data effectively, it is important to have some sort of statistical analysis package. The variety of software available for this is very wide. For the simplest requirements, a package like Epi Info may suffice. This software, which was developed by the Centers for Disease Control and Prevention in the USA, is particularly easy to use in analysing data from small-scale epidemiologic surveys, such as of disease outbreaks. It has a variety of tools to develop questionnaires, enter and analyse data, and produce tabular and graphic reports. Since it is a public domain package, it is also very reasonably priced. If large sample sizes and complex data structures are required, it may be necessary to use one of the costly mainstream packages.

Geographic information systems tools (see also Chapter 12)

An increasingly important form of analysis in health information systems involves the analysis of geographic distribution and trends in health service delivery. Geographic information systems software is helpful for mapping the spatial distribution and coverage of health services and as a tool to identify geographic areas to target for health service development activities. Tools available on the market offer a wide variety of options. High-end commercial systems represent a considerable investment but can perform extremely sophisticated analyses. Interesting software with similar features has been produced by the noncommercial sector, including IDRISI from Clark University, PopMap from the United Nations Population Fund and Epi Map from WHO and the Centers for Disease Control and Prevention. One of the key features of all this software is that it enables one to take data already entered into another database application and link it to points and/or regions on maps. In the past most of these packages have required most map manipulation and viewing to be done within the geographic information systems packages themselves, making it difficult to add mapping features directly within one's applications. The dynamic data exchange and object-oriented technology features of Windows-based mapping and viewing software should make this much more practical.

Presentation graphics

Graphical presentation of data analyses plays an important role in disseminating information. Although newer versions of spreadsheets, word processors, and even databases produce a wide range of graphics, you may want to consider a specialized graphics package. If you develop multimedia presentations and slide shows for training or conferences, a range of commercial presentation packages can make this work more effective.

Utilities

- *Antivirus.* Computer viruses have become a serious threat to computer use, particularly in developing countries where the illegal copying of software is widespread. Therefore, one of the most important software utilities to purchase is good antivirus software. This should be installed on each computer and loaded as the first line of the autoexec.bat file. A wide variety of packages are available, and some come loaded with the operating systems of most computers. Unfortunately, because new computer viruses are introduced all the time, it is critical to update your antivirus software regularly. Many antivirus software developers are now providing software updates over the

Internet or through public bulletin board services. Since many viruses load themselves into active memory when a computer first starts from its hard drive, it is very important that each computer be equipped with a write-protected, self-booting diskette with antivirus and other key utilities which are needed for trouble-shooting computer problems. (In some installations, this diskette is placed in an envelope and taped to the side of the computer processor unit.)

- *Other utilities.* A variety of other tools should also be considered. Software utilities are invaluable for hardware troubleshooting, data back-up, and hard disk maintenance.
- *Communications software.* If telephone and telecommunications systems are reliable, it is wise to invest in a modem and some sort of communications software. This will simplify data exchange with remote areas and can shorten the feedback loop considerably. Perhaps someday this will even cut down on the need for so many printed reports since some analyses could be distributed using electronic mail and viewed on the computer screen. Access to messaging and conferencing services such as the Internet has also expanded surprisingly fast in developing countries. This should prove very useful for everything from getting help and software updates to sharing information from analyses done on health information system data. With so much information being exchanged through the Internet, browser software, which provides built-in utilities for file transfer and electronic mail, is probably all that is required in most installations. If Internet access is not available, a variety of specific communications software packages are available to provide dial-up connections between two computers.

Hardware

Advances in production techniques and the widespread popularity of the microcomputer have resulted in dramatic decreases in cost/performance ratios. This is good news for health services investing in this level of technology. Unfortunately, the rapid evolution of the technology also means that there is a push to replace computers every 2–3 years to take advantage of new features. This flies in the face of traditional conventions to depreciate computer equipment over periods of 5 years or more. Below are some guidelines for guiding hardware selection decisions.

Microcomputers

Buy the most powerful personal computers you can afford. Key features to look for are processor speed, memory, and hard disk capacity. Look for computers with standard modular components that can be replaced or upgraded without sophisticated equipment. Hard disks, floppy disks, video adapters, and power supplies are key components which often need replacing. In a developing country setting, try to identify computer brands which are reasonably well supported by local vendors and standardize on as few brands as is practical. It is not a luxury to include a CD-ROM (compact disc read-only memory) drive now that some of the new software is being distributed almost exclusively on CDs.

Power supply

Make sure that computers get clean electric power. Invest in an uninterruptible power supply for each computer and use in-line surge suppressors with portable computers. Use battery-operated notebook computers where power is irregular, and consider solar panels to keep them charged. Many power outlets in developing countries are not

Table 36 *Choosing printers*

Printer type	Advantages	Disadvantages
Dot matrix	Only printer which will work with multipart forms which are used in some applications, such as inventory management and billing. It is also the only type of printer for printing onto stencils (remove the ribbon first). This is an inexpensive way to produce forms and reports for wide distribution if you have a stencil duplicating machine.	Slow, noisy, requires special paper for continuous form operation. Colour options give output of mediocre quality.
Ink-jet	Good-quality output. Low-cost colour models are excellent for geographic information systems and presentations.	Slower than lasers. Ink can smear. Sharpest printing with specially treated paper can be expensive, but will work well with most photocopy paper.
Laser	Best quality output. Fastest of 3 types and therefore necessary for long reports. Uses single-sheet plain paper like a photocopier.	Expensive to maintain and run. Colour option very expensive.

earthed. Be sure to install earth wires before using desktop computers and printers or you will risk burning out components or getting an electric shock.

Printers

There are three main types of printers that need to be considered. Table 36 suggests some of the key advantages and disadvantages of each which should help in the selection process. In developing countries, three issues make the choice somewhat more difficult:

- *Cost of consumables.* Laser printers are by far the most costly to purchase, maintain, and run—replacement toner cartridges can be very difficult to find. A dot matrix or ink-jet printer with ribbons or cartridges that can be re-inked are the cheapest.
- *Paper.* Continuous form paper which is often required for continuous dot matrix printing is often difficult to find and needs to be specially ordered. Ink-jet and laser printers will take a variety of qualities of single-sheet paper formats.
- *Power.* Laser printers are enormous power consumers and cannot be connected to any but the most powerful uninterruptible power supplies. As a result they are more susceptible to damage due to power fluctuations, which are very common in developing countries. Ink-jet printers are such low electricity consumers that many of them can run on rechargeable batteries.

Spare parts and consumables

Make sure that you maintain a stock of spare parts and consumables which are often difficult to find locally. This should include:

— floppy disk drives;
— power supplies;
— hard drives;
— network cards;
— cables;

— uninterruptible power supplies;
— keyboards;
— print heads, ribbons, ink-jet cartridges, laser printer cartridges;
— replacement RAM (random access memory) modules.

Networks

A wide variety of networking options are available, and there is increasing demand to link computers together to share data and expensive peripherals like laser printers and large hard disks. Most networks require considerable effort to set up and manage, so these costs must be weighed carefully before installing a computer network. If it is essential that a variety of users simultaneously input data into and update a shared database, a network will probably be necessary.

Perhaps the most popular option for personal computer local area networking available at this time is the thin Ethernet or 10Base-T cabling scheme. This is typically installed in a star configuration, with a telephone-type cable with modular jacks connected together through one or a series of concentrators. Thick Ethernet or fibre-optic cabling have advantages for certain applications, particularly where large distances are involved or very fast data transmission speeds are required, but they are somewhat more difficult to install and to maintain. Look for improvement in wireless local area networks to simplify network installation in the coming years.

Modems

With the incredible growth of the Internet, it has become almost indispensable to purchase a modem for any computer which has access to a direct-dial phone line. This allows a computer to send and receive electronic messages and faxes, transfer files, and access the Internet. Be aware that in many developing countries, however, it is often extremely difficult to obtain extra telephone lines for telecommunications. Sometimes government-run post and telegraph companies also impose serious restrictions on the use of telecommunications equipment which they have not installed themselves. Be sure to check local circumstances before making decisions and investments.

Data backup

Ensure a good mechanism for data backup and archiving. Stand-alone computer systems are particularly vulnerable in this sense, since few come equipped with tape drives or other high-capacity backup mechanisms, and hard disk capacities continue to increase. Consider investing in a portable tape drive unit or Bernoulli-type portable hard drive that connects through a computer's parallel port to back up individual stand-alone computers. Otherwise use some sort of file compression and backup utility to back up your data and important documents regularly onto floppy disks. Networked systems must have a reliable device for backing up and archiving data. Tape drives, optical drives, and recordable CD-ROM drives are all good options to consider.

References

Auxila P, Rohde J (1988). Microcomputers as a means to introduce effective management procedures in primary health care: the Haiti experience. In: Wilson RG et al., eds. *Management information system and microcomputers in primary health care*. Geneva, Aga Khan Foundation: 53–58.

Greenes RA, Shortcliffe EH (1990). Medical informatics—an emergency academic discipline and institutional priority. *Journal of the American Medical Association*, 263:1114–1120.

Sandiford P, Annett H, Cibulskis R (1992). What can information systems do for primary health care? An International Perspective. *Social science and medicine*, 34:1077–1087.

Wilson RG, Smith DL (1991). Microcomputer applications for primary health care in developing countries. *Infectious disease clinics of North America*, 5:247–264.

12 Geographic information systems

Rainer Sauerborn and Marc Karam

Why are geographic information systems a useful supplement to health information systems?

The spatial dimension of health and health care has been noted since ancient times (for a review see Monmonier, 1993, and Picheral, 1994). Most of the data contained in health information systems are spatial data, that is data that are tied to a specific area, such as the catchment area of a health centre, or a health district, or to a geographic point (a pharmacy, village, or hospital). In technical jargon, we say such data are "georeferenced". Typically, these data are maintained in a computerized database in which location is only one variable. We can therefore easily feed health information system data into a geographic information system. Doing so, we argue in this chapter, can enhance health information systems in four important areas:

- *Data communication*. Maps display existing data in a format which is easily comprehensible to decision-makers, health practitioners, laypersons, and the media alike. We have stressed throughout the book and particularly in Chapters 2 and 3 that data must be used for more effective action and decisions. As we will see, geographic information systems constitute a particularly useful tool in achieving this.
- *Data analysis*. Spatial analysis—for example calculating the population in a radius around a water point—can only be done using geographic information systems. In addition, the results of statistical analyses can be displayed in map format.
- *Decision support*. The intuitive grasp of maps and the ability to display both health information system indicators and the results of data analyses make geographic information systems a valuable tool for decision support. In addition, maps easily reveal (geographically bound) inequities in the allocation of resources, the performance of health services, and health outcomes.
- *Links to other sectors*. Maps are a generic platform for displaying information from all sectors: education, economic development, infrastructure, finances, agriculture, and so on. Thus they provide an opportunity to share data from different sectors and foster exchange and communication. A further advantage of the intersectoral use of geographic information systems is that investment and recurrent costs can be shared.

In this chapter, we begin by defining and describing what geographic information systems are, how they can be put to work, and how much they cost. We provide some examples of geographic information system applications from a wide variety of health sector applications. We then sketch a research agenda of how to evaluate their use and how to develop geographic information systems further in order to better accommodate the needs of health practitioners and policymakers. We conclude by weighing the pros and cons of adding a geographic information system to our health information system toolbox.

What are geographic information systems and how can we use them in the context of health information systems?

The elements of geographic information systems

Maps have been used for a long time to display what we know about space. Virtually all health managers, policymakers, and many health practitioners have maps in their offices on which they manually display information they need. They use maps in their zones to display the distribution of infrastructure, personnel, health service coverage, or of health events, such as the incidence of an epidemic disease and so on.

Thematic maps are maps that display the values of a variable, for example infant mortality, through colouring or hatching of the geographical areas to which they refer (Fig. 21). Such maps can be created manually. However, low-cost computer packages exist which can generate and update maps at little marginal cost. Apart from their ease of understanding, the main strengths of maps lie in their ability to illustrate comparisons, for example between districts or provinces, and to quickly spot differences and weak areas. Figure 21 displays differentials in infant mortality rates among the 101 provinces of Bolivia and graphically demonstrates the inequitable distribution of health status (Sauerborn et al., 1995b).

Linking an already existing, computerized health information system database to a digitized map can be done in a number of ways from the very simple geographical display of data ("mapping") to the very sophisticated geographical modelling (for examples, see Scholten & Lepper, 1991). We are now ready to define what exactly we mean by geographic information systems: geographic information systems can be defined as a set of elements that allow the computerized handling of geographically defined data, their entry, storage, analysis, and presentation (Eastman et al., 1993).

Typically, data for geographic information systems are of two varieties: the first is geographical data, that is the coordinates (latitude and longitude) which define the geographical location. This can refer to a point, such as a village or a water point; a polygon, such as the catchment area of a health facility; or a line, such as a river or a road. The second type of data is attribute data. These provide the characteristics of each data point, for example number of supervisory visits for a health centre or the number of HIV-positive cases for an area.

Geographical and attribute data are the core elements of geographic information systems. The way these two types of data are linked with each other and other elements is shown in Fig. 22. First, on the side of the attribute data, there is a link with the database software used for the health information system, controlling their entry, storage, and retrieval. This, in turn, can be linked to statistical software to perform more sophisticated analyses of the attribute data.

Fig. 21   *Bolivia, infant mortality rate (provincial level)*

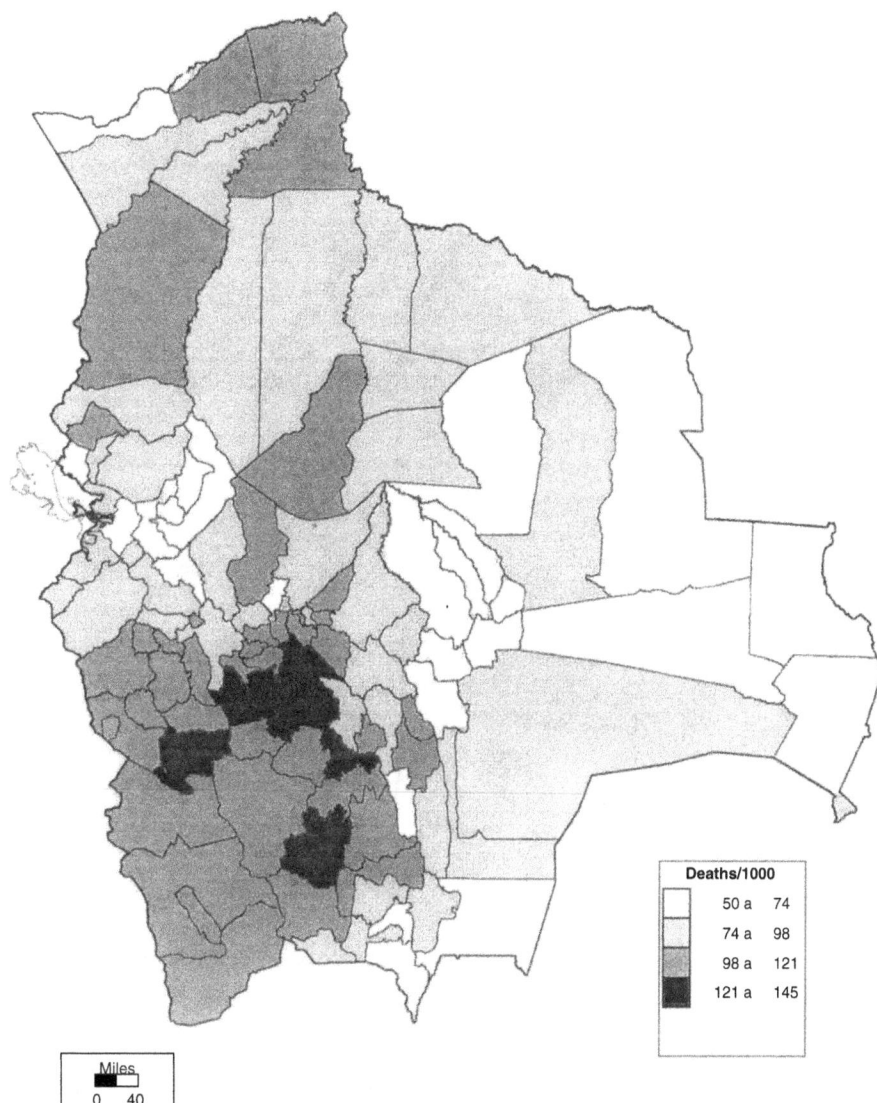

Legend:

Deaths/1000

50 a	74
74 a	98
98 a	121
121 a	145

Miles
0   40

Sources of geographical data

Paper maps can be digitized using a scanner or, preferably, a digitizing tablet. Paper maps are easy to obtain and perfectly appropriate for many purposes. However, especially in developing countries, maps are often outdated, omitting new villages or roads. They are likely to lack particular items of interest, for example health posts. Often they are also simply incorrect, for example situating villages wrongly.

It is possible to make maps (or to correct or complete paper maps) through surveys using global positioning systems. Here, each item of interest—villages, schools, health centres—can be positioned with a high degree of precision. This involves travelling to the location (e.g. a well, a

Fig. 22 *Elements of geographic information systems*

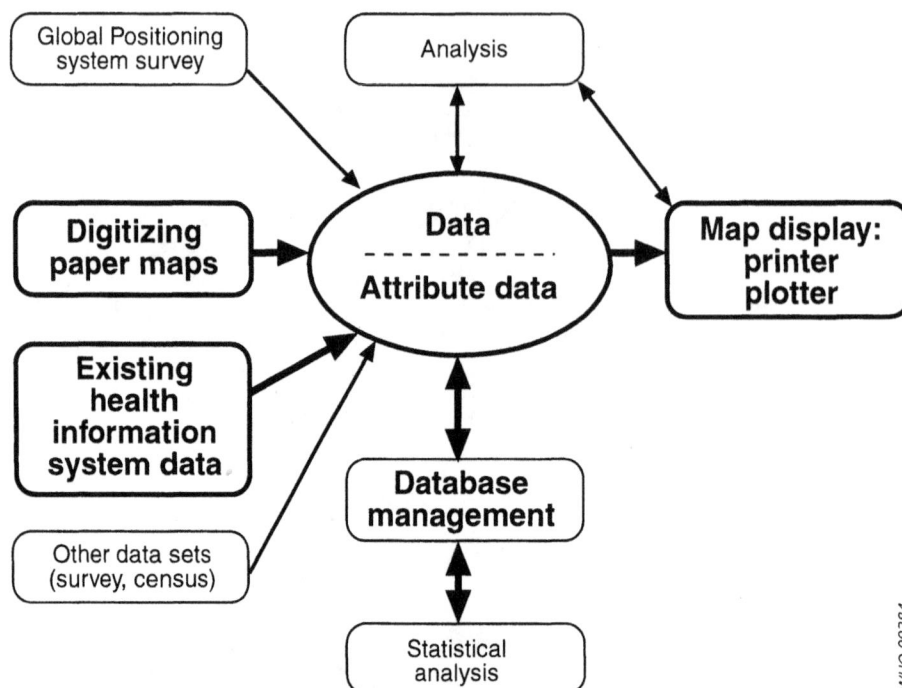

new hamlet which cannot be found on a map) and sending radio signals which are reflected by satellites. The global positioning system then calculates the exact coordinates from the signals received. A device the size of a cellular phone, costing around US$ 600, is precise to within ±30 metres. Given the low cost, high precision, and the fact that any geographical item of interest can be localized, it is no surprise that global positioning systems surveys are becoming more and more popular.

Finally, satellite images can be used as sources of geographical data. For example satellite information on climate dynamics can be used to model the movements of mosquito swarms.

Sources of attribute data

The primary resources for geographic information system applications within a health information system are listed below:

Routine health information system data
— health infrastructure, that is hospitals, health centres, village health posts, and any information related to them, such as staffing, equipment, and so on, which can be linked to the respective location;
— health indicators, such as cases of guinea worm or infant mortality rate (from census or vital event registration);
— performance indicators, such as immunization coverage, percentage of supervisions received or planned, percentage of recovery of non-salary recurrent costs, and so on.

> ## Box 37 Using geographic information systems to plan and monitor a guinea worm eradication programme
>
> The application of geographic information systems in the guinea worm eradication programme is a good example of the use of this tool in an intersectoral collaborative project. Facilities of various sectors are incorporated in base maps and displayed as single maps. Both health and education facilities are displayed, and theoretical catchment areas within a radius of 5 km (see Fig. 23) show at a glance the villages covered by the health infrastructure. One immediate observation is the absence of health coverage of a large number of villages. Officers responsible for health must therefore find ways of increasing their coverage to allow them to convey health education messages, for example.
>
> Geographic information systems make it possible to visualize what coverage would be if school teachers were also involved in guinea worm eradication activities, and in visualizing, it becomes clear that coverage can be dramatically improved if cooperation between the health and education sectors is established. Similarly, by displaying endemic villages and sources of safe water, the water sector and the health sector can easily visualize gaps, evaluate the need for wells, and effectively plan the development of water supply and sanitation.

Census data

A measure that is not contained in the health information system but which is extremely useful to include is the population size per village. This information can be obtained from census data or projections of census data.

Survey data

An example of special surveys carried out under the guinea worm eradication programme in Burkina Faso is given in Box 37.

Data from information systems of other sectors

Education, infrastructure, agriculture, and so on.

Analytical possibilities

Another feature of geographic information systems is their ability to perform geographical analyses based on different spatially defined data (more about this below). This feature, called "spatial analysis", is unique to geographic information systems and can be performed using neither a database management system alone nor with simple mapping software. These analyses can be geographic queries—for example, how many people live within a radius of 5 km from each water point? Or they can be sophisticated geographical models using overlays of several maps. The calculation of actual and theoretical catchment areas, displayed in Fig. 23, is an example of spatial analysis.

Display options

Geographic information systems contain a function for displaying attribute and geographic data together. It is possible to display primary

217

Fig. 23 *Actual and theoretical coverage by health centres, Sanmatenga, Burkina Faso*

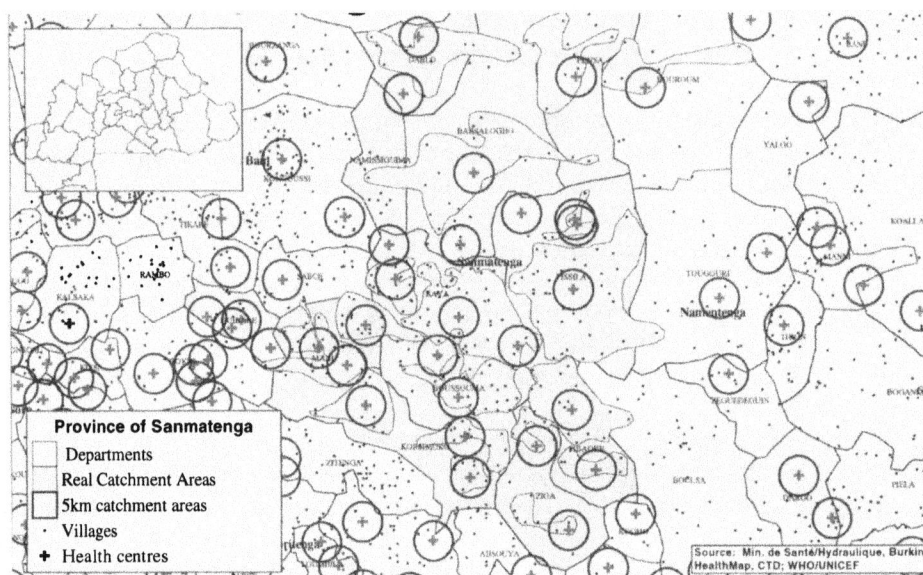

data or secondary data derived after statistical analyses or queries performed in both analytical elements. The display function therefore links both spatial and attribute information. These are several ways of displaying attribute data on a map:

- As symbols of proportional size. Examples are the display of the population size of villages or the number of cases of a given disease per village.
- As polygons of different filling or colours. Performance data can be displayed most conveniently through different colours and patterns in the catchment areas (polygons) of the health centre they belong to. Such a thematic map consists of areas of different patterns and/or colours reflecting range of values of the variable displayed.
- As superimposed tables displaying the raw data. All the data referring to a location on the map, such as a health centre (point) or a health district (area) can be accessed by just clicking on that point. This provides a window containing a conventional spreadsheet which can be searched, displayed, and printed in the usual way.

There is a growing literature on geographic information systems that describes system features and capabilities, hardware requirements, and software packages (for a general introduction, see Eastman et al., 1993). The following sections focus on the potential use of geographic information systems in health information systems and give examples drawn from our own experience.

How much do geographic information systems cost?

Because a geographic information system makes sense only once a computerized health information system is in place, it is fair to limit our consideration to its incremental costs following installation of the health information system. Moreover, we will consider the case of an initial implementation of a geographic information system. Sharing the cost of creating digitized maps across several sectors or programmes would, of course, reduce the costs for each sector or programme substantially.

Investment costs

In Bolivia, Burkina Faso, Cameroon, and Pakistan, system requirements were kept low: we used commercial geographic information systems software (about US$ 1000), a digitizing tablet for computerizing the maps (about US$ 500), and a low-end ink-jet colour printer (about US$ 600). In all countries, computers were already available to run the health information system. For all purposes presented in this chapter, a 486-MHz personal computer with 16 MB of RAM and a 700-MB hard disk will do the job. Digitizing a map of the detail of Fig. 26 will take approximately 2 weeks' time for a computer-literate person. This includes 4 days of initial training. In addition, and most importantly, those who are supposed to operate the geographic information system must receive thorough training of about 2 weeks.

The incremental costs of a geographic information system for a given country are therefore largely determined by two factors: the existing human and hardware resources and the number of geographic information system workplaces where spatial and attribute data have to be linked, analysed, and displayed. A single system centralized in the ministry is obviously much cheaper than a decentralized systems. In Cameroon, for example, the geographic information system workplace was implemented at the level of the province.

Maintenance costs

In the four countries from which our experience stems, technical assistance projects funded the cost of equipment, digitizing the maps, and initial training. As with all projects, but especially with computer applications in developing countries, the financial crux that determines sustainability lies in the recurrent costs: consumables, repair, maintenance, and depreciation. Although we are unaware of a rigorous costing of these line items as they pertain to running geographic information systems, it seems safe to say that they represent at least 30% annually of the initial investment costs.

Applications of geographic information systems within health information systems

We use the indicator concept, developed in Chapter 4, to structure this section according to input, process, output, and outcome. The examples presented here are certainly not exhaustive.

Health status (outcome)

The first documented use of maps of health outcome was probably John Snow's (1854) study of the link between the location of street water-pumps and cholera cases. Since then, a rich literature on displaying disease patterns on maps has evolved (examples are Kalipeni, 1993; Egunjobi, 1993; Ngatchou, Gubre & Ngwe, 1993; Salem, 1993). It is no surprise that, with the advent of computers, people have used digitized maps and appropriate software.

Fig. 24   *Bourasso: household illness density (per capita burden of chronic illnesses, April 1992)*

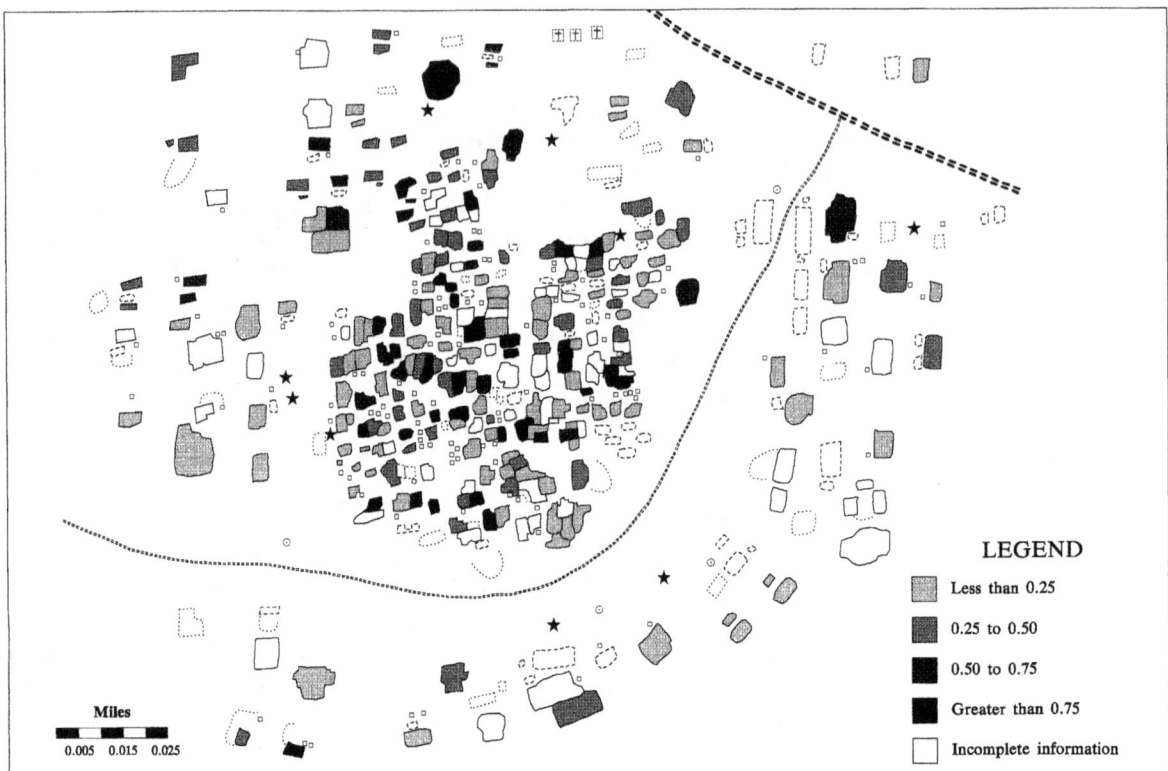

Figure 24 displays results of a health census on a village map. Here, each polygon represents a hut in the village of Bourasso in Burkina Faso (Sauerborn et al., 1995c). While these data were generated by a nonroutine method, namely a health census, it is conceivable that routine patient-based data that include the village of residence of patients consulting at the outpatient department could lead to a similar map.

Programme planning

A good example of the systematic use of geographic information systems in disease control is the WHO guinea worm eradication programme in 16 sub-Saharan countries. Overlays of access to safe water on maps of guinea worm prevalence assisted programme managers in planning safe water access for populations with a high prevalence of guinea worm (Box 37 and Fig. 23).

This map is an example of spatial analysis, which is one of the key features of geographic information systems. Three spatially referenced data sets were overlaid on the same map: population data by village (using routine national census data), cases of guinea worm disease (using nonroutine survey data), and health centres (using health information system routine data).

Planning health infrastructure and maintenance

It is obvious that health infrastructure is as inequitably distributed as health itself: using geographic information systems Akhtar and Izhar (1986) demonstrated just such inequalities in the distribution of health care resources in India and Zambia.

For health planners and managers it is important to explore ways by which health care delivery can be improved. It is important to analyse and understand the real pattern of health seeking as opposed to the theoretical catchment area. The map in Fig. 23 shows villages, health facilities, and their catchment area within a radius of 5 km and the actual catchment area. Some health centres have no catchment area, and some villagers seek care in a dispensary located at longer distance. Reasons for this can, for example, be better access by road, but it can also be an indicator of better performance of this facility as compared with a closer one, that is presence of a competent nurse, provision of drugs at that facility, presence of pharmacy in that village, and so on.

Displaying performance indicators

This is a relatively new field. By linking the database of the health information system with a digitized map showing catchment areas of health facilities, supervisors can easily spot performance outliers in their districts. Since both data and maps can be aggregated at the health centre, district, provincial, and national levels, each level of decision-makers can be provided with a thematic map that corresponds to their decision needs.

Displaying health care coverage

The most widespread use of geographic information systems is the display of coverage indicators, such as measles immunization for instance.

Intersectoral use of geographic information systems

Maps are used by virtually all social and economic sectors. This opens up two opportunities for intersectoral cooperation.

The costs of digitizing maps can be shared, both in terms of hardware and software, and of the actual creation of maps. In this case, each sector would be responsible only for creating the layers relevant to its own field: schools for the education sector, water points for the infrastructure sector, and various layers of infrastructure, performance, and outcome for the health sector. A true intersectoral view of development emerges when data sets of different sectors, such as health and education, are overlaid to explore synergies or disparities.

Who uses maps?

This section contains some illustrative examples of applications of geographic information systems. The list is by no means exhaustive, nor do we have enough information to analyse the full range of uses to which geographic information systems have been applied.

Operations managers and health practitioners

Health planners, supervisors, and practitioners are the typical users of geographic information systems. In Bolivia, geographic information systems will be used to plan facility and equipment maintenance. In Cameroon and Pakistan, geographic information systems are integrated into the routine feedback reports to health facility staff and district managers.

Policymakers

Senior policymakers have insisted on using the combined health and education geographic information system themselves from their own desks. To make this possible, a customized and especially user-friendly interface in Spanish was added to the existing software. In addition, geographic information system-generated maps of health and education indicators have been used in parliament and in planning commissions in Bolivia.

Media

In Bolivia and Cameroon, geographic information system displays have been used by the local and national media, including television.

Research agenda

We see three areas where research is needed to document and improve the usefulness of application of geographic information systems in the health sector.

Assessing the use of geographic information systems for decision making

The examples of actual use of the analytical and display features of geographic information systems, given in this chapter, are admittedly anecdotal. A thorough analysis is needed of the activities and decisions for which geographic information systems output is actually used, broken down by type of user, that is health practitioner, health manager, and policymaker. Ideally such an analysis should capture variables of the decision-making environment that foster or deter the use of the system. It is obvious that such an analysis has to include the use of the health information system in general. Such studies would test the assumptions underlying the role of information systems in health planning and policy, which we formulated in Chapter 3.

Cost analysis

It would be appropriate to determine the marginal costs of adding a geographic information system to an existing health information system. This would inform those who have to decide whether or not to introduce the geographic information system into the health sector. It allows them to better judge whether they can afford such a system, and more importantly, whether the benefits justify the costs.

Time series

Unless video display techniques are used, geographic information systems are notoriously weak at displaying temporal change. However, most routine data in health information systems are time series. To date, little is known about how we can display temporal change and spatial change in indicators at the same time without cluttering the display (see Langran, 1992).

Develop spatial analysis

To the best of our knowledge, there are only very few applications within an existing health information system where the full potential of statistical and spatial analysis of geographic information systems is brought to the fore. Research is needed regarding which types of these analyses might be useful for decision-makers to include in their health information systems.

Summary

- Maps are excellent, inherently appealing tools for displaying the geographic distribution of indicators of health information systems. Their use goes well beyond the professional health practitioner, health manager, or policymaker to the general public and the media.
- Maps reveal inequities (Curto de Casas, 1993; Sauerborn et al., 1995b), at least those that can be spotted on maps, which can be politically sensitive. On the other hand, this aspect allows those who take equity in health care delivery seriously to spot and remedy gross spatial inequities, for example in the allocation of resources or in health outcomes.
- Thematic maps can easily and regularly be updated. They allow easy access to databases related to health facilities by clicking on them. Further, they have a unique potential to assist health planners in certain tasks, such as monitoring disease control efforts or localizing new health infrastructures.
- The marginal costs of adding a geographic information system to an existing health information system infrastructure are relatively low, especially if they are shared by several sectors (ministries).
- The analytical capabilities of geographic information systems remain to be tapped, and appropriate applications need to be developed. Apart from area queries (how many inhabitants live in a radius of x km around a health facility), we are not aware of any modelling of planning scenarios based on geographic information systems. This is a challenge that lies ahead of us. Another challenge is to find ways to display temporal change on maps.
- One caveat is in order that applies to all computer applications in the social sector: that is the danger of developing a system that is not put to use for those who need it but rather remains within the circles of computer specialists for whom it is yet another gadget to play with (Sauerborn et al., 1995a).

References

Akhtar R, Izhar N (1986). The spatial distribution of health resources within countries and communities: Examples from India and Zambia. *Social science and medicine*, 22:1115–1129.

Curto de Casas S (1993). Geographical inequalities in mortality in Latin America. *Social science and medicine*, 36:1349–1353.

Eastman JR et al. (1993). *The GIS handbook.* Washington, DC, USAID/ARTS/FARA/SARSA: 1–66.

Egunjobi L (1993). Spatial distribution of mortality from leading notifiable diseases in Nigeria. *Social science and medicine*, 36:1267–1272.

Kalipeni E (1993). Determinants of infant mortality in Malawi: a spatial perspective. *Social science and medicine*, 37:183–198.

Langran G (1992). *Time in geographic information systems.* London, Taylor and Francis.

Monmonier M (1993). Maps in the humanities and social sciences. In: Monmonier M, ed. *Mapping it out—expository cartography for the humanities and social sciences.* Chicago, University of Chicago Press: 3–18.

Ngatchou R, Gubry P, Ngwe E (1993). Les inégalités géographiques de la mortalité au Cameroun. [Geographic variability of mortality in Cameroon.] *Social science and medicine*, 36:1285–1290.

Picheral HE (1994). Place, space, and health. *Social science and medicine*, 39:1589–1590.

Ruiz Mier F (1995). *Sistema de información geográfica sobre infraestructura social. [Geographical information systems and social infrastructure.]* La Paz, Ministry of Human Development.

Salem G (1993). Géographie de la mortalité et de la natalité à Pikine (Sénégal): intérêts et limites des données d'état civil dans les villes africaines. [Geographical variability of mortality rate and birth rate in Pikine, Senegal. Significance and limitations of the civil registration database in African cities.] *Social science and medicine*, 36:1297–1311.

Sauerborn R, Mendelsohn D (1994). *Design and implementation of a geographical information system for the social sector of Bolivia. Report for the UDAPSO project.* La Paz (for the Harvard Institute for International Development under USAID contract).

Sauerborn R et al. (1995a). *Geographical information systems—toy or tool for health systems research?* Workshop of the European Institutes of Tropical Medicine on Health Systems Reserch, Valbella, Switzerland, 29 January–1 February.

Sauerborn R et al. (1995b). Muestra de disigualdades en el sector social: el sistema de información geográfico de indicadores de salud, desnutrición, educación, vivienda y probreza en Bolivia. [Variability in the social sector: geographic information systems indicators of health, malnutrition, education, housing, and poverty in Bolivia.] Third Latin American Conference on Social Sciences in Medicine, São Paulo, Brazil, 8–12 April.

Sauerborn R et al. (1995c). *Stratégies d'adaptation des ménages aux coûts économiques de la maladie.* [Household strategies for adapting to the economic costs of illness.] Frankfurt, Lang.

Scholten HJ, Lepper MJC (1991). The benefits of the application of geographical information systems in public and environmental health. *World Health Statistics Quarterly*, 44:160–170.

13 The context of health information system reform

Theo Lippeveld

Introduction

In the previous chapters, we tried to create conceptual clarity and to define the structure and content of appropriate health management information systems. Although these concepts are integral to health information system reform, implementation goes far beyond them. Based on our experience and confirmed by other researchers and field workers (de Kadt, 1989; Helfenbein et al., 1987; Sandiford, Annett & Cibulskis, 1992), the task of health information system reform is both formidable and complex, particularly in the context of government bureaucracies in developing countries. Failures tend to be more common than successes. Designing and implementing "technically sound" systems involves not only technical expertise but also in-depth understanding of political, sociocultural, and administrative factors. This is well illustrated by the following description by Auxila & Rohde (1988) related to the implementation of a newly designed computerized information system in Haiti: "Resistance to any change in the [health information] system was predictable and high. For some employees, there was simply the fear that the computer would take their jobs, and for others, the inherent laziness at learning new tasks. For others, there was the clear desire to retain the existing system as the lack of knowledge and readily, retrievable data was in itself a power base for various people within the Ministry bureaucracy."

Identifying how these related factors positively or negatively influence the health information system reform process will permit policymakers and health administrators to develop appropriate strategies in designing and implementing a restructured health information system. Walt & Gilson (1994) propose a simple policy analysis model that, in addition to considering technical content, incorporates three other categories of variables that influence policy reform efforts: the actors involved in the reform process; the context within which the process takes place; and the process itself starting from policy formation, and ultimately leading to policy implementation (see Fig. 25). As Walt & Gilson clearly point out, the model is an extreme simplification of a "complex set of inter-relationships" among each of these components of the reform process.

In this chapter we apply this policy analysis model to health information system reform cases. First, we analyse how the specific technical content of health information system reform influences the reform outcome. Second, we identify the usual set of actors in such reforms, and discuss how, independently of the technical content, they can make or break the newly restructured health information system. Third, we focus on the role contextual factors play in health information system reform. And fourth, we examine the process of health information system reform

Fig. 25   *A model for health policy analysis*

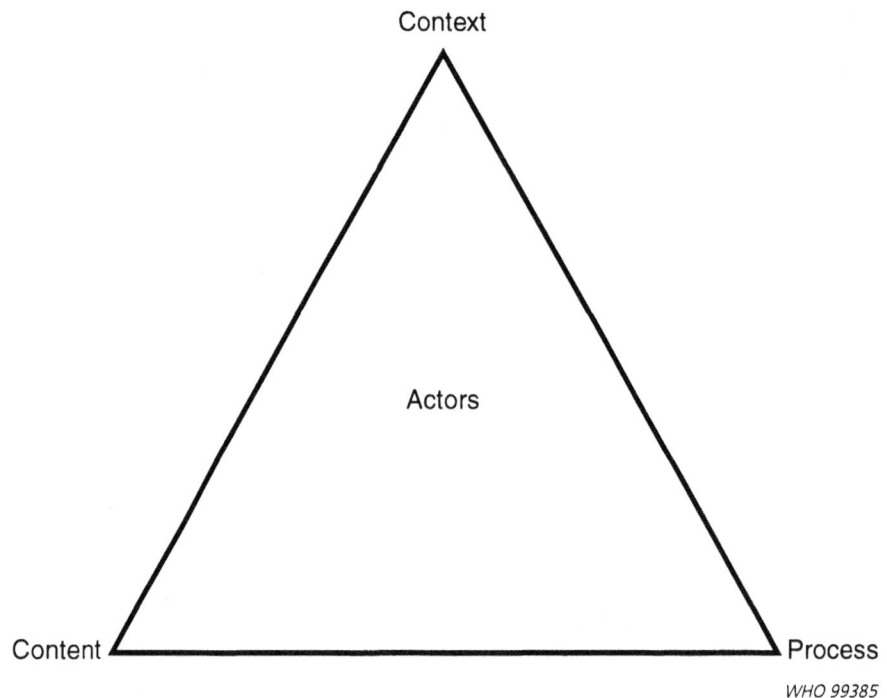

Source: Walt & Gilson, 1994.

itself, and how individual actors can influence it. Based on this analysis, we then present potential strategies for successful design and implementation of routine health information systems. Our experience and, consequently, most of our examples stem from health information system reform efforts at the national level. Yet the model of analysis as well as the proposed strategies can apply to health information system reform in other settings, such as within a nongovernmental agency, within one district, or even within one health facility.

Health information system reform: a policy analysis

The content: how is health information system reform related to other health sector reform efforts and what should its scope be?

If a health information system is a functional entity within the framework of the health services as a whole, clearly health information system reform should be narrowly linked with reform at other levels of the health care system. Frenk (1995) identifies four levels for reform: systemic, programmatic, organizational, and instrumental. Health information system reform fits into the category of "instrumental" health reform because it targets the improvement of various management systems. At the same time, it cannot be viewed separately from reform efforts at the systemic, programmatic, and organizational levels. For example, effective flow of information within the health care system depends upon the organizational structure of the health care system (organizational reform). Without a clear set of priorities (programmatic reform), managers and policymakers will find it difficult to agree upon a set of essential indicators for the health information system. And, of course, it is meaningless to restructure health information systems for health services that are not used by the population (systemic reform). This interrelationship was clearly demonstrated in Chad, where health information system reform was undertaken mainly because of pressure from USAID. During the consensus-building meetings in the Ministry of Health, it became clear that a broader organizational reform aiming at deconcentration of the health services system would be required to ensure effective use of the information generated under the newly designed information system. Health information system reform thus should be tied into a more general systemic reform providing universal access to essential care. Efforts to implement more accessible decentralized district health systems are now underway in several developed as well as developing countries. "Health information is not only an essential resource for the development of district health systems, but also an integral component of that development" (WHO, 1994).

What should be the scope of health information system reform? Obviously, from a technical viewpoint, the extent to which the existing health information system needs to be changed depends first of all on the status of the information-generating process (see Chapters 2 and 5). Do the indicators correspond to the real information needs at different management levels in the health services system? What is the quality of the data collection instruments? How effective are data transmission and processing? Do managers and care providers receive appropriate feedback on the reported data? And, most important, do they use the information for planning and management? Based on the answers to these questions, health information system reform can take any shape from partial to comprehensive restructuring. Health information system reform in Chad (Lippeveld, Foltz & Mahouri, 1992) was clearly comprehensive, whereas the Ministry of Health in Niger decided to limit health information system reform to changes in data transmission and processing through computerization at the national level (Ministry of Public Health of Niger, 1991). In the Philippines, the Field Health Services Information System initiated by the Ministry of Health was concerned only with first level care facilities, and limited reporting of information to the system management level (Ministry of Health of the Philippines, 1990).

But the technical requirements for change cannot be divorced from effects of the process of change itself. "The more radical or innovative the proposed change is in regard to the information system, the greater the implications for change in the organization" (Helfenbein et al., 1987, p. 64). Decisions about the scope of restructuring should therefore also take into account contextual and process factors as discussed below. The Ministry of Health of Pakistan decided not to include private health facilities in a first phase of the recently undertaken health information system reform process. Health officials determined that it would be difficult to impose the same type of standardized data collection system used for government health facilities on the private sector without a well-established regulatory framework already in place. Comprehensive restructuring is rarely feasible in the public sector, except for situations such as in Chad, where the unique political context immediately after the end of the civil war facilitated the consensus-building process (Lippeveld, Foltz & Mahouri, 1992), or more recently in Eritrea, where a new country is rebuilding its bureaucratic structures (Tekle et al., 1995). If possible, well-functioning elements of the existing system should be preserved. For example, in Pakistan it was decided not to change data collection procedures in major hospitals, because assessments had shown that the existing system provided satisfactory information to hospital managers

(Lippeveld, Foltz & Mahouri, 1992). The scope of restructuring can also be influenced in part by other ongoing reform efforts. For example, in Eritrea it was decided to link health information system reform with the overall process of administrative reform, which was intended to decentralize major decision-making powers to the regions.

Another heavily debated issue in recent health information system reforms, and one that shows the importance of both process factors and technical arguments in deciding the scope of health information system reform, is the appropriateness of creating national information systems. In the context of decentralized and community-based health systems, it is argued that health information systems should take into account the health problems of the community and be responsive to the information needs of local managers at the district level. Therefore, it cannot be imposed from the national level. Yet national managers claim they need standardized indicators and reporting procedures in order to make valid interregional comparisons for use in resource allocation decisions. The technical answer to this issue is embedded in the conceptual health services system framework presented in Chapter 2. Information needs can be derived from the specific functions and activities that exist at each level of the health services system. To the extent that they provide direct health care to communities, basic health services will need a certain number of indicators that are specific to these communities, particularly for facility and patient/client management. However, this should prevent districts from reporting a standardized set of data to the national level, so that national managers can make informed decisions related to their own functions and activities. Nonetheless, such data sets should only include data which can be used by the local managers and care providers, with data for the national level obtainable through other data sources. In order to make health information system design responsive to these objectives, it is important to include peripheral managers and care providers in the design process.

The actors: who has a stake in health information system reform?

Even something as technocratic as health information system reform has strong political dynamics. As Helfenbein et al. put it (1987): "Changing the way information is gathered, processed, and used for decision-making implies changing the way an organization operates. The objective of producing and utilizing information more effectively will affect the behavior and motivation of all personnel." Understanding what is at stake for each of the actors in the health information system reform process is therefore of utmost importance. As mentioned already, health information system reform is essentially taking place in the "bureaucratic arena"; thus, most of the involved parties are members of public or private bureaucracies. In most countries a tentative list of actors affected by health information system reform would include central level policy-makers, health planners, and administrators; national programme managers; health insurance administrators; regional and district level health administrators; health facility managers, such as hospital directors and those in charge of primary care facilities; selected staff from health-related sectors; donor agencies; nongovernmental agencies; staff from academic and health-training institutes; community leaders; and, ultimately, the communities at large. Each of these groups has different perceptions regarding the need for information and the information system itself. As an example, although presenting routine facility-based information on child health problems broken down by two age groups (e.g.

0–1 and 1–4 years) instead of one (e.g. 0–4 years) can improve the priority-setting decisions of health planners, it will double the data processing work of a clerk in charge of compiling monthly data in the health facility.

In their analysis of information systems for primary health care, Sandiford, Annett & Cibulskis (1992) identify at least three groups of actors strongly in favour of improved health information systems: health service managers, public health specialists, and information technology experts. However, each group has different expectations. Health service managers expect increased efficiency and more rational allocation of resources. Public health specialists are interested in both improved effectiveness and equity of the health care system. The information technology experts are convinced that computerized information systems will liberate health workers from "the drudgery of form filling". But as they point out, other influential groups do not necessarily share this goal of maximizing equity, efficiency, or cost-effectiveness. Managers often base their decisions on power relations and value judgements rather than on rational information, and improved information systems may be threatening for some of them. As an example, disease programme managers are generally accustomed to receiving information through vertical reporting systems and may strongly oppose efforts to integrate information systems. In other cases, the introduction of computers can mean the loss of jobs for certain employees. Another potential problem concerns health care providers, for whom a routine health information system is essential for high-quality information; nonetheless, they often show little interest in health information system reform, simply because it is not part of their "professional culture". Also, aid agencies could oppose health information system reform because they fear it would threaten their own particular information needs.

In their analysis of the introduction of a computerized personnel information system in the Kenyan Ministry of Agriculture, Peterson et al. (1994) point out the lack of organizational relationships within African bureaucracies. This finding implies that individuals can have significant impact with respect to the development of information systems. For information systems reform in the public sector to be successful, they stress that leadership (the "saint") is crucial in order to manage the "demons". In their terminology, the saint is a progressive senior government official who is willing to shoulder the reform effort, while "demons" are government staff or other concerned actors resisting the reform. Peterson et al. classify the latter group into two categories: destructive and apathetic demons. Although destructive demons can act openly or surreptitiously, it is the latter category that is most threatening, because they are difficult to recognize. The saint also needs support from technical experts (the "wizards"), but health information system reform can also fail because of "inappropriate wizards". Again, Peterson et al. classify them into two categories: the "high tech" wizards or "technoholics", who often create an information system that is overly sophisticated and inappropriate for meeting the information needs of the organization; and the "high tech" wizards, who will "deliver technology, training, and sensitivity seminars . . . but not the system required." We would argue that a systemic development effort as complex as health information system reform requires a "team of wizards", one that brings together experts from a variety of fields such as systems analysis, epidemiology, health policy and planning, human resource management, computer sciences, logistics management, and so on.

Reich (1994) developed a methodology for investigating how different actors might be affected by the envisioned health reform process. This method, called "political mapping of health policy", identifies and assesses groups that are likely to be resistant as well as their relative strengths and weaknesses.

The context: what is the environment in which health information system reform takes place?

Whatever perceptions the various decision-makers may have of the reforms, their influence on the design and implementation of the reform initiative is limited by the boundaries of the political, socioeconomic, and administrative context in which the reform takes place. A careful preliminary analysis of these contextual factors may shed light not only on the constraints these factors place on the reform process but also on potential strategies to cope with such problems during the design and implementation phase.

As already indicated, because health information system reform generally takes place within the public sector framework, *the administrative capacity of the government* is a critical determinant in the outcome of the reform. Unfortunately, government bureaucracies and, more particularly, health ministries in most developing countries are very weak. Their capacity to cope with change is also very limited, especially in countries with heavily centralized bureaucracies and ineffective service delivery systems at local levels. In fact, one of the factors explaining the success of health information system reform in Chad was the "underbureaucratization" of the Ministry of Health after the end of the civil war (Lippeveld, Foltz & Mahouri, 1992). One direct result of a management environment in which decisions are made on value judgements and power relations is an almost total lack of perception as to the link between information and management. This is certainly the case at the lower levels of the health care delivery system, where managers and care providers often have no control at all over the production and use of information. As Helfenbein et al. (1987) point out: "Information was generally something managers were obliged to send to a national office of health statistics or a planning department." This lack of "information culture" is probably the biggest constraint for any health information system reformer. The transformation of "data-led" information systems into "action-led" information systems will need substantial investments in training of health personnel or, as Sandiford, Annett & Cibulskis (1992) propose, "ritualization" of data analysis and interpretation procedures.

In Chapter 2, we described how establishment of a health information system must closely match *the structure of the health services delivery system* in order to fully support the decision-making process at different levels of the health system. Health care delivery systems may be situated on a continuum with three main management axes: centralized versus decentralized; vertical versus horizontal; and public versus private management. Understanding the actual and projected position of the health care system on this continuum is another crucial requirement for efficiently managing the health information system reform process. Health information systems should "fit" this health care system. A hospital administrator with no decision-making power over the promotion and transfer of his personnel is obviously not very motivated in keeping a very detailed personnel management record system. As Sandiford, Annett & Cibulskis (1992) state: "Where decision making is centralized, the information system must also exhibit some centralism, even though this may reduce its ability to detect and act on the patchiness within the system." Efforts to streamline reporting flows through line management channels in a health services system where national programmes have set up separate reporting systems will fail unless the proposed changes have the full support of the national programme managers. The move in several developing countries to decentralize and integrate health care delivery systems calls for concomitant changes in information support (WHO, 1994). District health information systems need to combine simple, efficient, and integrated data collection with the production of action-oriented information of acceptable quality, as was often the case under the "vertical" disease programmes.

Another contextual factor that can heavily influence the health information system reform process is *the political environment*. Even with a health information system reform that takes place mainly within the "bureaucratic arena", it is important to understand the influence of the prevailing political system in the country. An excellent example is provided by Foltz & Foltz (1991), who discuss health information system reform in Chad between 1985 and 1988. As the authors point out, "ministry business was often conducted on the basis of factional alliances, not bureaucratic position. Higher officials frequently blocked proposals or projects put forward by civil servants belonging to other factions, and called in extra-ministry allies to make their point stick". A direct result of politicized bureaucracies and, in our experience, a serious general constraint for systems development efforts, is the high transfer rate of civil servants. In most bureaucracies, whenever political constituencies change, the entire top management changes. Yet even under stable political regimes, high-level managers are frequently transferred to avoid the build-up of internal bureaucratic fiefdoms. During the 2-year design phase of the Pakistan HMIS/FLCF, consensus building between the provincial health departments was seriously hampered by the frequent changes of the director generals heading the delegations of each province.

Another part of the political context is *the international donor community* and the role it plays in health sector reform generally and in health information system reform more specifically. In the last decade, governments of developing countries have been under pressure from multilateral and bilateral donor agencies to increase the efficiency (less frequently the equity) of their health care delivery systems. Health care reforms have been imposed as "conditionalities" for further disbursement of funds. In several countries, such external donor pressure has been the real impetus for getting health information system reform on the agenda.[1] Although health information system reform in these countries is in actuality key for improving planning and management of the health services, it is obvious that without mobilizing internal support, such reforms ultimately cannot be sustained. This is well illustrated by the case of Pakistan, where health information system reform was initiated in 1991 with funding and technical assistance provided through USAID, but after the withdrawal of American aid in 1994, seriously suffered due to lack of government support.

---

[1] Recent examples of such "donor-driven" health information system reforms are Chad, Haiti, Malawi, Niger, and Pakistan.

Although the government sector is still the main health care provider in most developing countries, private providers increasingly manage health services. Should *the private sector* be included in health information system reform efforts? It is obvious that the incentives for private care providers to participate in a national health information system are not the same as those for civil servants. Certainly, they need information to follow up on individual patients and clients and to manage their health facilities. At the same time they are less likely to comply with burdensome reporting systems. The absence of well-established regulatory systems for the private sector in many developing countries exacerbates the situation. An important distinction also must be made between for-profit and nonprofit care providers. In several low-income countries, mainly in Africa, religious groups and nongovernmental agencies control a substantial portion of the health care delivery infrastructure. Such groups are often better organized than the private for-profit care providers and are also more willing to collaborate with government health services. In Chad, for example, reformers decided to include religious and voluntary groups in the health information system reform efforts. In Pakistan, on the other hand, where more than half of the health services are provided through private for-profit institutions, planners focused reform efforts solely on the government health services.

The process: how does it influence the outcome of health information system reform?

Unfortunately, without a well-managed implementation process, cognizance of all these issues is largely an intellectual exercise. In their analysis on public sector reforms in developing countries, Grindle & Thomas (1991) use a series of case studies to show that the policy decision to undertake reform is only the first step in a long process moving towards sustainable implementation. In analysing this implementation process, they consider the classic "linear model of implementation" (see Fig. 26) as insufficient to explain success or failure of reform. If the reform effort fails, a typical post-mortem is that there was "lack of politi-

Fig. 26 *The linear model of policy reform*

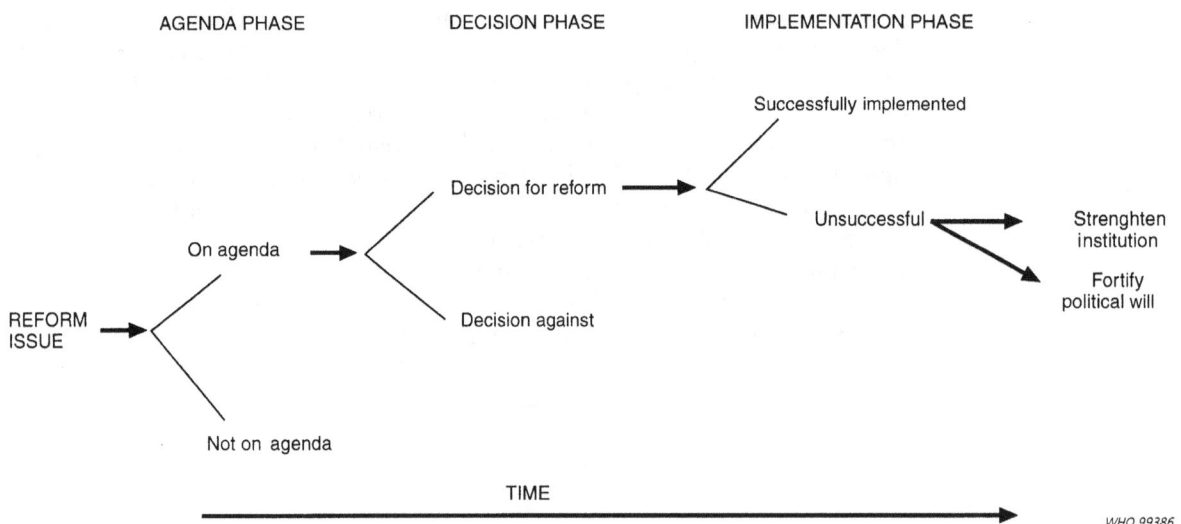

Source: Grindle & Thomas, 1991.

cal will", or "the implementing institution was not strong enough for the task". The authors propose an interactive model for implementing policy reform, in which "the process of policy change ... [is] shaped significantly by the actions of individuals in strategic locations to influence a particular change." These decision-makers and policy managers need to mobilize the political, financial, managerial, and technical resources necessary to sustain implementation of the reform (see Fig. 27). This interactive model permits a much more refined analysis of the health information system reform process, and also leads to the formulation of important health information system development strategies. In the following paragraphs we will apply this model to previous health information system reform experiences.

Throughout this book, the absence of an "information culture", particularly at lower levels of the health services system, has been identified as one of the main reasons that managers do not make decisions based on information. Experiences in Cameroon, Chad, and Pakistan have clearly shown that, while time-consuming, a broad-based involvement of future health information system users in the health information system reform process can be a powerful trigger for better use of information once the system has been operationalized. In all three countries, planners started

Fig. 27   *An interactive model of policy implementation*

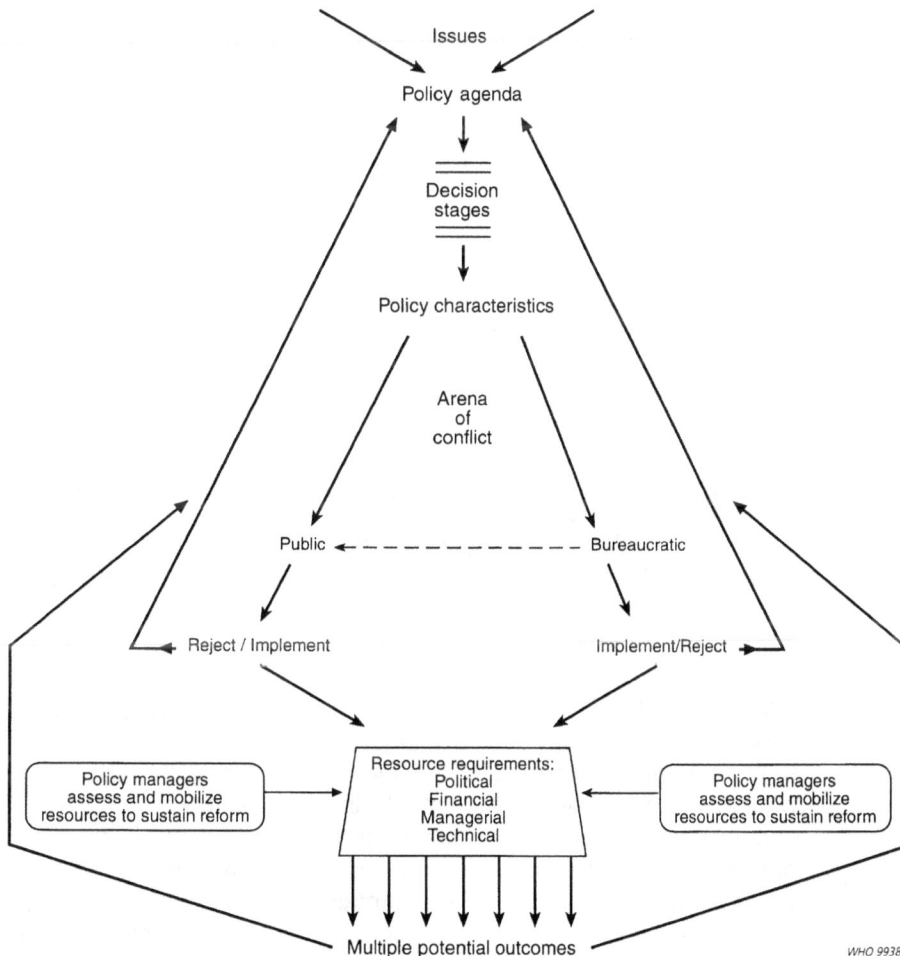

Source: Grindle & Thomas, 1991.

"health information system working groups", including policymakers, health managers, care providers, and, most important, potential opponents of the projected reform. These groups of future users met with the technical expert teams during a series of consensus-building meetings. The final form of the restructured health information system was based on compromises between various interested parties and reflected the particular information needs of the central as well as peripheral health services levels. WHO has adopted a similar consensus-building approach in recent efforts to advise countries on the selection and definition of a set of national health indicators (Sapirie & Orzeszyna, 1995).

Another successful strategy that has gradually changed the attitudes of health managers and care providers regarding the value of information has been to use extensive training activities during both the design and the implementation phase of health information system reforms. In most countries, curricula for doctors, paramedics, or other health-related professionals do not include courses on health information systems. Care providers frequently are not even shown how to fill out various data collection instruments when they begin their jobs. To address this problem, officials in Pakistan developed a 5-day training programme for district managers and care providers on their newly designed system. The trainees not only learned how to fill out forms, but also how to use, through case studies, the data of monthly reports in management decisions at the district and health facility levels.

The experience of Pakistan in designing and implementing a new "health management information system for first level care facilities (HMIS/FLCF)", as detailed in Box 38, also showed that, without the necessary resources, implementing the policy decision to change the health information system was very difficult. At various time periods during the implementation phase, the lack of financial resources and the premature withdrawal of the technical assistance team threatened HMIS/FLCF survival.

Time is another important resource that needs careful management during the implementation phase of health information system reform.

Box 38 Designing a health management information system for first level care facilities in Pakistan: is consensus building a worthwhile effort?

In May 1991, the Ministry of Health of Pakistan decided to transform its routine reporting system for first level care facilities into a comprehensive health management information system (HMIS/FLCF). During the design phase, an extensive consensus-building process was used both to win over potential opponents of the system as well as to ensure that the newly designed health information system would respond to the information needs of all health services levels. First, a series of meetings were held with national programme managers. Initially, Expanded Programme on Immunization managers were very worried that, by dismantling vertical information systems, health information system reform would disrupt effective programmatic and logistic management. Potential problem areas in defining indicators and information flows were openly discussed until satisfactory compromises could be found.

Then the Ministry of Health set up health information system working groups in each province. These groups included district managers, care providers, and statistical officers. During two workshops, the members of these health information system working groups discussed the content and structure of the future HMIS. A provisional list of indicators as well as a proposed macrostructure for HMIS/FLCF were presented by representatives from each province during a national workshop in January 1992. Representatives from the federal Ministry of Health, national programmes, professional medical groups, and the donor community also participated. Although the ministry would have accepted provincial differences in indicators and data collection procedures, all participants felt it more efficient to develop a national list of indicators and a uniform reporting system. It therefore took some heated debates and tedious compromises to reach that objective. The biggest stumbling block was disease reporting. Everyone agreed that the previous reporting on more than 100 disease categories was cumbersome and needed to be simplified, but what was the ideal number of disease categories and which ones should be chosen? The final list of 18 health problems mainly included those for which potential action programmes already existed, so that monitoring trends for these problems was important for programmatic decision making.

It was also decided to delegate the development of data collection instruments and the computerized data processing system to a team of experts. After a period of 6 months of design and field testing, during which the experts maintained close contact with the provincial workgroups, the final design and implementation plan of HMIS/FLCF was approved at the end of another national workshop. One of the compromises developed at this meeting concerned data transmission procedures. While vertical programme managers wanted to maintain parallel reporting procedures until HMIS/FLCF implementation was complete, district managers objected to the additional time and work burdens this would engender for care providers. The compromise solution was that all separate reporting would be discontinued as soon as a full district had been trained in using the new system.

Although this entire consensus-building process had taken more than a year, the benefits became obvious during the implementation phase. Managers at provincial and district levels who had been involved in the design phase started using preliminary computerized feedback reports in discussions with their staff on the implementation of maternal and child health services. Also, every time an attempt was made to change the content or the procedures for HMIS/FLCF implementation, members of the workgroups vehemently objected. For ammunition they cited the written agreements of the national workshop, which had been distributed widely throughout the country.

Unfortunately, after 1 year, during which time about half of the districts in Pakistan had worked with the new system. USAID's financial support stopped, and alternative funding did not become immediately available. Of course, this financial constraint slowed down the pace of implementation. As is the case in many bureaucracies, high staff turnover rates had resulted in the appointment of new managers to decision-making positions, and many of them had not been involved in the consensus-building process. Moreover, some of these decision makers started to question the new system, which further slowed the implementation process. Also, with the USAID technical assistance team out of the country, HMIS/FLCF implementation in most provinces could not be continued until the World Bank agreed to fund remaining training activities and bring in additional technical assistance.

"The longer the time needed to implement a reform, the more likely that potential conflict and resistance will emerge and that administrative capacity within the system will determine the sustainability of the reform" (Thomas & Grindle, 1990). Particularly in the case of routine health information systems, implementation over extended time periods can be very disruptive to system management. During the transition period in Pakistan, some health facilities began reporting under the new system, while the rest were still using the old reporting system. When resource constraints halted further implementation, data processing became very complicated, and channelling information to programme managers was delayed and incomplete. Certain opponents who wanted to prove the system's inability to respond to programmatic information needs exploited this situation.

Strategies for health information system reform

Thus far, we have emphasized that restructuring health information systems requires both a conceptually sound technical approach as well as in-depth understanding of the dynamics of the reform process. We used a policy analysis model proposed by Walt & Gilson (1994) to demonstrate, through previous experience, that the success of health information system reform depends not only on technical improvements of the health information system structure and of the information generation process but also on the various actors who have stakes in its outcome, the specific bureaucratic and sociopolitical context in which the reform takes place, and the process used to design and implement the change. The challenge, as Reinke (1988) states, "is to add rationality while still accommodating the interests of diverse constituencies and value systems."

Thus, given previous analyses, which strategies should reformers use to successfully guide health information system restructuring from the policy decision stage to the point at which the restructured system can achieve better planning and management throughout the health services system? For practical reasons we have categorized these strategies under the four main phases of health information system reform: (i) planning, (ii) assessment, (iii) design, and (iv) implementation. Be aware, however, that some of these strategies are not necessarily linked to a particular phase of health information system reform, but (especially planning phase strategies) are applicable to the entire health information system reform process. We also assume that for various reasons senior management of the organizations under consideration (usually the ministry of health) made the decision to undertake health information system reform.

Planning the health information system reform process

Establish a health information system development team
Based on the technical, organizational, and managerial complexities of health information system reform, a multidisciplinary team needs to be in charge of the health information system development effort. Ideally, this "health information system development team" will include a health planner/manager, a computer expert, and a skilled trainer. Because major health information system reforms are complex undertakings, they will probably also require external consultants for particular skill areas, such as systems analysis, epidemiology, policy analysis, manage-

ment systems development, computer programming, and so on. In addition, expatriate consultants will often participate in the reform efforts in developing countries. On the one hand, these consultants bring visibility to the reform process; on the other hand, they are not usually so well attuned to the cultural nuances of the organization as the local experts. In both cases, judicious management of consultants is required so that particular technical specialties are not overemphasized and do not disproportionately consume allocated resources.

Find a "saint": As pointed out before, health information system changes can encounter serious resistance. Health information system reform therefore needs leadership and protection, preferably a senior officer from within the organization, such as the director-general of the ministry of health. To effectively fulfil the role of system development protector, this person should (i) be committed to the reform, (ii) take the necessary risks, and (iii) have the right political connections (Peterson et al., 1994).

Ensure continuity of staff
Although staff transfers are a fact of life in most civil administration systems, all efforts should be undertaken to keep key staff in position during the entire health information system reform period, particularly the "saint" and members of the health information system development team.

Plan for time and resources
The worst that can happen to management systems reform is to run out of time or resources before the implementation phase is completed. Incomplete administrative reforms are not only failures but contribute to further deterioration of the management environment. Before undertaking any type of health information system reform, the health information system development team should obtain maximum assurance that enough financial and human resources are available to bring the reform within a given time period to a stage where the newly restructured health information system can be sustained without external resources. The required time period depends on the scope of the reform, but major reforms at national level can take easily up to 5 years before information is routinely used in management of the health services. The health information system development team needs to carefully time the various stages of the design and implementation phase. For example, if major administrative decentralization is planned to occur a year later, health information system reform should be postponed until then. Or, participatory design workshops are better not scheduled at the end of the fiscal year, when administrators have to close their books. As was mentioned earlier, the time period during which the health information system changes are implemented should be kept as short as possible, to avoid major managerial disruption.

Assessing the existing system and preparing options for reform

One of the first tasks of the health information system development team is to undertake an in-depth assessment study of the existing health information system. As explained in detail in Chapter 5, such a study first requires a detailed analysis of the health services system in general and the health information system more specifically. The team should utilize various data collection methods, such as a facility survey and interviews with health managers. Findings should be communicated through a written report identifying the most important weaknesses of current data generation and use.

Include policy analysis as part of health information system assessment

The health information system development team should not only assess the technical aspects but also the political environment, to ensure smooth implementation of the planned health information system reform. This requires a careful policy analysis, focusing on "winners and losers" and on the political and institutional context in which the health information system reform will take place. "Political mapping" (Reich, 1994) is one policy analysis technique that analysts could use in such assessments. Another method recently developed by Pinto & Mrope (1994) is institutional environment assessment. The institutional environment assessment is a diagnostic exercise to provide greater insight into contextual idiosyncrasies of public bureaucracies. The outcome of such policy assessments can give a clearer insight into the feasibility of the projected reform within the given political environment and based on the available administrative capacity and financial resources. For example, health information system reform is not likely to succeed within a weak bureaucracy, and with serious opposition against the reform from influential national programme managers, unless the designers build in persistent pressures, such as external financial commitments.

Prepare a series of options for health information system reform

This policy-oriented assessment study should also provide a better perspective on the scope and process of the intended reform. Is a major overhaul required (and feasible), or is it better to focus only on the data reporting and processing system? Should the private sector be involved in the health information system reform, and if so, to what extent? (For example, only for disease surveillance and reporting on preventive services?) How will care providers be involved in the design phase? Will a pilot phase be necessary to study the implications of the reform in a limited geographical area? Rather than providing straightforward answers to these questions in the assessment report, we suggest organizing the recommendations of the report in the form of options to be considered by decision-makers. This approach will help set the stage for a consensus-building process in the design phase.

Designing a new or restructured system

How will the new health information system be designed? To develop a technically well structured system delivered in a minimum time period, one might think that the easiest method would be to entrust the design to a group of experts. Unfortunately, it is also the most certain way to fail, because the new system, by ignoring attitudes and vested interests, will almost certainly be rejected by the future users. This is often the case with donor-driven health information system projects. For the sake of sustainable health information system reform, and based on various field experiences, we see at least four main strategies guiding the design phase.

Involve future users of the system

If the health information system is intended to improve information support to decision-making at all management levels of an organization, the health information system development team should make sure that representatives of all these management levels can have a substantial input in the design of the system. Indeed, future users, if they are top managers, or peripheral hospital directors, or community health workers, or officials from the Ministry of Finance, have different perceptions on what information is needed, on how to report data, and on how data should be presented for better use in decision-making. Care providers in particular, as the main data collectors, have strong opinions on data collection requirements that will directly affect their workload. How can all their different views be blended into an information system acceptable to most of the actors? It is obvious that some form of a consensus-building process needs to be used. To our knowledge, no standard formula is available. We suggest forming one or more "health information system working groups" that gather the main actors identified in the policy analysis. In order to have sufficient room for conflict resolution and active participation, groups should not have more than 30 participants. All geographical regions need to be represented. These working groups should then meet in a workshop setting in a time frame that allows them to reach consensus on all health information system design components. To encourage the participation of as broad a spectrum of care providers as possible, the consensus-building process should start from the periphery in the form of regional workshops. This is even more essential in the case of health services systems with a strong component of community participation.

Start from existing structures and tools whenever possible

The guiding principle throughout the design phase should be to keep changes to a minimum. Even small changes can be very disruptive to a smoothly running routine operation. Before a decision to change is made, system designers should carefully examine the trade-off between the benefits of the change and the risks of disrupting the status quo. This is particularly true for changes in data collection instruments. Also, designers should make sure that health information system changes are compatible with existing management systems and procedures. For example, a change in data collection on drugs can have a direct effect on drug management procedures.

Conceive the design process as continuous education

Creating attitudinal and behavioural changes leading towards an "information culture" is probably the most important act for building sustainable health information system reform. Although formalized training activities for that purpose will take place during the implementation phase, some significant on-the-job-training in the relation between information and management should have already taken place during the design phase. Participants in the consensus-building workshops can gain a better understanding of the basic concepts of information systems by becoming familiar with the initial steps of building a health information system: linking information needs to management functions and selecting a set of indicators for each management level. The format of the workshops can further contribute to create a "learning" environment by building in exercises that necessitate active involvement of all participants.

Introduce appropriate information technology

Successful health information system restructuring requires judicious use of computer and communications technology. Computer specialists should develop databases and software within the country. Health information system staff should be fully involved so that they can maintain and further develop the computer system. Designers should avoid imported software applications. If the project receives commercial support in the development of the software, local firms should be used to ensure that maintenance capability is on hand. Designers should expand computer use very gradually, particularly at subnational levels, and should first carefully assess institutional capacity. They should ensure that both computer and communications hardware have local sources of maintenance.

Implementing the proposed system

Obviously, the preceding phases are senseless without effective implementation. Effective implementation of the restructured health information system should demonstrate improvement of the information support to the health services and use of this information for decision-making at all levels. This is certainly not warranted by the mere technical content of the reform. The role of actors, context, and process during early implementation is more critical than ever. How can health information system development teams convince care providers that the restructured system will help them in improving quality of care? How can reporting requirements be enforced within the constraints of the civil service system? What should be the balance between a quality implementation process with judicious training of all care providers and a reasonable implementation time? The following recommendations and caveats will hopefully assist health information system development teams in achieving the objectives of health information system reform.

Marshal the necessary resources

As outlined above, the success of health information system reform is heavily dependent upon the capacity of the reformers to mobilize the required financial, managerial, and technical resources in a timely fashion during implementation. While donor resources can finance the initial development costs of the system, future funding of the necessary recurrent costs will ultimately determine the financial viability of the new system. As soon as health information system development teams have agreed on the macrostructure of the reform, we advise that they undertake a recurrent cost study, to ensure that the new system will not generate an unacceptable financial burden on the government. This study will also form the basis for negotiations with the Ministry of Finance to incorporate the new expenditures (if any) in the recurrent budget. Another main managerial challenge is the timely mobilization of technical assistance in areas such as data collection forms design, computer systems design, and the development of educational materials for the training programme. Finally, routine health information systems cannot function without the required data collection instruments. Health information system designers need to plan printing and distribution of these supplies well in advance, taking into account the implementation schedule of the training programme.

Provide intensive in-service training and supervision during the (early) implementation phase

Perhaps the most important resources the health information system development team should mobilize are the health information system users. To ensure full involvement of future health information system users, the team will have to set up an intensive in-service training programme combined with additional supportive supervision. The training programme will first teach all future users to fill in the new data collection instruments. An important part of the curriculum should subsequently focus on how the information generated can be used to improve health services planning and management, and the quality of the health care delivery system. The most practical approach is a "cascade" type of training, where the health information system development team first train health services managers and supervisors. They, in turn, will train the care providers. In district health systems, we advise a districtwise implementation of the system. The training team first trains all health facility staff in one district, provides them with the necessary printed supplies, and then moves on to the next district. Providing that sufficient "master trainers" are available, several districts could be trained simultaneously, to speed up the pace of implementation.

Ensure monitoring and evaluation as early as possible

Finally, no system can be perfect as first designed. Even with careful field testing, problems will arise with completing forms, data transmission, data processing, and feedback procedures. Close monitoring early in the implementation will permit most of these process-related problems to be solved. Later on, when the newly restructured health information system has been operational for at least 1 or 2 years, evaluation will focus on the outputs of the new system: how well the information produced by the system is used for decision making related to planning and management of the health services. The outcome of such an evaluation will help in adjusting the course of implementation. Ultimately, as a result of ongoing monitoring and periodic evaluation, a certain number of problems will remain which cannot be addressed without making changes in the overall system set-up. These problems will reach a critical level at a certain point in time. Health information system reform will then have to be put on the policy agenda again. At that stage, the reform implementation cycle starts all over again.

References

Auxila P, Rohde J (1988). Microcomputers as a means to introduce effective management procedures in primary health care: the Haiti experience. In: Wilson RL et al., eds. *Management information systems and microcomputers in primary health care*. Geneva, Aga Khan Foundation, 53–58.

de Kadt E (1989). Making health policy management intersectoral: issues of information analysis and use in less developed countries. *Social science and medicine*, 29:503–514.

Foltz A, Foltz W (1991). The politics of health reform in Chad. In: Perkins D, Roemer M, eds. *Reforming economic systems in developing countries*. Cambridge, MA, Harvard Institute for International Development.

Frenk J (1995). The power of ideas and the ideas of power: challenges to ENHR from health system reform. *Research into Action newsletter of the COHRED*, 1–4.

Grindle MS, Thomas JW (1991). *Public choices and policy change*. Baltimore, MD, Johns Hopkins University School of Hygiene and Public Health, Institute for International Programs.

Helfenbein S et al. (1987). *Technologies for management information systems in primary health care*. Geneva, World Federation of Public Health Associations: 1–70 (Issue Paper, Information for Action Series).

Lippeveld T (1995). *Evaluation of the health management information system for first level care facilities in Balochistan* (prepared for the Balochistan Health Department and for OBA Quetta).

Lippeveld TJ, Foltz A, Mahouri YM (1992). *Transforming health facility-based reporting systems into management information systems: lessons from the*

Chad experience. Cambridge, MA, Harvard Institute of International Development: 1–27 (Development Discussion Papers, No. 430).

Ministry of Public Health of Niger (1991). *The Niger national health information system*. Niamey, Ministry of Public Health: 1–34.

Ministry of Health of the Philippines (1990). *Field health services information system*. Manila, Ministry of Health: 1–70.

Peterson S et al. (1994). *Computerizing personnel information systems in African bureaucracies: lessons from Kenya*. Cambridge, MA, Harvard Institute of International Development, 1–25 (Development Discussion Papers, No. 496).

Pinto RF, Mrope AJ (1994). *Projectizing the governance approach to civil service reform: an institutional environment assessment for preparing a sectoral adjustment loan in the Gambia*. Washington, DC, World Bank (Discussion Paper, No. WDP252).

Reich MR (1994). *Political mapping of health policy: a guide for managing political dimensions of health policy*. Boston, MA, Harvard School of Public Health.

Reinke WA (1988). *Industrial sampling plans: prospects for public health applications*. Baltimore, Johns Hopkins University School of Hygiene and Public Health, Institute for International Programs: 1–36.

Sandiford P, Annett H, Cibulskis R (1992). What can information systems do for primary health care? An international perspective. *Social science and medicine*, 34:1077–1087.

Sapirie JA, Orzeszyna S (1995). *Selecting and defining national health indicators*. Geneva, World Health Organization.

Tekle DI et al. (1995). *Health information system assessment study: findings and recommendations*. Asmara, Ministry of Health.

Thomas JW, Grindle MS (1990). After the decision: implementing policy reforms in developing countries. *World Development*, 18:1163–1181.

Walt G, Gilson L (1994). Reforming the health sector in developing countries: the central role of policy analysis. *Health policy and planning*, 353–370.

World Health Organization (1994). *Information support for new public health action at the district level: report of a WHO Expert Committee*. Geneva, World Health Organization: 1–31 (WHO Technical Report Series, No. 845).

14 Approaches to strengthening health information systems

Theo Lippeveld and Steve Sapirie

Introduction

Information is crucial for decision-making at all levels of the health services. Policymakers need information for better allocation of scarce resources; planners for the design of more effective programmes; district managers for monitoring and evaluation of the health facilities under their responsibility; health unit managers to ensure the community equitable access to the services offered; and, most of all, care providers to provide quality care to their clients. In the last 2 decades, increasing need for efficient use of scarce resources has put information even higher in demand. Cost recovery, quality management, and the development of decentralized systems are all heavily dependent on well-functioning health information systems.

The focus of this book has been on routine health unit-based information systems. Routine health information systems, more than nonroutine methods such as surveys or rapid assessment methods, are the main data source in most countries. Yet they have the infamous reputation for producing a plethora of irrelevant or low-quality data. Therefore, most health managers, as a rule, do not use the information generated and make decisions based on "gut feeling".

By their nature, routine health information systems are intimately linked with the health services structure. The hypothesis that restructuring routine health information systems can have a direct impact on improved service delivery served as a major impetus for the authors to write this book. Routine health information systems, to live up to this potential, need to be more responsive to information needs of the health services at all levels—particularly at the service delivery levels, where the data are generated. This book, therefore, provides a health services model based on concentration levels, where, from the periphery to the centre, three types of management functions can be distinguished: patient/client management, health unit management, and system management. Restructuring of routine health information systems means better matching these management functions with the various components of the information-generating process and of the health information system management structure (see Chapter 2). Once routine health information systems fulfil their support role to the decision-making process at all levels, many expensive surveys can be eliminated, or at least redirected to generate data that are not captured by routine systems. In addition, such restructured facility-based systems can more easily be linked to population-based community health information systems as described in Chapter 9.

Although a clear conceptual model is helpful to the process of restructuring routine health information systems, it cannot provide all the practical approaches and strategies for successful health information system design and implementation. It is for this reason that in the subsequent chapters of the book, the authors integrate the text with country experiences in which they have been actively involved. This final chapter summarizes the lessons learned and sets an agenda for further development experiences.

Restructuring routine health information systems: what works and what does not work?

The materials in this book have been assembled by a number of experienced professionals who have worked within health information system development efforts around the world for over 20 years. Throughout the book, these authors make frequent references to the many difficulties that impede the development and successful use of routine health information systems or subsystems. Their collected observations confirm that a number of prerequisites must be satisfied to ensure that health data generation and use will succeed. Conversely, there are also a number of approaches and conditions that will almost certainly lead to failure. This chapter identifies both the prerequisites for success as well as the approaches that do not seem to work, and proposes alternative strategies that may increase the chances of success.

Preconditions for success

High-level interest and sponsorship: in search of a "saint"
All health development efforts require the support of senior managers and decision-makers, but nowhere is it more important than for the restructuring of health information systems. Health information system development touches all Ministry of Health departments, programmes, and institutions, both technical and administrative, as well as other government departments. High-level direction and coordination are imperative for the success of a health information system development effort. Eventually, a senior decision-maker, such as a director-general or deputy minister, should be identified as the project director, or, as Peterson et al. (1994) define him, as the "saint". In order to fulfil their role as "system development protectors" and to decrease resistance, directors should (i) be committed to the health information system restructuring process, (ii) be ready to take the necessary risks, and (iii) have the right political connections. The presence of a project director will facilitate participation and cooperation from all departments and programmes, which in turn will minimize duplication of data being recorded and reported, as well as help to establish systemwide data standards and procedures. In addition, distribution of a policy statement and strategy description can also give the development effort a certain legitimacy and clear definition of purpose.

Broad agreement with the principle of "information for action" at all levels
Early in successful health information system development efforts, managers and health workers at all levels must understand and acknowledge the importance of the linkage between management and information. One critical principle is that all information generated by

the new system must serve the process of action taking at all levels: within communities, for case management, for health unit management, for district management, for central level programme management, and for policy and planning at higher levels of the health system. Another principle is that no data should be requested from a service level which is not necessary and useful for managing the delivery of health care and performing other public health functions. This principle will help prevent the expansion of reporting requirements and ensure relevant monitoring and evaluation of the health status and service performance by higher health system levels.

Health information system development strongly linked to the overall health system development and reform process

If a health information system is a functional entity within the framework of the health services as a whole, it is obvious that health information system restructuring can only succeed if it is narrowly linked with reform at other levels of the health care system. For example, effective flow of information within the health care system depends upon the organizational structure of the health care system (organizational reform). Similarly, without a clear set of priorities (programmatic reform), managers and policymakers will find it difficult to agree upon a set of essential indicators for the health information system. And, of course, it is meaningless to restructure health information system for health services that are not used by the population (systemic reform).

Efforts to implement more accessible decentralized district health systems are now underway in several developed as well as developing countries. Health information system restructuring is part of this effort, as was stated by the WHO Expert Committee on Information Support for New Public Health Action at the District Level: "Health information is not only an essential resource for the development of district health systems, but also an integral component of that development" (WHO, 1994).

Availability of a core health information system development team

Successful health information system restructuring requires broad participation by future users at critical steps of the development process such as the selection of essential health indicators or the standardization of case definitions. However, successful efforts are always spearheaded by a small group of experts who carry out the staff work needed to develop standards, design criteria, and prototype databases. Moreover, high-level sponsorship and support as proposed earlier may not be available from the outset. The health information system development team may have to prove the worth of the proposed strategies by developing modest products early, even while the development plans are still being formulated.

Ideally, the health information system development team is multidisciplinary and includes, at a minimum, a health planner/epidemiologist, a computer expert, and a skilled trainer. Such staff may come from institutes of public health or epidemiological units, but placing such groups within the ministry of health during the entire health information system development process is usually an advantage. In this way, they can maintain communication with all services and programmes, and help ensure institutionalization of the restructured system. It is extremely important to keep the staff of the health information system development team in position during the entire health information system reform period.

Characteristics of health information system development approaches that are likely to fail

The folly of pursuing the grand design

Often the best-intentioned health information system projects fail because their managers and system designers are too ambitious, wanting to create an entirely new system that satisfies all user felt needs. The result is a health information system project that attempts to revise all data generation and reporting processes, whether they need improvement or not. Such efforts often attempt to integrate the generation and maintenance of health data at all levels, whether or not such integration is justified. These full system design efforts are intended to be systematic and efficient, because they are led by systems analysts who know how to normalize data. But the sheer difficulty of total system redesign and implementation normally exceeds the technical and management capabilities of most public sector health administrations. Such efforts are seen to be expensive and time-consuming, and often result in the operation of parallel systems of reporting, due to the difficulty and ineffectiveness of the new system and its procedures.

Health information system restructuring for central-level data accumulation

Traditionally, routine health information systems have been designed to provide epidemiological and statistical data to the central administration and programmes in the ministry of health. While it is true that central decision-makers need relevant information for policy and planning, the designers of such reporting systems often forget the important principle that all data to be recorded and reported should, first and foremost, be useful at the service delivery level. Even patient/client record forms sometimes contain data which have no use in the care process, but have been included because some central level office feels they need the data to monitor health or performance trends and produce annual reports. Often this practice is reinforced by international donor agencies which promote their own indicators while providing financial assistance in order to develop routine recording systems for capturing the necessary data. Such health information system restructuring methods wreak havoc on information use at all levels: not only do care providers, discouraged by the burden of data collection, make little use of the data for health unit and case management, but they also report incomplete and invalid data to higher levels, making them useless for policy and planning actions.

Forms review and revision without confirming the service information needs

Related to the previous issue, there is a tendency for many health information system development projects to review and revise registers, records, and forms used in service facilities, presumably to increase the validity, relevance, and completeness of reports to higher levels. Even if health information system developers start with proper identification of central level information needs, the result is usually only limited improvement of the information generated, in spite of the extensive resources and staff time consumed. Most important, these approaches fail to improve the relevance and usefulness of the information generated to support service staff in delivering clinical and outreach services to their patients and communities. Designers should place forms revision late in the health information system development plan of action, after the identification of information needs at all levels, and particularly at service delivery levels. Furthermore, they should only include those recording improvements which reinforce the performance of proper clinical and outreach procedures.

Information needs based on detailed decisions

New systems are often referred to as "management information systems" which are intended to support managers in decision-making. Designers therefore try to break down functions and activities into a list of decisions for which information needs are defined. For this purpose, senior service managers are carefully interviewed, but seldom do they know what data are most useful for decision-making. In truth, specific day-to-day decisions are rarely made consciously, and are often based on subjective feelings and experience. In any case, the designers' and planners' efforts generally produce long lists of data elements which are then incorporated into the new design. The result is an overly complex system which is even more burdensome to the care providers than the "inefficient" system it is intended to replace. One of the main assets of a well-designed routine health information system is a simple but essential set of indicators able to identify key problems. If needed, additional data and information to solve these problems can be generated through ad hoc data collection or nonroutine methods.

Mistaking computerization for health information system restructuring

One of the main objectives of many typical health information system development projects is the computerization of important data to be managed, monitored and analysed, and reported. In all countries, there are always numerous opportunities to apply computers in new or improved ways. However, whenever computerization becomes the primary objective of a health information system development effort, the more important purpose of serving the data needs of the care providers may be lost. Registers and records will be redesigned for facilitating data capture and entry, rather than reinforcing proper action for planning, management, and service delivery. Computers are, first and foremost, a support tool for data processing, data analysis, and data presentation and should be employed only if it is cost-effective to do so.

Donor-driven health information system restructuring

In the last decade, governments of developing countries have been under pressure from multilateral and bilateral donor agencies to increase the efficiency (and, less frequently, the equity) of their health care delivery systems. Health care reforms have been imposed as "conditionalities" for further disbursement of funds. In several countries, such external donor pressure has been the real impetus for getting health information system restructuring on the agenda. Although health information system restructuring in these countries is, in actuality, key for improving planning and management of the health services, it is obvious that without mobilizing national support, such projects ultimately cannot be sustained and may actually damage the existing routine health information system.

Most of these "donor-driven" health information system restructuring efforts include the redesign of the recording and reporting system, the development of integrated databases, the training of national staff locally and abroad, the abroad, the provision of computers, and the sponsorship of on-site expertise. Sometimes these projects succeed in getting a new recording and reporting system up and running within a 2-year period. But often, once the project is terminated, the situation rapidly deteriorates with accumulation of software and hardware maintenance problems, incomplete and delayed reporting, and the lack of continuity of national staff for managing the system. Part of the problem is the time constraint facing the donor agency. It must deliver its support within a fixed period of time, whether the necessary prerequisites such as national involvement and management capability are in place or not. A second problem is that such projects have to be planned in their entirety at the outset, with limited opportunity for revision in content and timing. A third problem arises when several agencies support the health information system development process. Each agency has its own approach and may find it difficult to collaborate with others. The national administration may find it difficult to act as the coordinator of the effort when most of the resources, both financial and human, are provided by the donor agencies, often as a grant. While external support can bring useful technical expertise and visibility from a political perspective, institutionalized and sustained health information system restructuring can only happen if the national administration "owns" the reform process, and therefore has full control over the content, the process, and the resources required.

Characteristics of health information system development approaches that are likely to succeed

Start every health information system development effort with the definition of indicators based on a conceptually sound health services system and specific management functions within the services

If the final outcome of health information system restructuring is to ensure better information support to the health services system, then the first requirement for any health information system designer is to have a clear understanding of how a health services system is structured and which management functions are involved. The model proposed in Chapter 2 categorizes management functions in three groups: patient/client, health unit, and system management. Management functions further vary according to the concentration level: from periphery to centre. They address curative, preventive, and promotional services, personal care as well as public health services. When restructuring is based on a conceptually sound health system model, information support can be more easily translated into relevant and appropriate indicators.

The first activity of health information system restructuring, therefore, is the selection of indicators for health services support, health services monitoring and management. This should be done through a consensus-building process involving health services managers at various levels, such as senior executives, programme managers, and district service staff. In countries where such a process has never taken place, the first step should be the development of a set of "essential" indicators. Such indicators address well-defined priority health problems, the services required to control those problems, and the resources critical for service delivery. They may also be used to monitor progress in health system reform and management.

Apply an evolutionary, problem-directed approach for improving the health information system

At the outset of a new initiative to strengthen the health information system, the health administration may not have a clear view of all the steps that need to be taken. In these cases, the early steps may involve different types of assessments that confirm where there are opportunities for improving the generation, use, and communication of important health data. Sometimes these assessments focus on specific types of data and communications processes, such as the disease surveillance system or the generation and use of clinic data. Planners and designers can undertake overall assessments of health information subsystems to uncover the cause of specific service and management issues or deficiencies. From such assessments, designers can use the findings to identify the information-related problems that most need early attention. They can then formulate short-term plans of action which include activities needed to address some of the problems found. As the implementation proceeds, they can extend the plan of action to include more of the components of the information system in need of strengthening. This evolutionary approach to health information system development allows for adjustment to accommodate new issues and opportunities for improvement.

Include policy analysis as a full part of health information system assessment

The success of health information system reform depends not only on technical improvements but also on in-depth understanding of political, sociocultural, and administrative factors. An essential question for health information system designers is how "to add rationality while still accommodating the interests of diverse constituencies and value systems" (Reinke, 1988). As described in Chapter 13, we suggest undertaking an in-depth policy analysis as part of any health information system restructuring process. Following the model proposed by Walt and Gilson (1994), such analysis includes (i) identification of all actors with stakes in the health information system reform (political mapping), and (ii) research on contextual political, socioeconomic, and administrative factors likely to influence the outcome of the health information system reform.

Enable broad participation in the health information system design process, but ensure technical soundness throughout by the use of a health information system design team

Everyone in the health sector cannot participate in all aspects of the design and implementation of health information systems, but based on careful policy analysis, the design team should at least ensure participation of key actors in the process and thereby foster their understanding and ultimate support during the implementation. Selected programme managers and service staff should be involved in the selection of essential health indicators. In addition, programme and service staff should participate in rapid assessments of health information system performance, as well as oversee specific functions such as disease surveillance and control, and clinic diagnosis and recording. The results of such assessments as well as options for improvement can be presented to larger groups of future users, and ultimately create broad ownership of the restructured health information system. This applies particularly to the establishment of standard case definitions and of standard treatment guidelines. Nevertheless, a considerable amount of health information system design and development work must be carried out by specialists belonging to the health information system development team. Report design, reporting procedures, database design, and the design of recording formats and registers need to be carried out by system analysts, epidemiologists, clinical specialists, and computer specialists, drawing on the inputs of programme and service staff.

Introduce information technology in an effective, efficient, and sustainable manner

Successful projects make judicious use of computer and communications technology at points in the system that will most benefit from this technology. The expansion of computer use, particularly at subnational levels, is undertaken gradually, and fully involves staff who will be required to enter data and use the resulting information. The development of databases and software is carried out within the country, with the full involvement of the staff who will be required to maintain and further develop the computer system. Hardware systems, even if financed by external sources, should take into account the local capacity to bear the recurrent costs generated by such systems. Imported software applications should be avoided. If commercial support is received in the development of the software, local firms should be used to ensure that maintenance capability is on hand. Both computer and communications hardware should have local sources of maintenance.

Attempt to produce useful, new information processes and products early in the development effort

The evolutionary health information system development strategy must insure that useful products are generated early in order to gain the confidence and support of senior managers, programme managers, and service staff. The confirmation of essential indicators is often one such product, and it leads naturally to others. Frequently, countries recognize that their clinicians are not applying standard case definitions in their recording of diagnoses. Sometimes such standard case definitions are not known or promulgated in the services. Establishing standard definitions for common and important health problems and conditions is a useful early product in health information system development. Frequently underuse of existing information is a major lacuna which can be addressed early through processes such as district or facility level problem-solving exercises. Before designers create solutions or interventions addressing these lacunas, they often request service staff to analyse their existing records and reports to assess performance and to understand the cause of operational problems. If carried out effectively, such activities inspire interest and ideas for further improvements of the information system.

An agenda for further health information system development experiences and research

While the experiences of health information system restructuring efforts in various countries have permitted the authors to propose a list of useful health information system development strategies, many questions regarding the development of relevant health information systems remain unanswered and need further experience and research. We conclude this book by inviting interested health system developers and researchers to address such questions through carefully set up health information system projects and research studies. The list of questions presented in Box 39 is certainly not exhaustive, but hopefully it will

Box 39   Future directions

General health information system development questions

- How can service providers and particularly communities as key information users be more actively involved in health information system development efforts?
- What is the ideal process and level for development of interdisciplinary social information systems, through which interactions between health, education, and economic development can be identified in an action-oriented manner?
- Given the benefits of a population-based community health information system, as described in Chapter 9, how can it effectively be linked to the facility-based routine health information system?
- Can health information system reform by itself have a direct impact on improved functioning of the health services, and if so, how?

Questions on indicator selection

- What are relevant and operational indicators for management support systems such as financial systems, personnel planning and management systems, building and equipment management systems (in addition to health problem and health services indicators for which extensive experience is available)?
- How can qualitative information be operationalized in a routine health information system (e.g. the quality of interpersonal relations between the care providers and the patients)?

Questions of data collection

- How can patient/client data recording be improved in order to help care providers to monitor and maintain the quality of their services?
- What innovative structural interventions can be proposed to better link routine service statistics with other nonroutine data collection systems (surveys, vital events registration, rapid assessments methods, etc.)

Questions of data transmission

- In hierarchical vertical transmission systems (still the most common data transmission system in many countries), how can the speed of data transfer be improved?
- What is the most efficient way to provide feedback to lower levels in systems where data are compiled at higher levels?

Questions on the use of information

- What is the relationship between the format in which information is displayed (maps, action-oriented graphs, etc.) and its use in management decisions?
- How can one design and conduct training that effectively improves the actual use of information for health services planning and management?

Questions on computerization in the health sector

- Is there an approach for determining where computerization is likely to pay the greatest dividends?
- What is an efficient strategy for designing and testing computer support for important components of the health information system such as hospital data, surveillance data, and various types of administrative information such as supplies, budget, and human resources management?

further contribute to establishing health information systems responsive to the management needs of effective and efficient health services systems in both developed and developing countries.

References

Peterson S et al. (1994). *Computerizing personnel information systems in African bureaucracies: lessons from Kenya.* Cambridge, MA, Harvard Institute for International Development: 1–25 (Development Discussion Paper, No. 496).

Reinke WA (1988). *Industrial sampling plans: prospects for public health applications.* Baltimore, MD, Johns Hopkins University School of Hygiene and Public Health, Institute for International Programs: 1–36.

Walt G, Gilson L (1994). Reforming the health sector in developing countries: the central role of policy analysis. *Health policy and planning,* 353–370.

World Health Organization (1994). *Information support for new public health action at the district level. Report of a WHO Expert Committee.* Geneva, World Health Organization: 1–31 (WHO Technical Report Series, No. 845).

Classes of indicators and their major attributes

The matrix below outlines the four classes of indicators, that is input, process, output, and outcome, and their major attributes. The definition and an example of an indicator are given for each attribute. Finalization of a set of indicators for a health management information system will require that the concise set of selected indicators be balanced as a set. As described by Bulatao (1995), "Balance in a set of indicators requires even-handed coverage of different [health system] goals and proportionate attention to key [health system] processes. Imbalance is often easy to identify, even in a large set of indicators: the 103 proposed by Bertrand et al. (1994), for example, lack any indicator relating to reproductive health outcomes or to program costs, though these are promised for later editions of their handbook. Balance is more critical, and often more difficult to achieve, the smaller the set of indicators. A small set cannot afford to overlook important attributes. This may mean relaxing some of the criteria highlighted . . . for the identification of 'good' indicators at points. Not all aspects of the [health system] are well-researched, and some weak indicators may have to be provisionally accepted".

Classes of indicators and their attributes	Definition	Example
INPUTS		
Availability of resources	Inputs are the human and financial resources, physical facilities, equipment, operational policies, and organizational arrangements that enable services to be delivered in the health system. This definition encompasses both the availability of resources, as well as the organizational structure of the system. The organizational arrangements, in turn, reflect authority–responsibility relationships, organizational design features, governance and empowerment issues, proximity of financial responsibility to operational accountability, the degree of decentralized decision making, and what kinds of decisions are delegated (De Geyndt, 1994). Donabedian (1980) considers structural inputs like physical inputs, staffing, money, and organizational arrangements as measuring quality of care.	• Indicator for availability of resources: trained nurses per 10,000 population.
Health determinants (risk factors)	Determinants refer to conditions that contribute to or are precursors of disease such as human behavioural factors or unhealthy environmental conditions. It includes factors such as cigarette smoking, alcohol use, obesity, low birth weight, and so on which have a negative impact on health.	• Indicator of risk factor: proportion of live-born infants weighing less than 2500 g at birth.
PROCESS		
Service delivery and support activities	Service delivery and support activities represent the bulk of the process indicators. In Cameroon, the information system provides indicators for the following support activities at the primary health care level: — community participation; — supervision;	• Indicator for support activities: proportion of health districts that have at least one trained professional for IUD (intrauterine device) insertion.

Classes of indicators and their attributes	Definition	Example
	— human resources (training, incentives); — financial management (public funding and cost recovery); — drug management; — maintenance.	
Quality of services and support activities	Quality of service indicators seek to address how well the staff perform their curative, preventive, and promotive tasks, as well as whether appropriate medical supplies and medications are available at the facilities. The quality of support activities is checked by measuring how well the support activities are carried out.	• Indicator of quality of services: proportion of women delivering at the health centre who are effectively immunized against tetanus. • Indicator of support activities: proportion of refrigerators in the district that are out of order.
Financial accessibility	Financial accessibility measures the extent to which people are able to pay for care. This is usually measured through a community-based willingness and ability to pay survey.	• Indicator of financial accessibility: proportion of people who are able to pay for a particular service, considering both personal contributions and health insurance.
Geographical accessibility	Geographical accessibility measures the extent to which services are available and accessible to the population. It is, of course, linked to the distribution of infrastructure in a given region but also to the actual offering of these services at these facilities. Geographical accessibility will vary according to local means of transportation, as well as the local topography. In developing countries, services are generally considered accessible if they can be reached within a 1-hour walk. Accessibility can also be expressed in terms of distance (population living less than 15 km from the facility).	• Indicator of geographical accessibility: proportion of the population living within walking distance of less than an hour from a health centre.
Cultural accessibility	Indicators of cultural accessibility consider whether access to health services are impeded by cultural taboos. Three examples are provided: (i) Can women use reproductive health services if all of the physicians in the facility are male? (ii) Will persons who belong to an ethnic minority use services that are staffed by the majority population? (iii) Will persons use health services for processes that are considered "natural", that is without the need for health intervention (such as pregnancy)?	• Indicator of cultural accessibility: proportion of pregnant women in a catchment area who can independently choose (and afford) to go to a clinic for treatment of a sexually transmitted disease.
OUTPUT **Use**	Use is the expression of the demand for services.	• Indicator of use: number of curative care episodes per 1000 population.
Coverage	Coverage measures the proportion of a target group that has received a particular service.	• Indicator of coverage: proportion of pregnant women who received at least two antenatal care visits of appropriate quality while pregnant.
Financial performance	Financial performance measures the financial viability of the organization.	• Indicator of financial performance: proportion of total costs actually recovered by the cost-sharing programme.
Acceptability (perceived quality)	Acceptability or perceived quality considers the extent to which patients are satisfied with the services offered. A patient's perception of the quality of care typically reflects the congeniality of the providers and waiting times, in addition to the technical competence of the facility staff.	• Indicator of perceived quality: proportion of patients who are satisfied with the service provided and would return to the provider for future care.

Classes of indicators and their attributes	Definition	Example
Behavioural changes	Indicators of behavioural output consider whether clients change their health-related conduct as a result of contact with a health-care facility or its information, education, and communication campaigns. It should be noted that Donabedian (1988) classifies behavioural changes as outcomes.	• Indicator of behavioural changes: proportion of mothers breastfeeding babies up to 18 months of age, before/after an intervention.
OUTCOME		
Health outcomes	These indicators measure the mortality and the morbidity (disability) for certain health conditions. Since facility-based health management information systems give only a limited perspective on the health status of a population, facility records should be supplemented with information from community-based surveys, vital registration, censuses, and other data collection instruments to fully understand health outcomes within a population. Health outcome indicators from a routine information system are important, though, because they monitor the conditions that impact on the management of health services and help managers to make resource allocation decisions.	• Indicator of health outcome: number of deaths from pregnancy-related and puerperal causes during a given year divided by the number of live births during the same year per 100,000 pregnant women (the maternal mortality ratio).
Effectiveness	Effectiveness is the extent to which objectives are achieved.	• Indicator of effectiveness: proportion of children under 1 year of age that are immunized against measles (compared with the national objectives of 80% coverage).
Efficiency	Efficiency is the extent to which objectives are achieved by minimizing the use of resources. Cost is a major concern in both developed and developing countries.	• Indicator of efficiency: cost per child vaccinated.
Sustainability	Sustainability is the ability or prospect to continue, prolong, keep something up (Wilson & Sapanuchart, 1993).	• Indicator of sustainability: proportion of donor funding to total funding.
Equity	Equity, or whether health services are provided "justly" within a population, is difficult to measure since it carries moral and political connotations. For this reason, few indicators have been unanimously agreed upon. Indicators include accessibility of health services, use of health services by demographic groups, inequalities in mortality and morbidity among different subgroups of the population, unequal distribution of health resources, and so on.	• Indicator of equity: proportion of selected categories of health personnel to the population in different provinces or districts.

References

Bertrand JT et al. (1994). *Handbook of indicators for family planning program evaluation*. Chapel Hill, NC, University of North Carolina at Chapel Hill.

Bulatao RA (1995). *Key indicators for family planning projects*. Washington, DC, World Bank (World Bank Technical Paper, No. 297).

De Geyndt W (1994). *Managing the quality of health care in developing countries*. Washington, DC, World Bank (World Bank Technical Paper, No. 258).

Donabedian A (1980). *Exploration in quality: assessment and monitoring*. Vol. 1: *The definition of quality and approaches to its assessment*. Ann Arbor, MI, Health Administration Press, School of Public Health, University of Michigan.

Wilson R, Sapanuchart T, eds. (1993). *Primary health care management advancement program*. Geneva, Aga Khan Foundation.

National lists of indicators: the trade-off between conciseness and completeness

We draw the attention of the reader to the fact that there is a need to make a trade-off between conciseness (limiting the number of indicators) and completeness (targeting all attributes) in the selection of indicators. As an illustration of conciseness, the following list of indicators was selected for assessing community health status and monitoring progress towards the year 2000 in the United States.

Progress towards the year 2000 objectives: consensual agreement by expert committees

Indicators of processes
- Proportion of children under 2 years of age who have been immunized with the basic series (as defined by the Immunization Practice Advisory Committee)
- Proportion of adults aged 65 years or older who have been immunized for pneumoccocal pneumonia and influenza
- Proportion of assessed rivers, lakes, and estuaries that support beneficial uses (fishing and swimming approved)
- Proportion of women receiving a Papanicolaou smear at an interval appropriate for their age
- Proportion of women receiving a mammogram at an interval appropriate for their age
- Proportion of the population uninsured for medical care
- Proportion of the population without a regular source of primary care (including dental services)

Indicators of health status outcome
- Race/ethnicity-specific infant mortality, as measured by the rate (per 1000 live births) of deaths among infants less than 1 year of age
- Death rates (per 100,000 population) for:
  — motor vehicle crashes; work-related injury; suicide; lung cancer; breast cancer; cardiovascular disease; homicide; all causes
- Reported incidence (per 100,000 population) of:
  — AIDS; measles; tuberculosis; primary and secondary syphilis; percentage of children under 5 years of age who are tested and have blood lead levels exceeding 15µg/dl; incidence of viral hepatitis B, per 100,000; proportion of children aged 6–8 and 15 years with one or more decayed primary or permanent teeth

Indicators of risk factors
- Incidence of low birth weight, as measured by percentage of total number of live-born infants weighing less than 2500 g at birth
- Births to adolescents (females aged 10–17 years) as a percentage of total live births
- Prenatal care, as measured by the proportion of children under 15 years of age living in families at or near the poverty level
- Proportion of persons living in countries exceeding US Environmental Protection Agency standards for air quality during the previous year

Indicators of risk factors (age-specific prevalence rates)
- Cigarette smoking; alcohol use; obesity; hypertension; hypercholesterolaemia; confirmed abuse and neglect of children

Source: The Nation's Health, *Journal of the American Public Health Association*, September 1991.

ANNEX 3

Health information subsystem: issue framework

HEALTH INFORMATION SUBSYSTEMS TO BE ASSESSED	HIS components of assessment							
	Use of Information — Decisions and Actions	Data Analysis — Transmission Reporting	Data Input — Recording and Collection	INFORMATION SYSTEM RESOURCES				Information Systems Management Coordination and Networking
				Financial Resources	Staff Availability and Capabilities	Material and Facilities	Computer Use	
Epidemiological Surveillance	Inadequate response to disease outbreaks and notifications	Inappropriateness of data processing and presentation of computer software Delays in report preparation and submission	Lack of standard case definitions	Lack of a regular budget for hardware and software purchase and staff training	Inadequate staff training in computer use and database development Lack of supervision of surveillance activities	Lack of established procedures for equipment maintenance	Inadequacy of computer facilities for surveillance data management and communication	HIS management and its support to epidemiological surveillance unclear
Service Reporting Case Monitoring Task Performance	Non-use of routine service reports for resource allocation	Problems of using standard computer applications for data management and analysis	Inefficiency of data collection procedures	Inadequate and uncoordinated funding for health activities	Inadequate staff training and job descriptions at all levels of the health system	Suboptional use of equipment	Lack of computer facilities for emergency management monitoring and performance analysis	Lack of a clear structure and function of the management information system Poor data communication among health care system levels

Examples of assessment questions and recording formats

Does the staff know or can they calculate the following population target groups?

	Yes	No	Size	Proportion of total	Purpose
Women of reproductive age (15–45)					
No. of pregnant women expected					
No. of births expected					
Infants 0 to 11 months					
Infants 0 to 23 months					
Infants 9 to 23 months					
Children 0 to 3 years					

What is the trend in the following three diseases over the past 6 months?

	Increasing	Decreasing	Variable (no trend)	True or False	Don't know
Diarrhoea					
Measles					
Meningitis					

Verify the trend in cases by extracting data from the registers

	Jan.	Feb.	Mar.	Apr.	May	June
Diarrhoea						
Measles						
Meningitis						

Determine whether the cases reported in the last annual report agree with the monthly registers

Disease	Number of cases		Percentage difference
	Total from monthly registers	Total in the annual report	
Malaria			
Diarrhoeal diseases			
Acute respiratory infection			
Meningitis			
Measles			
Anaemia			
Tuberculosis			

Awareness/availability of data on hospital personnel situation

Tables/registers are available with data on	Hospital Director	Chief Matron	Personnel Office
Sanctioned posts by staff type			
Filled and vacant posts by staff type			
List of in-service training received last year			
List of impending retirements by year			

Examples of assessment data tables

Staff knowledge of target population groups

Target groups	Health facilities						District/ Regional Office		Total			
	Dispensary		Health centre		Hospitals				Yes		No	
	Yes	No	Yes	No	Yes	No	Yes	No	No.	%	No.	%
Total population served												
Women of reprod. age												
Number of expected births												
Infants 0 to 11 months												
Infants 0 to 23 months												
Infants 9 to 23 months												
Children 0 to 3 years												
Children 0 to 5 years												

Availability and consistency of data on disease cases and trends

Variables	Health facilities						District/ Regional Office		Total			
	Dispensary		Health centre		Hospitals				Yes		No	
	Yes	No	Yes	No	Yes	No	Yes	No	No.	%	No.	%
Knowledge of disease trends												
Data available in monthly registers and reports												
Data from the registers and reports agree												

Data on malnutrition and security stock of supplies

Variables	Health facilities						District/ Regional Office		Total			
	Dispensary		Health centre		Hospital				Yes		No	
	Yes	No	Yes	No	Yes	No	Yes	No	No.	%	No.	%
Data are available on the number of children found to be malnourished during growth monitoring												
Staff are able to calculate the percentage of children 0 to 3 who are malnourished												
Staff are able to calculate the amount of security stock required for: FeS and folic acid												
Measles vaccine												

Mother health card, Chandigarh, India

Source: *Home-based maternal records: guidelines for development, adaptation and evaluation.* Geneva, WHO (1994)

गर्भ का रिकार्ड

Child health register

Source: Ministry of Public Health, Pakistan (1993)

CHILD HEALTH REGISTER (FR3)　　　　　　　　　　　Year __1992__

Serial No.	Registration Date	Name of Child & Father	Address / Village	Date of Birth	Age At Registration: Less than 1 Year	1 Year or more	Jan	Feb	Mar	Apr	May	Jun	Jul	Aug	Sep	Oct	Nov	Dec	High Risk
0025	03/07/92	Iraz s/o Inayat	Ghagen phatak	May 91		✓							M	M		N			
0026	08/07/92	Hauma D/o Hashmat	" "	23/08/91	✓								M	M	M				✓
0027	08/07/92	Sadiqa D/o Qasim	Qureshi Goth	15/05/92	✓								N			N			
0028	09/07/92	Lakhi D/o Ram	Raman Goth	June 92	✓								S	S	M		N		
0029	12/07/92	Huma D/o Rahim	Dina Shah	01/01/92		✓							M			N			
0030	16/07/92	Habib S/o JanDin	Baluch Goth	10/07/92	✓								N						
0031	22/07/92	Amina S/o Haji	" "	Dec '90		✓							M		M		M		✓
0032	25/07/92	Yousaf S/o Qasim	Achar Salar	Jan 91		✓							M	S	M				✓
0033	29/07/92	Karim S/o M. Bux	Ghagen Patak	19/05/92	✓								S			N			
0034	30/07/92	Khanum D/o Hanif	Dhabeji	26/08/92	✓									N		N			
0035	01/08/92	Nabi Bux S/o Shakeel	Achar Salar	01/02/90		✓								M			M	N	
0036	02/08/92	Lajvanti D/o Ram	Qureshi Goth	25/01/91		✓								N					✓
0037	05/08/92	Amina D/o Rasheed	" "	Mar 92	✓									S	M		M		✓
0038	10/08/92	Zainab D/o Rasool	Dhabeji	01/08/91		✓								M	M	N			
0039	11/08/92	Yaqoob S/o Karim	Achar Salar	08/08/90		✓								M	N			M	✓
0040	12/08/92	Sadiq s/o Amin	Qureshi Goth	09/10/91	✓									S	M	N			
0041	15/08/92	Shamim D/o Kazim	Dhabeji	23/08/90		✓								N		N			
0042	12/09/92	Taj Bux S/o Lal Bux	"	04/05/90		✓									N	M	M		✓
0043	15/09/92	Karam S/o Nyaz M	Achar Salar	05/06/91		✓									M		N		
0044	17/09/92	Rahim S/o Jan M	Qureshi Goth	06/07/92	✓										S	M	M	N	
0045	20/09/92	M. Khan S/o Qadir	Ghagen patak	09/06/90		✓									M		N	M	✓
0046	22/09/92	Nawaz S/o	" "			✓									M	N			
0047	25/09/92	Mohammad S/o Yamar	Jute Mill	02/10/91	✓										N			N	

Example of tally sheet

Source: Primary Health Care Management Advancement Programme, Module 3, Aga Khan Foundation, Geneva (1993)

Exhibit 16: CHW activity record

Name of CHW: _____ Village: _____ Month:_____

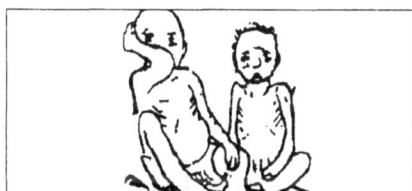

	Children identified malnourished this month	○○○○○○○○○ ○○○○○○○○○ ○○○○○○○○○
	Children suffering from ARI	○○○○○○○○○ ○○○○○○○○○ ○○○○○○○○○
	Number of referrals made	○○○○○○○○○ ○○○○○○○○○ ○○○○○○○○○
	Children born this month	○○○○○○○○○ ○○○○○○○○○ ○○○○○○○○○
	Children who died this month	○○○○○○○○ ○○○○○○○○ ○○○○○○○○ ○○○
	Mothers who died this month	○○○○○○○○○ ○○○○○○○○○ ○○○○○○○○○

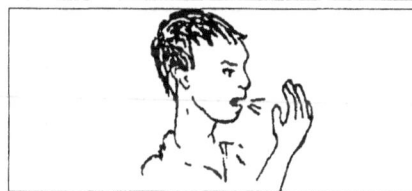

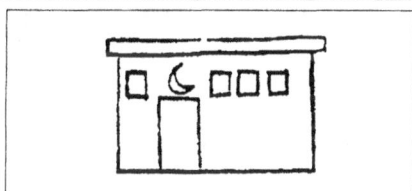

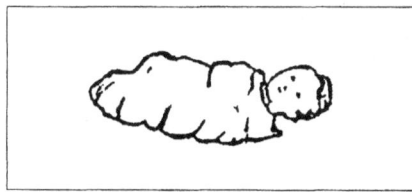

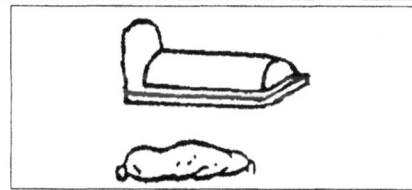

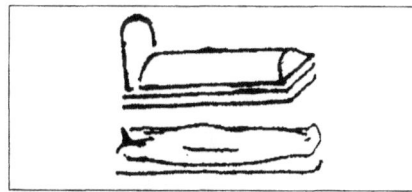

INSTRUCTIONS: Fill one circle for every case seen.

Hospital daily attendance sheet

Source: Ministry of Health, Republic of Chad (1986)

REPUBLIQUE DU TCHAD
MINISTERE DE LA SANTE PUBLIQUE
SECRETARIAT D'ETAT
DIRECTION GENERALE
BUREAU DE STATISTIQUES
PLANIFICATION ET ETUDES

FICHE DE PRESENCE JOURNALIERE
SERVICES D'HOSPITALISATION

MOIS : _DECEMBRE_

ANNEE : _1986_

Nom de Formation/Localité _CENTRE MEDICAL DE BOUSSO_

SERVICE _PEDIATRIE_   (B) TOTAL LITS/PLACES: _20_   (A) NOMBRE DE JOURS: _31_

DATE	1	2	3	4	5	6	7	8	9	10	11	12	13	14	15	16	17	18	19	20	21	22	23	24	25	26	27	28	29	30	31	TOTAL
(C) NOMBRE PRESENTS	17	15	16	17	16	15	18	19	15	18	18	17	20	20	18	16	14	13	13	15	17	18	19	18	17	17	17	15	17	16	18	519 (C)
(D) ENTRANTS	2	3	4	4	3	3	4	2	6	0	4	3	4	1	2	2	0	1	2	4	3	2	4	1	0	0	4	3	1	2	3	77 (D)
(E) SORTANTS	4	1	2	4	3	0	2	5	1	0	4	0	4	2	3	2	1	1	0	2	1	1	5	1	0	0	6	0	2	0	3	60 (E)
(F) DECEDES	0	1	0	1	0	0	1	1	2	0	0	0	0	1	0	1	0	0	0	0	1	0	0	1	0	0	0	0	0	0	1	11 (F)
(G) EVADES	0	0	1	0	1	0	0	0	0	0	0	1	0	0	0	1	1	0	0	0	0	0	0	0	0	0	0	1	0	0	0	6 (G)

(H) OCCUPATION MOYENNE = $\dfrac{C \times 100}{A \times B}$ = $\dfrac{519 \times 100}{31 \times 20}$ = 83.71 %

(I) SEJOUR MOYEN = $\dfrac{C \times 2}{D + E + F + G}$ = $\dfrac{519 \times 2}{77 + 60 + 11 + 6}$ = 6.74 jours

Source: Ministry of Public Health, Pakistan (1993)

POPULATION CHART OF CATCHMENT AREA

(FR11)

Institution: **BHU BHANPUR**   I.D. No.: **345617** Year: **1992**

Union Council: **BHATKELA**   District: **GUARA**

1	2	3	4	5	6	
Sr. No.	Name of Villages	Population	Distance from Facility (Km)	No. of CHWs	No. of TBAs	
					Trained	Untrained
1	Sunjural	474	5	0	1	0
2	Gariwala	1,438	3	0	1	0
3	Haji Golti	836	8	0	1	0
4	Bhanpur	2,847	0	0	2	0
5	Ghais	1,371	7	0	0	1
6	Guju	931	13	0	1	0
7	Dhabeiji	1,749	21	2	2	0
8	Gori bazi	372	14	1	0	1
9	Karampura	1,699	12	0	1	0
	TOTAL >	11,717		3	9	2

% of population living more than 20 km. from Institution: **14.9** %

TARGET RISK GROUPS	STANDARD DEMOGRAPHIC PERCENTAGES	ESTIMATED POPULATION
Expected Pregnancies	4.5	527
Expected Births	4.0	469
0 - 11 months	3.8	445
0 - less than 3 years	11	1,289
CBAs (15 to 44 years)	21	2,461
Married CBAs (15 to 44 years)	16	1,875

Example of supervisory checklist

Source: Primary Health Care Management Advancement Programme, Module 6, Aga Khan Foundation, Geneva (1993)

PHC service quality checklist
18. Treatment of minor ailments

This checklist is intended for use in the observation of treatment of minor ailments. Before using it, the local treatment protocol should be reviewed in order to adapt the tool to the local situation if necessary. It is also recommended that you review the checklist carefully before using it to be sure that you understand the questions and know how to use the form. For observation of service delivery, mark "yes" if the service provider carries out these activities during service delivery. For interview questions, mark "yes" if the respondent answers correctly.

1._____ Health facility
2._____ Service provider
3._____ Observer/supervisor
4._____ Date

Medical history
Did the service provider:
5. YES_____NO_____ Ask about the chief complaint (fever, pain, cough, etc)?
6. YES_____NO_____ Determine the present history of the illness?
7. YES_____NO_____ Determine condition-related past and family history?

Physical examination
Did the service provider:
8. YES_____NO_____ Check vital signs (blood pressure, temperature, pulse, respiration rate etc.)
9. YES_____NO_____ Conduct a related physical exam?

Diagnosis
Did the service provider:
10. YES_____NO_____ Make differential diagnosis (e.g., cough, TB, pneumonia, bronchitis, abdominal pain, gastroenteritis, acute cholestitis, appendicitis, etc.)?

Laboratory diagnosis
Did the service provider:
11. YES_____NO_____ Order condition- or preliminary diagnosis-related diagnostic tests (laboratory tests, x-ray studies, etc)

Treatment and follow-up plans
Did the service provider:
13. YES_____NO_____ Provide appropriate treatment according to the condition?
14. YES_____NO_____ Provide information to the patient about the condition and treatment plan?
18. YES_____NO_____ Discuss the importance of compliance with the drug therapy?
21. YES_____NO_____ How often will you take this medicine?
22. YES_____NO_____ What is the dose you will take?
23. YES_____NO_____ For how long will you continue treatment?

HMIS/FLCF monthly report: section on mother care activities

Source: Ministry of Public Health, Pakistan

8. MOTHER AND CHILD CARE PREVENTIVE ACTIVITIES

A. Pre-natal Care

(From Mother Health Register)

Expected New Pregnancies this month (CA Population / 270) ☐ (1)

Number Newly Registered (2)		Newly Registered During 1st Trimester (3)		Haemoglobin under 10 gm% at 1st measurement (4)		Total Visits (5)	
% of Expected New Pregnancies (2) / (1)	%	% of Total Newly Registered (3) / (2)	%	% of Total Newly Registered (4) / (2)	%	No. of Re-visits (5) - (2)	

B. Deliveries   Expected Deliveries this month (CA Population/300) ☐ (1)

(From Mother Health Register)

C. Post-natal Care
(From Mother Health Register)

Total Number of Deliveries (2)		No. of Deliveries by Trained Persons (5)		% of Expected Deliveries (5) / (1)	%	Number of Deliveries in month previous to reporting month (7)	
Number of Stillbirths (3)		No. of Deliveries in your Facility (6)		% of Deliveries by Trained Persons (6) / (5)	%	Rec'd at least 1 Postnatal Visit (8)	
Number of Abortions (4)						% of Deliveries in previous month (8) / (7)	%

D. Maternal Deaths   Number: ☐   *(From Mother Health Register)*

Source: Pakistan Child Survival Project, 1993

HEALTH MANAGEMENT INFORMATION SYSTEM
FIRST LEVEL CARE FACILITIES

DATA COLLECTION INSTRUMENT PRE-TEST REVIEW FORM

Name of Register/Form : _____

Name of Person/Institution providing comments :_____

Date :_____ Signature :_____

Instruction:

Please fill out one of these forms for each data collection instrument for which you have comments. For those participating in the pre-test, these should be completed at the end of the pre-test period.

If you have specific comments about changes or improvements to the layout of the registers or forms, please attach a copy of the draft form/register with your comments marked on it.

Please circle the number on the scale of 1 to 5 which best describes your answer to the following questions:	Circle a number for each question						
1. How appropriate do you consider this instrument for the data collection purpose described in the instructions?	Unsuitable	1	2	3	4	5	Very Suitable
2. How clear and easy to follow were the instructions accompanying the data collection instrument?	Unclear	1	2	3	4	5	Very Clear
3. How difficult (i.e. time and effort) was it to complete the data collection instrument?	Very difficult	1	2	3	4	5	Very Easy
4. How suitable is the layout of this form/register for efficient data collection, aggregation and/or facility management?	Unsuitable	1	2	3	4	5	Very Suitable

General comments and suggestions for improvement (Please continue overleaf):

The Pakistan Child Survival Project was financed by the United States Agency for International Development under Project number 391-0496-C-00-0769-00